You and Your Aging Parent

You & Your Aging Parent

A Family Guide to Emotional, Social, Health, and Financial Problems

FOURTH EDITION

BARBARA SILVERSTONE
HELEN KANDEL HYMAN

WITH COMMENTARY BY BOB MORRIS

AND WITH SPECIAL CONTRIBUTIONS BY KIM WALLER AND PENNY SCHWARTZ

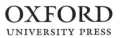

OXFORD
UNIVERSITY PRESS

2008

OXFORD
UNIVERSITY PRESS

Oxford University Press, Inc., publishes works that further
Oxford University's objective of excellence
in research, scholarship, and education.

306.874
Si39y

Oxford   New York
Auckland   Cape Town   Dar es Salaam   Hong Kong   Karachi
Kuala Lumpur   Madrid   Melbourne   Mexico City   Nairobi
New Delhi   Shanghai   Taipei   Toronto

With offices in
Argentina   Austria   Brazil   Chile   Czech Republic   France   Greece
Guatemala   Hungary   Italy   Japan   Poland   Portugal   Singapore
South Korea   Switzerland   Thailand   Turkey   Ukraine   Vietnam

Published by Oxford University Press, Inc.
198 Madison Avenue, New York, NY 10016
www.oup.com

Oxford is a registered trademark of Oxford University Press

Library of Congress Cataloging-in-Publication Data
Silverstone, Barbara, 1931–
You and your aging parent: a family guide to emotional, social, health, and financial
problems / Barbara Silverstone, Helen Kandel Hyman; with commentary by Bob
Morris and with special contributions by Kim Waller and Penny Schwartz.—4th ed.
    p. cm.
Includes bibliographical references and index.
ISBN 978-0-19-531316-1
1. Aging parents—Family relationships—United States.   2. Middle-aged
persons—Family relationships—United States.   3. Old age assistance—
United States.   4. Older people—Psychology.   I. Hyman, Helen.   II. Title.
HQ1064.U5S54 2008
306.874084'6—dc22   2007029755

Please visit this volume's companion website at
www.oup.com/us/youandyouragingparent

9 8 7 6 5 4 3 2 1
Printed in the United States of America
on acid-free paper

To the Memory of—

Janet Sainer
1918–2007
A Pioneer in Services for the Aging

and

Helen Kandel Hyman
1921–2006
Co-author of You and Your Aging Parent

Contents

Preface

You and Your Aging Parent, first published in 1976, was the first trade book to focus on the relationship between adult children and their aging parents. It turned the spotlight on the challenges faced by many adult children—now known to us all as the "sandwich generation"—as they attempt to cope when elderly relatives need increasing support. *You and Your Aging Parent*, updated in 1982 and 1989, has been referred to by gerontologists as the "bible" of the sandwich generation.

The book enjoyed steady sales for 25 years but was once again out of date and in need of revision. Programs and services for older adults and their families have changed significantly, a new generation of adult children and their parents face the challenges of aging, and recent research findings have deepened our understanding of the aging process and later life. This revised edition of *You and Your Aging Parent*, the planning of which began during its 30th anniversary year, addresses the changes that have taken place.

Perhaps the most dramatic change in the years since the last edition was published in 1989 has been the increased attention paid by the research, policy, and service communities to the families caring for their aging relatives. We are proud if our book played a role in this dramatic awakening. However, given the abundance of helpful books for family caregivers now on the market, we asked ourselves if a fourth edition of *You and Your Aging Parent* was needed. An affirmative answer to this question reflected our observation that most of these books are focused almost exclusively on the caregiving situation and the adult child as caregiver. In contrast, in each of its editions, *You and Your Aging Parent* has told an enduring story about adult generations negotiating the challenges of later life that extend beyond the caregiving relationship. More than a "how-to" book for younger family members, this book again tries to engage not only adult children but also older persons themselves. We bring the personal perspective of the aging parent closer to home than perhaps was possible in earlier editions.

In this fourth edition, much of what has made *You and Your Aging Parent* an invaluable resource for so many families (as well as students, professionals, and service providers) has been retained, including, for the most part, the organization of the book and our observations of the intangibles in family relationships that rarely change. The table of contents does not differ markedly in structure from that of previous editions, but various chapters have been updated to incorporate new information on the practical aspects of growing old in America, from finances to housing to medical care to social services, and on the challenges that parents and their adult children face today as they navigate the aging process. Because of the abundance of helpful information now available for families from other sources, however, we have been selective about the content of this fourth edition and have focused on issues and information requiring more public attention, including adding a new chapter on a recent phenomenon—the widespread use and misuse of prescription and over the counter drugs by older adults. Also new to the book is commentary by Bob Morris—playwright, columnist, and author—who brings to the end of each chapter his own perspective on today's middle-aged child as he experienced his own parents' aging.

Although diagnosed with lung cancer, Helen Hyman was eager and able to collaborate on the outline of this fourth edition, and a proposal was submitted to Oxford University Press in the fall of 2005. Responding well at that time to the chemotherapy she was receiving, Helen felt well enough to move ahead with our collaboration, and we signed a contract with the publisher in January

2006. But her condition worsened, and she died 2 months later. It was with a heavy heart, then, that I moved ahead with this edition, but I am gratified that Helen's voice, and much of her original contribution, have been retained in the pages that follow.

B.S.

Acknowledgments

My appreciation extends over the past 31 years to those we acknowledged in earlier editions, especially the late Charlotte Kirschner. Her research contributions and sensitivity to the challenges faced by older adults and their families were invaluable to all four editions.

The exciting new additions to the fourth edition would not be possible without the fine contributions made by stellar writers Bob Morris and Kim Waller, and I thank them. I am also very grateful to geriatrician Dr. Harrison Bloom for his expert advice and to Dr. Penny Schwartz, social worker and advocate on behalf of older adults, for her guidance and permission to publish her Personal Papers Inventory. My assistant, Alexis Bortone, deserves heaps of praise and gratitude for her adeptness in helping me update and organize a vast array of new information.

The encouragement of senior editor Marion Osmun, was indispensable to moving ahead with the fourth edition, and I deeply appreciate her expert guidance over the past year and her good humor, which lightened my load. I thank the children of Helen Kandel Hyman for their confidence in my carrying on with the fourth edition after their mother's death. And, last but not least, to my husband, Stanley, for his patience, insight, and love over the past 45 years and being a staunch supporter through four editions of *You and Your Aging Parent*.

B. S.

You and Your Aging Parent

Introduction

We always had Thanksgiving dinner at my parents' house: my brother and his family, my husband, and my children. Year after year, it was always the same—the polished silver, the good china, the wonderful cooking smells. But last year something was different. My father's hands shook so badly that he could barely carve the turkey. My mother looked frail, almost shrunken, at the other end of the table. Suddenly, for the first time, it hit me: my parents were getting old.

Mary Lewis was 55 years old. Her father was 82 and her mother 80. She knew their ages well. Hadn't she always celebrated their birthdays with them? But she'd never admitted that they were getting older with each celebration. It came to her as a shock.

It was my mother's funeral, but I couldn't think about her at all. I kept watching my disabled father and thinking about him. What would happen to him now? Who would take care of him? Where would he live? How would we all manage?

Barry Richards was 38 and his wife was pregnant again. Their apartment was barely big enough for another child, and they couldn't afford to move yet. There was no way Barry's father could live with them. But he certainly couldn't live alone. Where would he go now?

I called my mother last night and I let the phone ring and ring, but she didn't answer. The same old panic started. Was she sick? Had she fallen and broken something? Was she unconscious? Maybe a heart attack? A stroke? I told myself she was probably out at the store—but I couldn't be sure. I'm never sure. I live 500 miles away and I go through this every time she doesn't answer her phone. Why does she make it so hard for me?

Frances Black's mother insisted on staying on in her old house long after her husband's death, even though the neighborhood had changed and was no longer pleasant or even safe. She stubbornly refused repeated invitations to move in with Frances and her family or to move closer to them. So Frances worried constantly, phoned several times a week, and prayed each time that the phone would be answered. She continually felt guilty and inadequate. But that was nothing new—she'd felt that way most of her life. Somehow, Jerry, her younger brother, had always seemed to do everything right. He still did—even though Frances was the one who phoned regularly.

M ARY, BARRY, AND FRANCES ARE THREE SEPARATE people, living in different parts of the country, with different lifestyles, different careers, and different incomes. They have never met, nor are they likely to. But if they were to meet, they would find that they have one thing in common: they all belong to the special generation caught in the middle—men and women pulled in three directions, trying to rear their children, live their own lives, and care for their aging parents—perhaps even their grandparents—at the same time. Some are facing the immediacy of their own aging. These sons and daughters, commonly referred to as the "sandwich generation," need to have their title revised. Their sandwich is now, in many cases, a triple-decker.

This painful three-way pull is not experienced by everyone in the middle generation. Some people have no reason to feel conflicting loyalties if their parents remain active and self-sufficient into their 70s, 80s, and 90s. Many older adults take old age surprisingly easily. Far from needing help from younger relatives, vigorous old men and women are often the ones who do the helping, encouraging their children and grandchildren to turn to them in times of trouble. Research findings reveal that there is a great deal of exchange of "goods and services" between the generations—as much flowing from the older to the younger generation as vice versa.

Despite the popular image, being old is not necessarily synonymous with being weak or helpless or finished. Old age can be a time of enjoyment, contentment, and productivity—even creativity. Because of prevailing prejudices, younger generations are rarely aware that all kinds of people—writers, artists, politicians, musicians, philosophers, scientists, businesspeople, craftspeople— often keep right on working for decades after their 65th birthday, sometimes making major contributions in their 70s, 80s, and 90s. The young tend to assume that life must be dreadful for the old, but the old themselves, who are experiencing old age firsthand, take a far less negative view of their own lives. As the columnist Russell Baker once wrote, "Wrinkles are just as natural a part of life as diaper rash and adolescent acne and a lot more comfortable, to boot."

A survey commissioned by the National Council on the Aging and conducted by survey expert Louis Harris as far back as 1974, dramatizes the gap between the feelings of the older and the younger generations. The sample of respondents 65 and older were asked about their own lives; the sample of respondents 18–64 were asked about their beliefs about the lives of old people. A few of the findings selected from the Harris tables (Table 1–1) are enough to illustrate how false the prevailing assumptions are (similar findings have been reported by subsequent studies).

These figures can be deceptive. It has been said that statistics are "people without tears." While life may have seemed easier for most older people than was generally assumed, there were substantial numbers for whom life was tragically difficult. Assuming the numbers are similar today, the 12% who feel lonely represent only a small minority of the total, but in the USA, with more than 35 million people over 65, that small percentage translates into over 4 million lonely old people. The 21% who rate their problem of poor health as "very serious" translates into over 7 million ailing old people—one

TABLE 1–1

	Percentage of aged reporting they themselves have a very serious problem with:	Percentage of those under 65 believing most people over 65 have a "very serious" problem with:
Not having enough friends	5	28
Not having enough to do	6	37
Not feeling needed	7	54
Loneliness	12	60
Not having enough money to live on	15	62
Poor health	21	51

out of every five! Nor does it help much to read the statistics and find out that other people's parents are getting along pretty well if our own parents are getting along pretty badly. If we care about them at all, we usually want to do something to help them get along better, and most of us don't know what to do. Few of us have even vague plans about how to proceed if the day ever comes when they cannot manage alone.

The statistics show us that the odds are in our favor—the day may never come. Many of us escape the problem completely. In the back of our minds we may think, "Why plan for something that may never happen—if we're lucky?" Our parents may not live to be old; they may never need help; or, if they do, they may turn to someone else in the family—not us. A brother or a sister may offer to take in both of them, or whichever parent is left alone, widowed or divorced. We can sidestep the problem. But there is always the possibility that the very problem we have refused to think about will one day descend on us, disturbing our lives, our emotions, and our finances.

Even the most careful planner is taking a gamble. Plans that we make may be systematically foiled by the very unpredictable nature of the aging process. No one can sit back complacently in middle age and proclaim, "It's all set; I'm ready to take over when my parents need me," because except in certain special situations it is impossible to predict what aging parents will need and when.

Clare Fowler thought she was facing the future honestly and intelligently. She had begun thinking about it after her 50th birthday, when the younger of her two children got married. She knew that women usually outlive men in the United States—she had read the statistics. In addition, she was 12 years younger than her husband, who was already in his 60s. It seemed likely that she would be widowed at some point in the future; naturally, she hoped it would be the far future. Mr. Fowler was willing to discuss the likelihood with her, and they went over the financial picture. They both agreed that Mrs. Fowler should try to live an independent life and under no circumstances should live with either of their children. They even discussed some of their ideas with the children themselves, who—like most children—were not too eager to listen.

But things didn't go according to plan. Mrs. Fowler died suddenly of a stroke at the age of 56, and her 68-year-old husband, who had never for a moment contemplated his own widowerhood, was left so emotionally helpless that he seemed incapable of living alone. To pull himself together, he made his home "temporarily" with his son and daughter-in-law and their children. There he stayed for the next 17 years, until he died at the age of 85.

Just as the future is unpredictable, the aging process itself does not follow any uniform calendar. Parents of young children know what comes next in early childhood development. Within a reasonable period, we know when our children will walk and talk, when their first teeth will come, and when they'll be likely to start kindergarten or high school. We can anticipate some of the emotional stages: the negativism at 2½, the rebellion in adolescence. The stages of growing old have no such predictable pattern. We can't look at our 60-year-old parents and announce, "Okay, 5 years to go until you're over the hill." One man's father may be beginning to decline at 65, it's true, but the next man's father may still be capably running his own life at 85—and still trying to dominate his son's, too, for that

The stages of growing old have no such predictable pattern. We can't look at our 60-year-old parents and announce, "Okay, 5 years to go until you're over the hill."

matter. One young woman of 25 is currently concerned, not about her mother or her grandmother but about her great-grandmother. This nonagenarian adamantly lives alone in a somewhat isolated house, stoking her own coal furnace, warming water on her stove, and letting her well-heeled descendants agonize over her welfare—but from a distance.

Vigorous elders are no longer a rarity. Many, less prominent, though all wearing that rather meaningless identification tag "65 and older," function just as well as their younger brothers and sisters still in their prime. Thanks to medical advances and widely followed regimens of healthy eating and regular exercise, millions of men and women are not only living longer but also feeling healthier and stronger, playing tennis, running marathons, climbing mountains, continuing their careers, or starting new ones. Some gerontologists even suggest that the upper age limit for middle age, formerly considered to be 65, be changed to 75, with 75 now the point at which the term "old" may be more appropriately applied. This shift seems to be quite logical, particularly since professionals involved with the lower end of the life cycle are suggesting that adolescence currently lasts until age 30.

In addition to the irregular and unpredictable calendar of physical aging, emotional and personality problems intervene and confuse the picture. Failing eyesight or severe arthritis may be overcome by sheer willpower and personal vitality by one elderly individual, who continues to live and function independently and even productively. By contrast, a similarly afflicted contemporary may retire quickly into invalidism and total dependency.

Apart from the passage of the Social Security Act in 1935, the later stages of life did not receive much attention, either from professional experts or from the public at large, until the 1960s. Society's interest was focused mainly on the earlier stages: infancy, youth, and middle age. Since then, however, aging has captured more and more of the limelight and is attracting long-overdue public and professional attention. This mounting concern about life in the later decades is well deserved. The elderly segment of the population has been steadily growing over the past century and increasing faster than any other age group. A disproportionate leap in the numbers of the elderly is anticipated in just a few short years, when the oldest baby boomers turn 65.

TABLE 1–2

	Population over 85
2000	4 million
2035	7 million
2050	19 million

Within the over-65 population in the United States, the over-85 group is increasing the fastest and will continue to do so, according to projections (Table 1–2). The size of this age group is especially important, because these individuals tend to be in poorer health and require more services than younger people.

Average life expectancy—which was 18 years in the days of ancient Greece, 33 in the year 1600, 42 in the Civil War period, and 47 in 1900—is now over 77. This dramatic change has taken place within the lifetime of many older adults. As Ronald Blythe points out in *The View in Winter:*

> If a Renaissance...man could return, he would be as much astonished by the sight of two or three thousand septuagenarians and octogenarians lining a South Coast resort on a summer's day...as he would be by a television set. His was a world where it was the exception to go grey, to reach the menopause, to retire, to become senile...

The 35 million men and women over 65 today represent over 12% of the population of the United States. The total population has increased threefold since 1900, but the ranks of the elderly have increased tenfold. By the year 2030, the older population is expected to reach 71.5 million. For the weight of its numbers alone, both present and future, that is a group to be reckoned with. The reckoning has been accelerating in recent years, although not nearly fast enough.

In the 44 years from the first White House Conference on Aging in 1961 to the fourth in 2005, major efforts were made to improve the welfare of older Americans. The year 1965 saw the passage of the Older Americans Act and the creation of a central federal office, the Administration on Aging, now under the Department of Health and Human Services. A network of area and local offices on aging has expanded throughout the nation, and today there are offices on aging in every state and territory, providing a wide range of services.

Medicare, social health insurance for persons over 65 and disabled persons, also adopted in 1965, has broadly expanded to provide coverage and services for over 35.4 million adults over the age of 65, including most recently coverage of some prescription drug costs. Social Security, adopted in 1935 to provide income maintenance to what was then a relatively small population of older adults, now provides benefits to over 33.2 million. For two thirds of the elderly population, this program provides the majority of income, and for one third, it provides nearly all of their income. Legislators over the years have paid close attention to the needs of older adults, and this consideration has not been without some amount of self-interest. The over-65 segment of the population, far from being disengaged socially or politically, is a powerful and articulate interest group, likely to register its opinions at election time. Studies of voting patterns consistently show that the turnout at the polls is higher for older voters than for very young ones.

The rising interest in the older population is not limited to legislative circles. Programs for older adults are featured in the popular press. TV and documentary films are showing the many faces of old age and are making the general public stop and think about the needs of older adults. Advice books addressed to older adults and their families have proliferated, and titles such as *geriatrician, gerontologist,* and *geriatric care manager* are now part and parcel of our vocabulary. Social planners are contemplating more comprehensive long-term care services and suggesting second careers to make the retirement years more meaningful. Even the building and architectural fields are dreaming up new communities geared to the lives of older people. Thanks to the virtual explosion in its field, gerontology is expected to be one of the fastest-growing career opportunities in the years ahead.

In recent years, the families of older adults have also moved into the limelight. Once written off as uninvolved and uncaring, families, including spouses and life partners, are recognized as the major caregivers of older adults. An abundance of research has documented the burden and stress experienced by family members, especially when caring for severely impaired older adults, and support services to assist them have increased dramatically in the last decade. Even if they are not playing a hands-on caregiver role, younger family members continue to be involved with their older relatives. They tend to prefer separate homes. So do their elderly parents. But that does not mean that they prefer separate, independent lives. Far from it.

Most of these families continue some involvement—often a close one—with the parent generation. Of the nearly 35 million men and women over 65, more than three quarters have at least one living child. Some time ago, a series of surveys made over a 20-year period with national samples of the over 65 population all reported that older people and their children (at least one child) usually maintained ongoing contact. Furthermore, despite the assumption that children these days grow up, move far away from their parents, and then do not visit much, the studies reported that 85% of the older adults with living children had at least one child who lived less than one hour away and that 66% of the elderly respondents had seen one of their children the very day they were interviewed or the day before; only 2% had not seen any of their children within the past year. Similar findings today generally support this picture.

Many families are willing and eager to help when aging parents, or even grandparents, are in trouble. These grown-up, usually middle-aged children, often over 65 themselves, may be motivated by a sense of responsibility, duty, or guilt; they are motivated just as often by genuine concern and love. But when elderly parents become more dependent and the problems of daily living multiply, their children soon discover that "love is not enough."

But if love is not enough, what else is there? Millions of sons and daughters are asking this question. These millions will increase steadily in the future as extended longevity creates a further abundance of three-, four-, and even five-generation families, resulting in what sociologist Vern Bengston has dubbed "the bean pole family." The millions of people concerned about their aging parents can be found anywhere and everywhere. Their problems are not limited to any one geographical location, any one socio-economic class or cultural group. Some are only in their early 30s, others much older. Some may even be in their 60s or 70s already, concerned about their own futures while still trying to help their parents, their children, and perhaps even their grandchildren. They have low, middle, and high incomes, because although money helps, it rarely provides the complete solution. They may be blue-collar or white-collar workers, a corporate CEO or an administrative assistant, a primary bread-winner or a couple holding down two or more jobs. They are found in every ethnic group (with variations); they are urban, suburban, ex-urban, and rural. They are highly educated or barely educated. Today the "sandwich generation"—or the "triple-decker"—is talked about, analyzed, and probed on TV panels and documentaries and on radio talk shows, as well as in seminars and conferences, frequently with titles such as "You and Your Aging Parent."

This book is primarily addressed to that large middle generation—today's baby boomers—who are facing the challenge of aging in their parents and maybe their grandparents as well as themselves. The book may also be helpful to older family members who are facing the challenges of their own old age and caring for a spouse or partner and maybe even a parent. It cannot pretend to cover every situation, touch on every problem, or list all of the resources available today. An abundance of information is available in many online and offline publications, some of which are listed in Appendix A. The chapters that follow are intended to help readers to think through their own personal situations more realistically and to begin to figure out more effective solutions to their own individual problems. The book takes no position on what this solution might be. Among the many types of families and the varying situations they face, there are multiple ways of caring.

While many of the solutions can be found in the outside community if families know where and how to look, other solutions may be found much closer to home. Sons and daughters naturally must understand their parents' needs before they can help them, but they must also understand themselves and their own feelings. Their own emotions are likely to con-

Sons and daughters naturally must understand their parents' needs before they can help them, but they must also understand themselves and their own feelings.

fuse the picture, hinder communication, and perhaps even prevent them from helping effectively.

֍

This book is therefore divided into three parts. Part I, "Taking Stock," presents an overall view of the range of problems that may complicate life for the older adults themselves and for their children: the emotions, conscious and unconscious, that color relationships between generations, the feelings between brothers and sisters that help or hinder when families try to work together.

The situations faced by older adults themselves will also be discussed: the "normal" losses of old age—physiological, psychological, and social—and the way some of them learn to compensate for these losses and relish the gains that are possible in later life. Marriage in the later years will be examined, as well as widowhood and widowerhood, the possibilities of remarriage, and the continuing sexual life of the older adults—an issue raised frequently by professionals but often viewed with uneasiness or alarm by the younger generations. The equally difficult and often unmentionable subject of death and the period before death is included, a logical final step in the process of taking stock.

Part II, "Taking Steps," analyzes available solutions to the problems raised in the earlier chapters. It considers first the ongoing relationships between children and elderly parents who are still managing fairly independently. How much communication is necessary? How much is expected? How much visiting? Phoning? Is it possible to have too much communication? How can older people be encouraged to plan for future emergencies, such as a disabling illness or accident? A chapter is devoted to the financial challenges of later life. Two chapters are devoted to the help and care required by older adults who cannot manage their own care to greater or lesser degrees and the varying capabilities of families to provide or manage this care. In addition to elders with seriously impairing mental and physical conditions who require around-the-clock care, attention is paid to the "in-betweeners"—those who suffer intermittent health crises and may need some help in their daily lives. The resources available in the community to help older adults and their families manage are described as well as in-home and nursing home solutions when both older adults and families cannot manage. The role that family members can play in easing the transition from home to nursing home and other stressful relocations is discussed. Because the family serves as the basic support system for older adults, Part II includes a chapter that describes how family members can work together to take more effective action on behalf of their elders.

Part III, "Extra Steps," includes a chapter new to this edition on the critical issue of medications and the knowledge required to be informed consumers. A glimpse of the future will be offered, including what it holds for those who will grow old in the years ahead and the proactive role that older adults and their families need to play in the political and policy arena. Finally, the epilogue discusses the issue of looking back after our parents have died.

The appendices include some of the resources available to older adults and their families both online and offline. While it is not comprehensive, the information here will point the reader in the right direction. Two checklists are also included: one for evaluating nursing homes and home health care services, and the other for keeping a personal papers inventory.

❧

When *You and Your Aging Parent* was first written in 1976, the authors were members of a generation struggling with the challenges faced by their aging parents. They could speak for adult children. But just as the elderly of today are different from yesterday's older generation, the middle generation is different as well, and so an important contribution to this fourth edition is the commentary of playwright, humorist, and *New York Times* columnist Bob Morris, one of today's baby boomers (albeit a late one, born in 1958). Bob brings an essential voice to this edition as he describes his own perspective as an adult child of elderly parents and his experiences with them during their declining years.

Very much in touch with his own feelings, and a keen observer of family relationships and his parents' experiences with failing health, Bob tells a story that is not atypical of his generation. He takes a sharp view of his baby boomer peers, who, like their parents before them, often do not confront the looming vicissitudes of aging:

I'm part of a huge demographic. Everybody's facing aging, or will be soon. But we'd like to avoid it as long as possible, keep it on the shelf, away from our fabulous little lives. Everybody's so scheduled now, so style conscious and exercise obsessed. But you have to wonder, how do parents fit into that?

Bob, with his older brother, grew up in a middle-class suburb of New York. While remaining in touch with his family, he chose a very different lifestyle as an adult, but was pulled back fully into the family circle when his mother became seriously ill and died, followed by his father's death 2 years later. These were wrenching emotional experiences for Bob, but he brings humor and pathos to his vivid recollections. More of his commentary follows each chapter and concludes as part of the epilogue.

Part I
Taking Stock

2

Facing Up to Feelings

Mary Graham was a devoted daughter—everyone said so. All her friends were amazed at the way she treated her old mother. . . . Such loving concern—such patient understanding! They knew that Mary phoned her mother every day, visited her several times a week, included her in every family activity, and never took a vacation without her. Her friends also knew that Mary's husband and children had learned to accept second place in her life years ago.

Mary herself knew that she had always done her best for her mother. Why did she always worry that her best was never good enough?

IN TIMES GONE BY, CHILDREN WHO SEEMED LOVING AND attentive to their parents were labeled "good" children, just as parents who seemed loving and attentive to their children were labeled "good" parents. The quality of the love and attention was not usually examined, nor was the cost to the giver or the effect on the receiver. Things are no longer so black and white.

The behavior of family members toward one another is viewed today as a complex process governed by a wide range of feelings. In this context, even traditionally "good" behavior is open to revaluation and tends to become suspect when carried to an extreme. "He

"He gave up his life for his old mother" may have been considered the highest form of noble sacrifice several generations ago, but today such a sacrifice might be questioned.

gave up his life for his old mother" may have been considered the highest form of noble sacrifice several generations ago, but today such a sacrifice might be questioned. *Why* did he do that? Didn't he have a right to a life of his own, too? A 60-year-old daughter still cowering in infantile submission before the rage of an autocratic 90-year-old father may have symbolized the supreme example of "dutiful affection" to the Victorians, but current thinking would make us wonder about the deeper reasons behind such behavior.

It is important that sons and daughters take stock of their feelings about their aging parents if they want to find some comfort for themselves and become better able to communicate with them and help effectively. Enough concrete obstacles can stand in the way when sons and daughters want to help. They may live too far away. They may have financial, health, career, or marital problems that legitimately prevent them from taking a supportive role in their parents' lives. But sometimes there are no such concrete obstacles—life may be going along quite smoothly—yet a daughter may be incapable of reaching out to her mother, and a son may wonder why his friends seem able to help their parents more than he can help his. Such children often excuse themselves by playing the "it's-easy-for-them" game:

> "They have so much money—*it's easy for them* to help John's parents."

> "With that big house—*it's easy for them* to find room for Mary's father."

> "Jane doesn't have a job—*it's easy for her* to visit her mother every day."

> "All their children are grown—*it's easy for them* to spend so much time at the nursing home."

All these statements have the same unspoken implication: "I would be just as good a son [or daughter] if only my life were different." But the unspoken implication would probably have greater validity if it substituted the words "if only my feelings were different." Un-resolved or unrecognized feelings can affect a child's behavior toward a parent, blocking any attempts to be helpful. Those feelings can also serve as catalysts for unwise, inappropriate decisions that hinder rather than help efforts to solve the older person's problems. Last, but equally important, unresolved feelings about parents can be very painful—sometimes really oppressive—for children. The well-being of both generations may improve, once these feelings are understood, accepted, and acted on appropriately.

Feelings That Spark an Emotional Tug of War

It is self-evident that human beings are capable of experiencing and acting on a wide range of feelings. Different people and different situations obviously arouse all sorts of different emotions. It is less self-evident that one human being can experience an equally wide range of feelings toward another human being. That is exactly what happens, however, when a substantial bond exists between any two people. A whole variety of different (and often conflicting) feelings can be aroused at different times. When people are important to us, we love them when they please us, hate them when they disappoint us, resent them when they hurt us. Love is not a 24-hour occupation, and even in the warmest relationships there can be moments of ir-ritation, envy, and frustration.

It might be easier if our feelings toward someone we love were more clear-cut and consistent, particularly when that person is old and perhaps helpless, but consistency and clarity are rare qualities denied to most of us.

All feelings do not have the same intensity. The minor annoyance we feel toward someone we love can easily be controlled, just as the occasional, though surprising, moments of affection we feel toward someone we dislike can also be tolerated. When contradictory feel-ings coexist with equally high intensity toward the same person, however, a painful conflict results. "I wish I didn't love my mother so much; then I could really hate her," a daughter cries in anguished frustration. She is deserving of sympathy for her emotional tug of war. Her struggle might be less painful if she realized that both the anger and the love she feels for her mother may be closely related and can sometimes last a lifetime. She might also be relieved to know that she is not alone and that many people are offended and angered most by someone they love very much, although they may try to remain unaware of their less acceptable feelings toward their parents. When intense feelings are pushed out of our own awareness, they only rise again—sometimes in a disguised form. Once admitted and accepted, these feelings can more easily be placed in perspective, and the person who bears them freed to behave more effectively.

Many of the feelings we have about our parents in their later years are the same old ones we always had about them.

Many of the feelings we have about our parents in their later years are the same old ones we always had about them. They were formed in childhood, and a pattern was established and carried through life. The intensity and immediacy of these feelings may have changed somewhat as we grew into adulthood. By moving out of our parents' house we also moved away from daily contact and interaction. Emotional and physical distance provided a wide buffer zone. While our parents remain active and self-reliant, they live their own lives, with greater or lesser involvement with ours. The relationship with them may be pleasant and gratifying or frustrating and abrasive.

Old feelings from the past can rise up to plague us again when our parents get older, feebler, sicker, or poorer, and are in need of our help, as we were once, long ago, in need of theirs. We can no longer so easily maintain an emotional distance, even when physically separated, and too easily fall back into old patterns, both pleasant and unpleasant: old affections may rise again, old wounds reopened, old loyalties remembered, old debts revived, and old weaknesses exposed once more.

In addition to bringing old feelings into play again, our parents' aging—especially if they become dependent on us—may intensify feelings and attitudes that we developed later because of experiences in our own separate adult lives. Some of these newer feelings, like the older ones, may seem unacceptable, and we may prefer to ignore them. But ignoring them won't make them go away.

Because such a variety of feelings, some less comfortable than others, enter into the relationships between grown children and their aging parents, it may be helpful to examine a number of the most common ones: love, compassion, respect, tenderness, sadness, indifference, and then fear, anger, resentment, hostility, contempt, and shame. Finally, we turn to the most uncomfortable feeling of all—guilt—which today is worn like the scarlet letter by so many adult children of aging parents.

Love, Compassion, Respect, Tenderness, and Sadness

When some or all of these feelings are present in a relationship and are not too complicated by the simultaneous existence of powerful conflicting feelings, they serve as a vital source of support and strength for both generations. They provide comfort for the older generation and enable the younger generation to reach out willingly to help. When feelings of love and respect have always existed between parents and children, they usually reflect a strong bond developed by a longstanding pattern of mutual caring.

When feelings of love and respect have always existed between parents and children, they usually reflect a strong bond developed by a longstanding pattern of mutual caring.

While growing up, children look to those closest to them for models of behavior and tend to copy what they see. If one or both parents show a young child love, care, unselfishness, and consideration, it is likely that the child as an adult will find it natural to show some of these feelings to his parents when they are old. Children who have never witnessed giving, reaching out, sharing, or tenderness in action often have no models to copy and never learn how to feel or show these emotions. Your parents' behavior toward others, as well as toward you, may have provided additional models. You may have seen them behave with respect and consideration to their own parents—your grandparents. Family traditions and patterns of behavior are often passed on from generation to generation.

But behavior is a complex process, and many other factors besides family tradition and models established in early childhood can influence the positive feelings we have toward our parents when they are old. Their treatment of us as children may have been far from tender and warm. We may have seen them as distant, cold, and punitive and thought them unfair and unreasonable while we were growing up. But later in life, when time, distance, and our own experiences put a different perspective on past behavior, we may come to understand, as adults, what we could not understand as children: why our parents acted the way they did. Mistakes they made in the past may continue to rankle in the present, but the intensity of the resentment may be counteracted by a new respect we develop for the way they cope with life as old people. "He was a domineering tyrant when we were young," a son says of his father, "but how he's mellowed! He's great to be with now, even though he's so sick—no complaints, no self-pity. I really admire the guy, and I hope we'll do as well when we're his age." A daughter remembers her deprived childhood: "We had to fight for everything we had. Mom and Dad seemed like misers—penny-pinchers. But now that I've got my own family, I can understand what they went through to raise five kids. I'd do anything to make things easier for them now." Strong feelings of love, compassion, tenderness, and respect are likely to be accompanied by sadness, as members of the younger generation realize that their elderly parents are no longer the people they used to be and that death is coming closer every day.

Indifference

Love, affection, respect, compassion, and concern can all exist simultaneously in any relationship between grown children and their aging parents. These emotions may have equal intensity, or some may be stronger than others. It also may happen that one of these emotions may exist alone, without any of the others. A son may respect his parents and be concerned for them—and because of these feelings, he may be extremely helpful to them. But he may never have loved them, liked them, or felt much real affection for either one; instead, he may have felt apathy and indifference. That lack of feeling may be quite painful, and he may experience considerable remorse because of it, but even so, he may feel responsible for their welfare and concerned about their problems. While love and affection are often effective catalysts to a helping relationship, they are not essential.

While love and affection are often effective catalysts to a helping relationship, they are not essential.

Fear

"She lies there like a fragile little doll—she couldn't lift a finger to hurt me. How can I still be scared to death she's going to be mad at me for something?" asked a middle-aged woman on one of her regular visits to her mother in a nursing home. She laughed as she spoke because she realized how ludicrous it seems to fear an 80-lb, bedridden invalid. But she was serious, too. Some children live in fear of either or both of their parents, even when these parents are weak, helpless, frail, or terminally ill. Children may fear so many things— disapproval, losing love, death, the irrevocable loss of the older person, and also losing out on an inheritance. Chronic, irrational fear or anxiety in relation to a parent is likely to have its roots in dimly remembered early childhood experiences. Small children are totally dependent on their parents; without them, they feel stranded, abandoned, alone. The parents, being bigger and stronger, are also the ones who set the rules and enforce the dictates of society. Thus, a child can fear his parents on three levels: abandonment, loss of love, and punishment. Children who never resolve or shake off the vestiges of that close, dependent relationship may continue to suffer fearful or anxious feelings in relation to their parents in one form or another throughout life.

Older parents themselves are often responsible for reinforcing fearful feelings in their grown children, unconsciously or even deliberately continuing to nourish old childhood dependencies. Weak old men and fragile old women often somehow find the strength to retain command, directing their children's lives from wheelchairs and sickbeds. A son may long for freedom from a domineering mother while simultaneously suffering constant anxiety that he will do something to displease her. A child may also grow up in fear that he will not live up to his parents' expectations for him in terms of career, worldly success, or material possessions. He may also be afraid that he will never be the kind of person they want him to be— someone they approve of. "I've got a good business going," a middle-aged man complains. "I put three kids through college, I'm president of our Rotary Club, but my father thinks I'm a failure—his only son was supposed to be a lawyer. And you know what? Whenever I'm with him, I feel like a failure, too."

Anger, Resentment, Hostility, and Contempt

Large-scale upheavals and tragedies obviously have an emotional impact on children that often affects their future lives. Death or chronic illness of a mother or father, divorce, neglect, abandonment—such events can determine the kind of feelings children have for parents, feelings that can last a lifetime. "I hated my mother when she remarried" or "Our family fell apart after my father's business failed" or "My father walked out one day and left us alone." Such statements pinpoint causes and serve to explain the rise of hostile feelings. But even without such dramatic events, the development of angry feelings in childhood is often unavoidably stimulated through the early years of day-to-day family living.

Just as the comfortable feelings of love and tenderness, as well as the uncomfortable feelings of fear and anxiety, are associated with close ties, so, in many cases, are angry, hostile, and resentful ones. These feelings are often most intense between the persons most closely attached to each other. There are subtle differences between them. Anger is a transitory feeling, but if it becomes chronic, it is usually referred to as *hostility*. Contempt describes the way a person feels toward someone he considers worthless or immoral. Children are likely to have moments, even longer periods, of all these uncomfortable emotions while growing up. Few relationships are free of them. But when occasional flare-ups become solidified into permanent attitudes, a complex relationship develops.

Oscar Wilde wrote in *The Picture of Dorian Gray:* "Children begin by loving their parents; as they grow older they like them; later they judge them; sometimes they forgive them." He implied that the judgments are not always so favorably resolved. Childhood may seem an eternity away as people grow older and many memories are left behind, both pleasant and unpleasant. But the feelings developed in that period are not so easily left behind; they tag along through life.

Once a resentful child begins to live his own adult life, he may forget how angry he used to be with his parents. But just as the helplessness and disabilities of their old age can awaken feelings of tenderness and compassion untapped for years, their new dependency can rekindle old feelings of anger and resentment long thought to be dead and buried. Buried—yes. Dead—never. Sons and daughters may remember all over again the way their parents neglected them as children, the way they punished them unfairly or too harshly, the way they scorned their abilities or belittled their accomplishments, and especially the way they favored another sibling. Forty years later, we can still be angry and resentful about our parents' failures in the past. The fact that they are now old and frail may not diminish these feelings, particularly if they continue to behave in the infuriating manner we have disliked for so long. Our failure to help them now may be a form of subtle retaliation: "You need me now. Where were you when I needed you?"

Shame

This uncomfortable feeling comes in several forms and with varying degrees of intensity. Everyone knows moments of shame; they come and go throughout life in response to an endless number of causes. For the sons and daughters of elderly parents, shame can sometimes be an ever-present feeling. The simplest and most common form of shame comes when children feel they do not do enough for their parents. Perhaps a son doesn't visit his parents enough; perhaps he is unable to give them financial help; perhaps he allows a brother, a sister, or even a stranger to provide solutions to problems he feels he should be handling himself. He may have his own reasons for behaving the way he does, but nevertheless he feels deep inside that if he were a better person he would be doing a better job. Sons and daughters who feel ashamed for those reasons have plenty of fellow sufferers.

A second form of shame is involved when sons and daughters are ashamed, not of themselves for their own failings, but of their parents for their failings. A self-made man may be ashamed of his poor, illiterate parents and keep them in the background because he does not want his world to know where he came from. An intellectual

A second form of shame is involved when sons and daughters are ashamed, not of themselves for their own failings, but of their parents for their failings.

woman may be ashamed of her uneducated father, a sophisticated city-dweller of her small-town parents. A son may want to keep an alcoholic father hidden—like other family skeletons—in the closet. When we are ashamed of our parents, it is usually because we fear that their shortcomings will reflect badly on us in the eyes of other people whose opinions we value: our friends, neighbors, colleagues, church groups, social clubs, employers, even in-laws.

In his memoir *Lost in America: A Journey with My Father*, Sherwin Nuland speaks of the shame he felt as a young man about his father's disabilities, feelings that did not diminish as his father grew old.

> And, so, I did not become less embarrassed by my father as I grew older and thought I was growing more mature. If anything, his steady deterioration and my increasing involvement with the world outside of the Bronx (where I grew up) only increased my discomfort when he and I were with strangers. My shame—for it *was* shame— became more severe as my circle of friends came to include young people and older ones, too, who had never encountered anyone like him before.

A third level of shame is a combination of the first two: we may be ashamed of ourselves because we are ashamed of our parents. This is probably the most painful form of shame and the most difficult to cope with. It stirs up great emotional conflict in sons and daughters, prevents them from offering constructive help to their parents, and forces them to bear a continual and heavy burden of guilt.

And Finally—Guilt!

Guilt has been left for last because it is usually the end result or the prime mover of many of the other uncomfortable feelings from the past and present.

> John Wilson is ashamed of his parents. He feels ashamed of himself because he is ashamed of them and guilty because he is not helping them more. He then feels angry and resentful of them because he has to feel guilty and then anxious and fearful that some unknown punishment will be dealt out to him be- cause of his anger.

Poor John. Because of one uncomfortable feeling, shame, he has to suffer the entire gamut of other uncomfortable emotions. This is a frequent occurrence; rarely does one single emotion stand alone. The whole mixed bag of feelings is interrelated, one capable of setting of another. Guilt can evoke resentment, resentment more guilt, and guilt more fear—an endless, self-perpetuating cycle. Pity the unfortunate human being caught in the middle!

Guilt is a hidden or exposed emotion that signals to us our own sense of wrongdoing in words, deeds, or even thoughts. It is often accompanied by lowered self-esteem and a wish for punishment. Conscious feelings of guilt are not the same as unconscious guilt, which may be experienced as a need for self-punishment.

> Phil had planned for some time to spend his only day off with his bedridden father. When the day came, it was so beautiful that he decided he had to go fishing instead. On the way to the lake, he got lost twice on what had always been a familiar route and dented his car when leaving a gas station. When he finally arrived at the lake, he found he had left his fishing tackle at home. That night he slept fitfully and dreamed that his father had died.

But guilt is not always so buried. People can also feel very guilty for things they have actually done or not done: objective sins of commission or omission. In that respect, guilt means an acceptance of responsibility for action taken or action evaded and, within reasonable limits, can be a sign of emotional maturity. Our guilt may stem from the uncomfortable suspicion that we have not behaved responsibly toward our parents, and then, the more guilt we feel, the more difficult we may find it to behave responsibly. Responsible behavior usually flows more easily when we understand not only our parents but also ourselves and our feelings toward them.

A 50-year-old man put this understanding into action as he carefully inspected a well-known nursing home and discussed his situation with the administrator.

> My mother and I have never had an easy or a pleasant relationship. She's always been a difficult, cold, resentful woman. I can't forget the way she treated me when I was young . . . and I only had superficial contacts with her when I grew up. But she

needs someone to take care of her now, after her stroke. I certainly can't bring her to live with my family and me—none of us could take it. But she is old, and she is my mother, and I want her to be as comfortable and as protected as possible.

Such cool, objective understanding is rare. The guilty feelings of grown sons and daughters are so primed and ready these days that they can be set off by the most insignificant stimulus. A sentence, even a gesture or a shrug, from an elderly mother or father can easily do the trick. Some statements are heard so frequently that they are included in comedy routines because they strike home universally. "You young people run along and enjoy yourselves. I'm perfectly fine *alone* here by myself," or "I know how busy you are. I understand that you forgot to call me yesterday. Of course, I *did* worry." Shakespeare's King Lear pointed to the guilt of past, present, and probably future generations when he cried, "How sharper than a serpent's tooth it is to have a thankless child!"

Any discussion of guilt should include at least a reference to the guilt sons and daughters feel when they wish that an elderly mother or father would die. Most people who feel it also consider it too terrible to admit, particularly if they are angry with their parents. The death wish comes in two forms: the more acceptable form is reserved for a parent who is terminally ill, in constant pain, with no chance of recovery. A daughter says in genuine sorrow, "I hope Mother dies soon. I can't stand to see her suffer anymore."

A less acceptable death wish is directed toward a parent who is not terminally ill but is merely difficult or incapacitated, sapping the physical and emotional strength of the family. A son or daughter who is closely involved may feel (but rarely admit), "I wish she would die and then I'd have some life for myself at last." There are many instances in which both these wishes are understandable, but since it has traditionally been considered "wicked" to wish death to another person, particularly a parent, these wishes usually involve some burden of guilt.

In addition to the specific guilt suffered by individuals, there may also be a pervasive guilt generated by the uneasy knowledge that we cannot provide for our elderly parents as they provided for us when we were young. We have a sense that we are welshing on a debt. But in present-day society, paying that debt is often impossible. Because of inadequate facilities within the family and inadequate services outside in the community, well-intentioned children may have to suffer the guilty burden "We are not caring for those who cared for us."

A fable of a father bird and his three fledglings seems to wrap up the subject. It appeared in a book written in 1690 by a widow in Germany for her children. Glückel of Hameln's message still rings true in 2008.

We should, I say, put ourselves to great pains for our children, for on this the world is built, yet we must understand that if children did as much for their parents, the children would quickly tire of it.

A bird once set out to cross a windy sea with its three fledglings. The sea was so wide and the wind so strong, the father bird was forced to carry his young, one by one, in his strong claws. When he was half-way across with the first fledgling the wind turned into a gale, and he said, "My child, look how I am struggling and risking my life in your behalf. When you are grown up, will you do as much for me and provide for my old age?" The fledgling replied, "Only bring me to safety, and when you are old I shall do everything you ask of me." Whereat the father bird dropped his child into the sea, and it drowned, and he said, "So shall it be done to such a liar as you." Then the father bird returned to shore, set forth with his second fledgling, asked the same question, and receiving the same answer, drowned the second child with the cry, "You, too, are a liar." Finally he set out with the third fledgling, and when he asked the same question, the third and last fledgling replied, "My dear father, it is true you are struggling mightily and risking your life in my behalf, and I shall be wrong not to repay you when you are old, but I cannot bind myself. This though I can promise: when I am grown up and have children of my own, I shall do as much for them as you have done for me." Whereupon the father bird said, "Well spoken, my child, and wisely; your life I will spare and I will carry you to shore in safety."

Special Reactions to Aging

While many of the feelings we have about our parents can be traced back to childhood sources, it is never too late to experience new ones. Successes and failures in adult life can also strongly affect the way we feel about our parents.

While many of the feelings we have about our parents can be traced back to childhood sources, it is never too late to experience new ones. Successes and failures in adult life can also strongly affect the way we feel about our parents. Their plight itself or some new understanding of our own can stimulate unaccustomed feelings of love and compassion we never knew before. New stresses can produce angry or fearful reactions we would never have believed we were capable of feeling. While the intensity of some feelings persists unabated through life, the intensity of others can fade through the years, leaving room for new ones, although it is often difficult to figure out where the new ones come from. Men and women may seem quite puzzled by their changing feelings: "I used to get along so well with my parents; why are they driving me up the wall all of a sudden?" or "I don't have any patience with them anymore," or "I'd give anything to skip visiting Mother this week—I can't understand why she depresses me so much these days." Clues to the roots of these troubling feelings may be found in how the younger generation answers the following questions.

Can You Accept Your Parents' Old Age?

As old but active men and women begin to undergo mental and physical changes, their children can react with mixed emotions: shock (if there is sudden physical and mental deterioration), denial (if the deterioration is a slow slide downhill), anger, shame, fear, and resentment, as well as the more expected feelings of sadness, sympathy, and concern. We may be surprised at our own reactions to our parents' decline and wonder how we could possibly be angry with them when we ought to be sympathetic. Yet anger is not as inappropriate as it may seem.

Most of us, as children, viewed our parents as immortal—strong enough to protect us forever. As we mature, we learn we can take care of ourselves and in the process find out, with some regret, that our parents are not quite as perfect or infallible as we once thought. Somewhere inside us, however, remains a trace of the old conviction that our parents could still protect us if we needed them to, so their physical and mental deterioration is shocking. On an intellectual level, we keep telling ourselves, "It's understandable—they're getting old; they're fading." But on a gut level we can still be sad, frightened, and resentful, as if they have broken a promise to us—a promise that was never actually made. Every time we see them, we have to be reminded of their mortality—and our own. The deterioration of a vigorous mind—confusion, disorientation, loss of comprehension, loss of memory—can be even harder to accept than the deterioration of a vigorous body in those families in which intellectual activities and verbal communication are particularly meaningful. Nothing can be more painful than the realization that a parent no longer understands us, or even recognizes us. Why should we be so surprised that the realization makes us angry or that we try to deny it?

Can You Accept Your Own Aging?

So far this chapter has focused on relationships between children and their aging parents, and the feelings generated by these relationships. But another set of feelings can be aroused independently of interpersonal reactions: the feelings people have about old age in general, their own old age, and their own mortality. The behavior of children toward their elderly parents can be profoundly affected by these feelings.

Many people, including today's baby boomers, are reluctant to talk about their old age and mortality; some even prefer not to think about either one. Our attitudes vary, depending on whether we admire old people or secretly despise them, whether we feel older people deserve respect or consideration, whether we believe they can remain sexually or creatively active, and whether we dread the day when we will be old or the day we will die. Not everyone can agree with the poet Walt Whitman:

Many people, including today's baby boomers, are reluctant to talk about their old age and mortality; some even prefer not to think about either one.

Youth, large, lusty, loving
Youth, full of grace, force, fascination.
Do you know that old age may come after you
with equal grace, force and fascination?
—"Great are the Myths," #317 from *Leaves of Grass. 1900*

The feelings we have about our own old age often have a direct bearing on how effectively we can help our parents during their old age, and how constructively we can plan for our own.

People who tend to have a positive attitude toward old age in general, including their own, are more likely to be able to reach out to their elderly parents with concern, compassion, and constructive support. If old age appears as a time to be dreaded—and many features of modern society would suggest to us that it is—then our parents' decline may seem very threatening. Their aging seems to toll the bells for our own aging and our inevitable death.

At the funeral of an 85-year-old man, his gray-haired daughter was overheard saying sadly, "There goes our last umbrella." She explained later that she had always thought of the parent and grandparent generations as umbrellas, because even when umbrellas are broken and threadbare they can still give some form of protection and shelter from the elements. When her father, the last of the older generation, died, she mourned him because she felt, "Now we have no shelter left. There's nothing anymore between us and what lies ahead for us. We're next in line."

Being next in line, of course, means being next in line for death. If we cannot contemplate our own mortality, how can we contemplate our parents'? It can be really painful, yet every time we see them, we are reminded of the very thing we'd prefer to avoid thinking about.

An interesting parallel can be drawn between the way people look at childhood and the way they look at old age. For many parents, one of the pleasures of watching their children grow involves the reawakening of childhood memories and the chance to relive the pleasures they knew when they were young. Similarly, as we watch our parents grow old, we may see the shape of our own old age lying in wait for us. We may resent them because they force us to "pre-live" our own old age and death long before we need to. A Pakistani tale (similar versions of which are found in the folklore of other cultures) makes this point clearly:

> An ancient grandmother lived with her daughter and her grandson in a small but comfortable house not far from the village. The old woman grew frail and feeble, her eyesight became dimmer every day, and she found it hard to remember where she'd put things and what people had asked her to do. Instead of being a help around the house she became a constant trial and irritation. She broke the plates and cups, lost the knives, put out the stove, and spilled the water. One day, exasperated because the older woman had broken another precious plate, the younger one gave some money to her son and told him, "Go to the village and buy your grandmother a wooden plate. At least we will have one thing in the house she cannot break."
>
> The boy hesitated because he knew that wooden plates were only used by peasants and servants—not by fine ladies like his grandmother—but his mother insisted, so off he went. Some time later he returned, bringing not one but two wooden plates.
>
> "I only asked you to buy one," his mother said to him sharply. "Didn't you listen to me?"
>
> "Yes," said the boy. "But I bought the second one so there will be one for you when you get old."

Special Reactions to Caregiving

The caregiving provided by adult children to their aging parents covers a wide range of support, from the common intergenerational exchanges within and between generations to around-the-clock support and hands-on care when an older relative is very frail and disabled. These latter circumstances place a burden on the family caregiver that is managed with relative equanimity by some and experienced as very stressful by others. Although many family caregivers report that they gain much satisfaction from providing care to their aging relatives, even they deal with feelings that are sometimes troubling. Some of these feelings relate to the change in roles experienced by the caregiver; others relate to situations in which the caregiver feels overburdened.

Can You Accept a Different Role?

Although few old people return to "second childhood," which Shakespeare describes as the last in the seven ages of man, they frequently, because of increasing helplessness, need to depend on people who are stronger. When the family is young, the parent plays the independent, strong role and the child the dependent, weak one. When some parents age, they may be willing to abdicate the power they once had, glad to pass it on to more capable hands. The "gift" may weigh heavily on some sons and daughters, who prefer their old, familiar dependent roles. Others take the gift and use it well, but resent being forced to accept it. The acceptance in itself symbolizes the end of one long-standing relationship and the beginning of a new one.

A teacher in her 40s described how shocked she felt one day when she heard herself speaking to her ailing mother in the cheery tones she used in kindergarten: "Now, let's hurry up and finish this nice soup." Later she commented wryly, "I have three children at home and 20 in my class at school. I certainly don't need another one. What I need is a mother, and I'll never have one again." She knew that she and her mother had, to an extent, changed roles forever, and accompanying this new relationship were feelings of anger, resentment, fear, and sadness, all mixed up with love.

In *The Caregiver's Tale: Loss and Renewal in Memoirs of Family Life*, Ann Burack-Weiss comments on a common theme expressed in the memoirs of children who have lived relatively separate adult lives from their parents. She notes the equilibrium between the generations that is shattered when the parents become more dependent.

Years, usually decades, have passed since the authors spent so much time in their parents' company or so much time thinking about them when they are apart. The authors are no longer the children they were; they have spent some time out in the world, learning about others and about themselves. Their parents too have changed. However strong their personalities remain, the ravages of aging and illness have reduced their power.

Most important, the relationship itself has changed. It is not as some suggest a "role reversal." Rather it is a new kind of intimacy, one infused with a need to know their parents as individuals in their own right, to see them "whole." (p. 73)

Are You Overburdened?

Children who are beset by a multitude of concerns in their own lives—health, finances, career, children, grandchildren, even their own retirement worries—may be so drained that they cannot begin to shoulder their parents' problems as well. They may try to do their best, feel ashamed that they are not doing better, and more likely than not, resent the older generation for giving them additional burdens to bear. The following phone call dramatizes this situation— a conversation between a mother and daughter, including the younger woman's unspoken thoughts:

Daughter: Hello, Mother. How are you? *[Don't let there be anything wrong today! I just can't take one more problem.]*
Mother (small, shaky voice): I nearly died last night.

Daughter (solicitously): Was your leg bad again? *[Oh, God! It's going to be one of those days again. I hope she doesn't keep me on all morning. I've got to get down to talk to Janie's teacher. Why is that child getting into so much trouble this year?]* Are you using the heating pad?
Mother: The pain was like a knife. I said to Mrs. Forest this morning—

Daughter (cutting in, a little impatiently): Didn't you take that new medicine Dr. Croner gave you? He said it would help.
Mother: Don't talk to me about doctors! What do doctors care about an old person? It was a waste of my time going to him.

Daughter: But you said he was such a genius. *[A waste of whose time! Does she have any idea what I went through to take her to that doctor? I changed my whole week*

around. Janie missed her dentist appointment, I got a
parking ticket, and Jack was furious. Jack's always furious
these days.]

Mother: Mrs. Forest said he was a genius. Mrs. Forest
cares about how I feel—she listens to me. You're so busy
all the time—you don't really want to worry about me.
You have your children and your husband to think
about.

Daughter (guilty, but exasperated):   Oh, Mother, stop saying
things like that. *[Why does she always do this to me?*
I wonder if she'd care if she really knew what's going
on with us now. One of these days, I'll tell her. Why
shouldn't she know that Jack and I are fighting all the time,
Janie's doing terribly in school, and we have to borrow
money to get the car fixed?] You know how much I care
about you!

It is never easy to take on another person's burden, even when
things are going smoothly, but there are some periods in life when
it's almost impossible. Ironically en-
ough, it very often happens that older
people begin to need more support just
at the point when their children's lives
are the most complicated and their responsibilities are heaviest. A middle-
aged woman is likely to have to deal
with her children's adolescent crises and
her parents' geriatric ones just as she is
going into menopause herself. Her husband may be going through
the same midlife crisis. A middle-aged man may struggle to provide
money for his children's college tuition and his parents' necessary
medical expenses just when he has been passed over for a long-
awaited promotion, which he now realizes will never come. His wife,
if she is working, may have similar financial and career pressures.

If, in establishing their life's priorities, sons and daughters have
not been able to assign first—or even second or third—place to their
parents, they may never forgive themselves. But if they try to
shoulder their parents' burdens as well as their own, they may feel

continually resentful, wondering, as the days go by, "When is there going to be time for me?"

What Untouchable, Unresolved Feelings Can Produce

Earlier in this chapter, we stressed that there is room for all kinds of feelings in interpersonal relationships. Many people recognize this on an intellectual level, but even so find it difficult to express or admit feelings that have traditionally been considered immoral or "bad," tending to disavow unacceptable ones, pushing them out of awareness. However, these feelings keep right on existing and struggling for expression. Lock them up and throw away the key—they'll still struggle to get out. The struggle can distort our perception of ourselves and our relationships, and make it difficult to communicate effectively and to arrive at appropriate decisions. It does not necessarily follow, however, that every wrong decision is the result of unresolved feelings. Plenty of mistakes can be made from simple ignorance, and sons and daughters admit these mistakes every day.

> "We thought John's father would love the country and being with us, but he just sits and looks out the window. We forgot what a city person he is."

> "I made my mother give up the house much too soon after Father died. I didn't realize she needed more time."

Errors can reflect a lack of knowledge about an unfamiliar situation. They can also reflect a family's inability to work together effectively. But well-meaning mistakes aside, it is important to explore some of the typical pitfalls lying in wait when unresolved feelings direct our relationships with our parents and the decisions we make with them. Some of the most common ones are reviewed next.

Withdrawal

Mel Brooks's "2,000-Year-Old Man" character could always draw laughter from his audience when he said, "I have 42,000 children and not one of them comes to visit me." That statement strikes home for many listeners. Lack of attention from children is a familiar parental complaint.

Children avoid their parents for many reasons, and great numbers of them suffer only occasional twinges of guilt. Some want to be more attentive, but despite their conscious desire, find it difficult to visit, phone, or write, and sometimes to keep in touch at all. It may be that they are avoiding a confrontation that would arouse uncomfortable feelings. It may be that they prefer to keep under wraps feelings of anger, resentment, irritation, or jealousy. They may wish they could behave differently and condemn themselves regularly—"What's the matter with me? Why can't I do better with them?"—and then withdraw still further.

Oversolicitousness and Domination

This pattern is at the opposite pole from withdrawal. Instead of removing themselves, some children may come even closer, choosing a more acceptable type of involvement. By hovering over his parents, spending an abnormal amount of time with them, letting them become completely dependent on him before they need to be, a son may think he is acting out of love and devotion. This could be true, but it could also be his way of blocking out angry or guilty feelings.

Just as withdrawal may disguise fear, oversolicitous behavior may serve the same purpose. In that situation, the fear lurking in the background may be fear of loss. It is not easy for an adult to accept the fact that he is still very emotionally dependent on his parents, that he has not grown up yet or proven to himself that he can stand alone. Such anxiety can be very painful, and an adult child may attempt to palliate it through overprotective behavior, which implies, "As long as I'm with them, nothing can happen to them," or conversely, "If I leave them alone for a minute, they may slip away from me."

Fault Finding

Sometimes there is a job we feel we should do, and we cannot manage to do it. Conscious of our own inadequacy, we may feel angry with ourselves as well as guilty. If we have to face the fact that we are shortchanging our parents, uncomfortable feelings may flow in still another direction. What a relief it may seem to blame, not our parents or ourselves, but a third party!

When someone else is shouldering the responsibility for our parents' welfare—siblings, other relatives, favored housekeepers, or nursing homes—a little voice may keep reminding us that we are not doing our share. That voice can be successfully drowned out by an endless barrage of criticism of those who are doing *our* job for us. We may accuse these "stand-ins" of being inconsiderate, inefficient, and inept, and point out how they are not showing the right kind of care or concern. Certain criticisms, especially those of nursing homes, may be valid, and it is wise to keep a close, watchful eye on anyone who is providing for the welfare of frail older adults. But if *nothing* is right—*no* way, *nowhere*—then could it be that deep down inside we feel that something is wrong with us?

People frequently distort their view of the world around them to make themselves feel better. These games are popular with many sons and daughters. By placing the blame elsewhere, they give themselves the momentary comfort that they have removed the blame from themselves. The comfort provided by fault finding is almost invariably offset by angry feelings from other family members and the paid or volunteer helpers older adults are depending on.

Denial

It is not uncommon for children to deny that their parents have problems or need help. Sometimes the denial is so successful that these children are able to disbelieve what is going on right in front of them. If they cannot accept weakness in themselves, they may deny the realistic symptoms of frailty in their ag-

Children deny that their parents have problems or need help. Sometimes the denial is so successful that these children are able to disbelieve what is going on right in front of them.

ing parents. In Joseph Heller's book *Something Happened*, the hero, Bob Slocum, describes his behavior toward his mother:

> My conversation to my mother, like my visits, was of no use to her.
> I pretended, by not speaking of it, for my sake as well as for hers (for
> my sake more than for hers), that she was not seriously ill and in a
> nursing home she hated, that she was not crippled and growing older

and more crippled daily. I did not want her to know, as she did know (and I knew she knew), as she knew before I did, that she was dying, slowly, in stages, her organs failing and her faculties withering one by one. . . . I pretended she was perfect and said nothing to her about her condition until she finally died. I was no use to her.

Denial is also closely tied in with fear of losing parents. A daughter may feel that if she can ignore the warning symptoms of her mother's physical deterioration, perhaps they will go away. The most dangerous part of this kind of denial is that the older person may not get medical help until it is too late to do any good. But even when doctors are consulted, denial leads many children to have unrealistic hopes for miracles from the medical profession.

Outmoded Role-Playing

Many children discover at a very early age that certain types of behavior produce enjoyable responses from their parents. Since these responses are so gratifying, they may repeat the behavior, assuming a role that comes to be expected of them. A role can be assumed by a child to get along in the family, but a role may also be assigned to a child. Listen to parents discussing their children with friends: "Jim's the dependable one," or "June's the emotional one," or "Fran's so easygoing," or "Susie's the clown." All these qualities may be found in the various children from time to time, but every child has more than one emotional color and will be in trouble if expected to function only in one role.

If roles are perpetuated as part of family fun and tradition, they are not necessarily harmful. A gentle family joke kept alive through the years may be a warm and tender reminder of past closeness. But if roles are perpetuated out of anxiety or fear—if a daughter feels she must cling to hers to remain acceptable to others—then she may find it hard to step outside it, be herself, and deal constructively with problems affecting her parents' lives and therefore her own. Thus, if she still clings to the outgrown role of being the "child" to her parents, she may see herself as still dependent on them, when in reality they are the ones who now need to lean on her. Her behavior is therefore inappropriate to the real circumstances. On the other hand, she may cling to an old role of being "the dependable one" in the family, the child who always did the most for her parents. She may be afraid to give up this role and may make unreasonable demands on herself, even when her brothers and sisters are perfectly willing to share the burdens involved in caring for their parents. This kind of self-martyrdom will be explored in chapter 3.

Protracted Adolescent Rebellion and Blind Overinvolvement

When grown-up people are still angry and rebellious toward their parents, it is legitimate to wonder if they ever as adolescents had a period of healthy rebellion that permitted them to mature successfully and assume separate adult roles. Normally, there comes a time when children need to break away from close parental control, give their parents a hard time, disagree violently, try their own wings, and make their own mistakes. This breakaway period has varying degrees of intensity, depending on the individual adolescent. The upheaval gradually quiets down, the struggle for independence is resolved, and eventually the adolescent joins the adult world. But some children make rebellion a way of life. The skirmishes continue through the years, no decisive battle is won, and adult maturity remains elusive. A son who is still in constant conflict with his parents may also, in a perverse way, enjoy blaming them for preventing him from growing up. He may even project onto his parents tyrannical motives that he can rebel against. The anger he feels toward them may blind him to the fact that they are getting old and need him to grow up at last.

Those who never go through any adolescent rebellion at all are even more vulnerable. A daughter who has never been able to break away from one or both parents may never be able to see himself as a separate individual. The result, often masked as a loving, devoted relationship between parent and child, can in reality reach a point where the child cannot separate his or her feelings from the parents'. This process may be particularly painful to bear, especially if the parents seriously deteriorate as they grow old. What a burden it can be for a daughter to live through her parents' old age with them and then have to face the same problems a second time when she gets old herself! Overinvolvement by an adult child can force an older person to be unhealthily stoic to avoid causing a child pain, or a mother or father may be stimulated to demonstrate more exhibitionist suffering by the knowledge that a child secretly enjoys being allowed to share the pain.

Scapegoating

The burdens and problems of our own lives, as mentioned earlier, can lead to an unfortunate type of behavior toward our parents: the process of scapegoating. Human beings often find it difficult to face up to the real things that trouble them: illness, failing resources, marital problems, troubles with children or careers. It is sometimes convenient to blame a totally innocent source (or person) for these problems, and direct anger and resentment toward something or someone else. Even if the older person is not actually blamed for the problems, he or she may have to bear the emotional outbursts generated by them. A campaign of television commercials for a well-known headache remedy in the 1960s centered on the scapegoating of an elderly relative by a younger one. The series included a line that became famous: "Mother—I'd rather do it myself." It ended with the gentle reminder, "Sure you have a headache, but don't take it out on her." Substitute the words *unfaithful husband, bankrupt business, unloving spouse, disturbed child,* or *bad investment* for *headache,* and the possibilities for scapegoating are endless—in every family.

Scapegoating is not usually done deliberately. It is a very human type of behavior, but when carried to an extreme, it can be very destructive to everyone, particularly to the elderly.

Feelings That Can Persist and Those That Change in a New Context

It's often difficult to understand our own feelings and our own behavior. Some people are able to discover insights for themselves and move ahead to work effectively on family problems. Others may find themselves in an emotional quandary, unable to mobilize themselves. Or they may overreact and behave inappropriately. These emotional quandaries can result from relationships with an aging parent in much the same way as they result from relationships with a husband, a wife, or a child. Just as we may turn to a counselor or psychotherapist when in turmoil about our marriage or our children, we can find similar help with our mixed-up feelings about our aging parents. Many people find it helpful to talk to their family physician, priest, minister, or rabbi. Others prefer to consult mental health professionals (see Appendix A).

It would be unrealistic to suggest that aging parents and their grown children will live happily ever after, even when their feelings toward each other are open and accepted. The best that can be hoped for is that problems will be faced directly and the most helpful solutions found—*under the circumstances.* But the circumstances of old age are sometimes unhappy. Many old people carry into the later years the personal traits that colored their relationships in their earlier years: selfishness, greed, cruelty, bigotry, or hostility. And even in the best relationships, there will inevitably be pain and sadness. It is natural for children to feel these emotions when they watch their parents deteriorate and move every day closer to death.

However, there can be pleasure and comfort, even in these final days. This can be a time for looking back and looking ahead. The younger generation has one last opportunity to relive family history with the older one and understand—perhaps for the first time—the continuity of the life cycle. Some look to elderly relatives as precious sources of soon-to-be-lost information and eagerly listen to old stories and older memories. There is a chance for enjoyment and peace of mind, even in the midst of sadness, and a chance to know one's parents as individuals in their own right. This reward eludes children who continue to struggle with unresolved troubled feelings until their parents' death—and afterward.

> Death ends a life . . . but it does not end a relationship which struggles on in the survivor's mind . . . towards some resolution which it never finds.
>
> —Robert Anderson, *I Never Sang for My Father*

Bob Morris on the Emotional Tug of War

By nature, I am a selfish person. I know that and admit it. So when it comes to looking back on the responsibilities and worries I had about my parents when they were struggling in the last years of their lives, I am not as inclined as some might be to keep my ugliest feelings to myself. I'm more willing to let you know the truth about how I felt when faced with the fact that neither of my parents would have the easy deaths I had wanted for them so that it would also be easier for me. Many kids have parents who suffer more. But I still felt under siege in the last years of both my parents' lives. It was a total downer to know people I loved so much were suffering.

Ultimately, like so many things are in retrospect, it was tremendously gratifying to help them through their last years. My brother and I went through, in total, maybe 6 or 7 years in the role of worried, saddened sons. In those years, I always made it my goal to be able to keep serving my parents while serving myself. I tried to show them a good time that made me feel happy about doing so. And as a writer, of course, I could write about my travails with them in my *New York Times* column and as commentaries on *All Things Considered* on National Public Radio (NPR). I even wrote a one-man show about my father's year of dating after my mother died that I later sold as a memoir to be called "Assisted Loving." So I took advantage of the situation in my own way.

The emotional tug-of-war was about feeling that I wasn't good enough. Maybe a couple weeks had passed and I hadn't been to visit my parents, or maybe I didn't get down from New York for that visit to Florida one winter as I had intended. Maybe I should have been more patient. Maybe I should have been more on top of their medications and getting them to install safety rails in the bathroom. That kind of thing. Now that they're both gone, I look back and realize that I was good enough. But I will say that the motivating factor of guilt probably put me at my best with them—or made me a lot better than I might have been without it. I mean, guilt is a tremendous motivator. Mixed with love and humor, it can get you through the roughest patches with aging parents. That's what my brother and I had going for us. Yes, I was lucky not to have to tend to my parents alone. My brother and I were a fabulous team for them and for each other. We found ways to laugh through all of it.

But then, we never had major bones to pick with our parents. I know there are probably all different kinds of childhood experiences boomer kids have. My only complaint was that, as a writer, I never had any big issues with them to write about. We weren't running with scissors growing up. We were running with tennis rackets. So any childhood conflicts that arose were so superficial as to be laughable. They were very superficial. Why weren't my parents more stylish? Why weren't they more ambitious? My mother was a librarian. She was parsimonious. And she took her Judaism pretty seriously. My father, a small-town lawyer who later became a New York State motor vehicles judge, was full of opinions, even though he wasn't very well read. Is that anything to complain about? Probably not. He spent all his time on the tennis court. People loved him. He had a talk-show-host personality, better at talking than listening. And both his fashion sensibility and his table manners always left something to be desired.

My mother, from a working-class family in upstate New York, had made her way to Long Island after college in the early 1950s. She was a very pretty woman. She met my father—who had some wealth in his family, but by the time he was 10, had no mom or dad and was kind of shuffling from place to place. He was a young small-town lawyer. And I'm sure, to my mom, that was pretty glamorous. So in 1956, they bought what they thought was their dream house in West Islip, a suburb of Bay Shore in Long Island, if you can imagine such a thing. It was one of those cookie-cutter post-war neighborhoods on the Great South Bay. I can still remember, well into my 30s, visiting them and walking around that neighborhood, trying to imagine it as I would prefer it—older, you know, with bigger plots and more trees—rather than as it was. Sometimes I think about that in the context of how I thought about my parents for too many years. I was trying to envision them as I wanted them to be, not as they were. But they loved their house, both the one on Long Island and their rental in Palm Beach. And I was petty enough to complain about both.

But again, in terms of my childhood, I can't say that there were big complaints. I'm gay. They were okay with it. I wanted to be a writer, despite the instability of such a thing. They were encouraging. By the time I went off to college—which was expensive and they paid for it in full without question—I pretty much divested myself of them and Long Island. Some children call their parents every day or see them for dinner once a week. That blows my mind. I would call about once a week when they were well—that's all. I always thought of myself as a person who needed lots of personal space—with both family and lovers. My life was pretty antiseptic.

So the process of their aging was a big growth inducer for me.

3

The Family Merry-Go-Round

Martha Willis never fully recovered from the severe bout of flu she suffered the winter before her 80th birthday. Although she stayed on in her own little house, she could no longer take care of it or herself alone, even with the help of a homemaker who came in several times a week. Her oldest daughter, Sylvia, who lived closest and whose children were teenagers, took on the major responsibility for her mother's care. Eventually, Sylvia found that she was spending more and more time in her mother's house and less and less in her own.

In the beginning, everyone pitched in to help—her younger sisters, her husband, and her children—but as time went on, Sylvia noticed that her sisters seemed less available, her husband less understanding, and her children more resentful, often accusing her of being more interested in Grandma than in them. Tensions built throughout the family and erupted frequently. In one typical week, Sylvia screamed at her favorite sister over the phone, accusing her of "never doing anything for Mother." She had an ugly fight with her husband, who stormed out of the house and the next day forgot her birthday. In the same week, her younger son was suspended from school for cutting classes and her older son had an asthma attack. "Mother's the least of my worries," Sylvia complained bitterly to her friend. "Since she got sick, the whole family's starting to fall apart."

O F   T H E   N A T I O N ' S   A P P R O X I M A T E L Y   3 5   M I L L I O N   C I T I-
zens over 65, too many have no families to care for them or about them. In sickness, in trouble, and in poverty, they have to go it alone, and their very aloneness makes their situation even more tragic.

But millions of older adults are not alone. When their ability to manage independently seems threatened, plenty of relatives may be concerned, not only sons and daughters but also sons- and daughters-in-law, brothers and sisters, stepchildren and foster children, nieces and nephews, and grandchildren. Concerned friends and neighbors may also become involved. In times of serious crisis, a few close relatives usually assume the real responsibility, but any number of others—all of whom have some connection with the older person *and* with each other—may be drawn into the act, offering help, suggestions, advice, and criticism. Their offers can be constructive and valuable, or in some cases, misguided and destructive.

It may seem to you, if your own mother is deteriorating, that it is impossible to find a solution satisfactory to everyone—to her, to you, and to others in the family. Some situations undeniably defy solution. But it may be a mistake to jump too quickly to the conclusion that your own situation is hopeless. Just as your feelings about your mother may make it easy for you to help her or may stand in the way of helping her, other relationships can similarly facilitate or block effective behavior: your feelings about your brothers and sisters, theirs about you, and everyone's feelings about your mother.

Family Harmony or Family Discord

Throughout history countries have mobilized their efforts to deal with threats and disasters such as wars, famine, or disease, rallying together with greater unity than ever. And so with families. A shared crisis—a father's stroke, a mother's loss of vision—can bring out the best in every member, drawing everyone closer together. At such times brothers and sisters may get to know one another again as adults and be gratified by the new relationships. Husbands and wives may find hidden strengths in each other and be pleasantly surprised by the discovery.

> "I got married and left home when my brother was a teenager. I never realized what a great person he'd turned into until I spent all that time at home when Mother was sick. We're real friends now."

> "Jennie was such a helpless crybaby when we were little—who'd believe she'd be the one we all depend on now that Dad needs so much care?"

> "I really talked to my brother when we visited my mother at the nursing home—we hadn't talked that way in 20 years."

> "Lizzie's sense of humor saved us. She could always make us laugh, even when everything looked terrible."

> "My husband was always so quiet and unemotional. But he had what we needed when Mother got cancer. He was the one who kept things going—the rest of us just fell apart."

There are hidden benefits for everyone when members of the younger generations rally together to help the older ones. Older adults benefit if their relatives work together with them to find the best possible solutions to painful problems. The younger family members benefit if the crisis brings them all closer together again; old and valued relationships are often re-established, and new relationships may emerge, setting a pattern for the future.

There are hidden benefits for everyone when members of the younger generations rally together to help the older ones.

But those benefits are enjoyed only in some families. The crisis that brings unity to one may lead to civil war in another, and the problems of an older adult may be further intensified by family conflict.

We tend to speak of families as homogeneous units. We refer to the Jones family and the Smith family and the Brown family as if each one had a single mind and personality: "Oh, you can't count on the Davidsons," or "The Katers are so generous," or "The Phillipses are loud." But every family is made up of a number of individuals with a variety of personalities, capabilities, needs, ambitions, and frustrations. To function as a unit, family members, even when they are adults, may develop a certain balance in their relationships.

Frequently, the unifying force in such families is the older generation, which maintains the balance, perpetuating ties between children. Elderly parents often serve as the family news agency: "Mother told me about your promotion—we're thrilled," a sister may e-mail her brother, or "Dad wrote to us about your car accident, so I had to call," says another sister, making phone contact for the first time in months.

When a sudden crisis reduces an independent elderly woman to helplessness, or slow deterioration finally disables a formerly self-sufficient old man, the news agency closes down. Brothers and sisters are thrown together again and must deal with each other directly, without a parent as intermediary. They may once again need to function as a unit, as they have not done since childhood. The successful balance they may have achieved may be out of kilter. The family is forced to realign itself to absorb the changes.

Similar realignment may be necessary in marital relationships. A husband who has taken a back seat, staying carefully removed from his wife's family, may be forced by a crisis to take a more active role and contribute time, concern, advice, and even money. A wife who has managed a wary, though polite, involvement with her mother-in-law may eventually, because her husband needs her, be forced into an intimate, supportive relationship with a woman she never really liked.

Is Your Sibling Rivalry Still Showing?

The roles children assume or are assigned in childhood influence their relationships not only with their parents but also with their brothers, sisters, and other relatives. Some roles are accepted and admired by everyone and make for affectionate relationships that last a lifetime.

Many roles, however, while accepted or even encouraged by parents, are branded by others in the family as phony. A brother, aware of the admiration his sister always receives for being "the easygoing one," may always have been able to see through the role to her "real" self, which is actually fearful and manipulative. He may brand her as a fake and despise his parents for being so blind. "Don't pull that act with me," he may have said many times while they were growing up. "You'd like to stand up to Dad just the way I do, but you haven't got the guts!" Thirty years later, he may still suspect her motives when she hovers anxiously over their ailing father.

A highly competitive group of brothers and sisters may continue to compete later in life, although not quite as directly with each other. But when their mother begins to age, they may resume open competition with each other over her welfare, particularly if she was the original source of their competitiveness. Each sibling may claim to be considering Mother's well-being, but the underlying motivation is winning out in a final family contest.

Sibling relationships can also be affected by the position held by each one in the family structure, and by the age differences between them. The oldest may have always been expected to shoulder greater responsibility when everyone was young, and that expectation may continue into adulthood. But the opposite may happen. The oldest may marry first, and by making an earlier separation, leave the younger ones to deal with problems that remain. The youngest, as "the baby" in the family, may be seen as the one who is let off scot-free, while more was expected of the older ones. Conversely, the youngest, being the last to leave, may be left holding the bag because everyone else has gone. The varieties and mixtures of old relationships between brothers and sisters are endless.

These relationships do change and shift through the years. You may be amazed, when your parents are old, to find yourself depending on the sister who was the most scatterbrained or the brother who was the most self-centered. Such switches may pleasantly surprise you, but you may be even more astonished to find out how few changes have taken place since childhood. What a shock to discover that your 40-year-old sister is just as selfish as ever, or that your 60-year-old brother is still trying to boss everyone around. Don't forget that they may be equally shocked that you haven't grown up much either. Even though you have all come together again to try to help Mother, she may be pushed aside while family history repeats itself.

A particularly crucial childhood role—and one that often affects relationships years later—is the role of "the favorite." When they are growing up, children often wonder about their parents' feelings, asking themselves, "Do they love *me* best?" or "Which one of us do they love best?" In some cases, the favored relationship can be limited to one child and one parent: "Joey's always been closer to Mother, but Dad loves me best." In other families, the role of favorite is conferred on one child and then passed on to another, depending on the stage of development of each. That unstable state of affairs can lead to further tensions as children compete for the prize, never knowing exactly where they stand. Parents usually loudly deny having favorites and honestly believe they love *all* their children equally, but their behavior may reveal their true feelings. "Look, Ma, no hands!" a triumphant 4-year-old may shout, balancing for the first time in his life on a two-wheel bicycle. If his mother's response to this dramatic accomplishment is merely, "Be careful! Don't scratch your brother's bike!" the 4-year-old may wonder what further act of bravery he will have to perform to gain the maternal spotlight. He may keep trying all his life, hoping that one day he will do something to make his mother's face light up for him the way it does for his brother. Like eager scouts, less-favored sons and daughters often push themselves through life to do more and more good deeds, hoping for just that reward. But sad to say, no brownie points are given out to middle-aged daughters and no merit badges to graying sons.

Favoritism is particularly hard to bear if the favorite seems to hold the crown for no valid reason. A 10-year-old sister (in second place) may wonder, "Why is it always Connie? Why never me? Why can't they see how pretty and clever and kind I am?" Years later, she may be asking the same questions: "Why do they always turn to her for advice—can't they see how greedy, cold, self-centered, and neurotic she is? Don't they realize how much better off they'd be if only they listened to me?"

Overly solicitous behavior toward elderly parents may mask the anger a grown child feels for having to take second place, but it may also be a way of saying, "Look how good I am to you. *Now* won't you love me best?" or "By God, I'm going to be your favorite child *just once* before you die!" Indifferent, uncaring behavior may also be a way of saying, "You always loved Jack the best—he got the most—now let *him* take care of you." An uncaring son may be accused by others of taking a back seat and not coming forward to help his parents when they are old and need him, but he may merely be continuing to stay in the exact place they assigned to him when he was young.

Who's in Charge?

Your mother may have said over the years, "I will never be a burden to any of my children," but unless she has made some prior arrangements to cover all emergencies, as she grows older, she may have no choice. She may be forced to turn to someone in her family for help. In families where there are several children, however, the big question is: *Who will that someone be?*

Your mother may be forced to turn to someone in her family for help. In families where there are several children, however, the big question is: Who will that someone be?

If you are the only daughter in the family, the chances are that it will be you, rather than one of your brothers. If there are several daughters, the chances are that it will be the one living nearest to their parents. Experts in family relations report that daughters (usually middle-aged) are more likely to take on the major responsibility for their parents' care. They and other female relatives are normally the ones who contact outside sources of support—family and community agencies—when they cannot cope with the responsibility alone. Even when their parents are getting along well and do not need help from anyone, daughters are usually thought of as keeping in closer touch than sons, who are more likely to become involved on special occasions or with major decisions and financial arrangements.

This pattern of caregiving is continuing into the twenty-first century in spite of the fact that increasing numbers of women have entered the labor force and have careers of their own. Many business executives are aware that a significant number of their employees have ongoing responsibilities for elderly relatives. Some women must leave the labor force to care for an ailing parent. The middle generations are often forced to juggle the demands of children, career, and caregiving. These three Cs often add up to a fourth: conflict.

The Caregiver May Be Chosen

When there are two or more children in any family, one may be chosen by the parents to take care of them. Their preference may have always been known. One particular daughter (or son) may have always been called when problems arose—one who could always be counted on to respond to any emergency, who kept in touch on a regular, even daily, basis. That relationship is often mutually gratifying and supportive to both generations over the years, with giving as well as receiving on each side. In the later years, when her parents have greater needs, that daughter may be willing, because of these strong mutual bonds of affection, to make sacrifices in her own life to make her parents' lives easier. The child who is singled out by the parents as their main source of help may be the oldest, the youngest, the strongest, the weakest, the favorite, or the least favorite.

Most often, however, it is the daughter (or son) who lives close by who becomes the "primary caregiver," and that very proximity makes it natural for the parents to turn to her and her family. She may not even realize what is happening, but little by little she may assume more and more responsibility for her parents' welfare, until one day she may wake up and realize that she is the caregiver. If she is in a long-term relationship, her partner may share the role to some extent, but she may bear the brunt of it. In other families, as one by one children grow up and move into their own lives, one particular child (usually a daughter, but sometimes a son) may be expected to stay around, all future plans constantly influenced by the thought, "I'm the only one left—I can't leave them now." The unmarried daughter, mainstay of her parents' old age, was seen more frequently in the past, but she has not gone completely out of style today. Her life may become a series of postponements. She may hope to travel, to work in a foreign country. She may consider marrying Joe or Frank or Tom, but only "after Mother gets well," or "when Mom and Dad sell the house and move south."

"I was always in the right place at the right time," an unmarried career woman explained. Specifically, her statement meant that whenever there was a crisis in her parents' lives, she "happened" to be conveniently on the spot, while her brothers and sisters were conveniently (for them) miles away. After a number of years, everyone began to take it for granted that she would always be there and any plans for marriage or career advancement would always be indefinitely tabled. It never seemed to occur to the absent ones that they should disrupt their own lives and come home to help out. It *did* occur to their "dependable" sister as more and more years went by, but she was unable to extricate herself from a pattern everyone had allowed to develop—herself included.

This pattern may not be as outmoded it may seem. In a May 2006 article, the *New York Times* reported on a trend among high-powered career women to give up their careers to return to their childhood homes to care for aging parents.

A potentially explosive situation exists when parents divide their needs, accepting help and care from one child and advice and guidance from another.

A potentially explosive situation exists when parents divide their needs, accepting help and care from one child and advice and guidance from another.

"I spoke to Larry last night. He doesn't think Dr. Parker's doing a thing for your father's arthritis. He thinks we ought to go to Dr. Larribee over in Beechwood Center," Mrs. Fuller said to her daughter Kate.

"But you've always liked Dr. Parker. He's known Dad for years. And Beechwood Center's miles away," replied Kate, who always drove her father for his regular treatments. She tried not to show the resentment she always felt when her brother had one of his "great ideas."

"Larry wants us to try Dr. Larribee," continued her mother.

"Then let Larry drive. He lives around the corner from Beechwood," snapped Kate, knowing exactly what her mother's next words would be.

"Oh, Kate. You know how busy Larry is. Surely you want to do what's best for your father."

Of course Kate wanted to do what was best for her father. Didn't she always follow through whenever Larry had a great idea? She dutifully took her father to Dr. Larribee, driving the extra 30 miles to Beechwood Center and back, gritting her teeth and hissing at herself, "Here you go again—doing Larry's work for him!"

The Caregiver May Volunteer

The caregiver may ask for the job. A son may realize that he is in the best position to help; a daughter may feel she can take care of her parents as well as her children. When their parents begin to deteriorate, these volunteers are ready to help out or to take over completely. But sometimes they are ready too soon, and take control of their parents' lives long before this is necessary. "Premature volunteering" by one of their children may accelerate an older couple's decline and make them dependent long before they need to be. The volunteer may then be suspected of assuming control more to satisfy his or her own needs than out of concern for his or her parents. In this case, the volunteer may have been waiting a lifetime for just this opportunity.

The volunteer may be the son who has always felt least loved and hopes finally to gain recognition and approval from everyone. For this reward, he may be willing to make painful sacrifices in his own personal life—in his relationships with his wife and children, and in his career.

The favorite son (or daughter) may also volunteer. He may feel forced by his parents' expectation that he will return to them the concern they have always shown him, or he may volunteer out of guilt that he has received so much more than the other children in the family and feel obligated to make it up to everyone. Or he may always have had a lurking worry that he did not really deserve his favored position—that he was unworthy of it, that it was conferred on him by mistake, or that he would never live up to it. When his parents are old, he finally has a chance to convince them and himself that they were right to favor him after all.

Occasionally, a son or daughter volunteers as caregiver, but functions in name only, assuming the title but performing none of the duties.

The Pseudo-Caregiver

Occasionally, a son or daughter volunteers as caregiver, but functions in name only, assuming the title but performing none of the duties. Like a good general or clever executive, he is able to delegate responsibility to the lower ranks. He may use phrases like "Just this once" when he asks someone to pinch-hit for him, as if asking for the first time. "You *will* call Mother every day while I'm on vacation, won't you?" a pseudo-caregiver may say earnestly to his sister. She would be justified in replying, "What difference will it make if you *are* away? Don't I call her every day anyway?"

A son (or daughter) who acts as pseudo-caregiver usually has his own motives: to establish himself firmly in first place in his parents' affections, to gain admiration from the outside world, or perhaps to inherit the most from his parents—even if they have very little to leave behind.

Brothers and sisters sometimes seem to conspire to help the pseudo-caregiver retain the title, knowing that efforts to unseat him or her would be futile or would cause pain to the parent who needs to perpetuate the masquerade. "I'm the meat and potatoes in my parents' lives, but my brother's the champagne," a sister admitted honestly. "I'm around all the time, but I don't do anything exciting or dramatic—just the ordinary, little, everyday chores that everyone takes for granted. But he breezes in and whisks them off to the country for the day—brings them some special treat or takes them to a restaurant or a show. He breaks that awful monotony for them. They can live on one of his visits for weeks. They even look younger afterward. I can't do that for them. I guess they need both of us."

The Caregiver as Martyr

Some aging parents place unreasonable demands on their caregivers. In many cases when other relatives are really unable to help or simply prefer to keep a safe distance away, the caregiver is genuinely overburdened and justified in feeling that there is just too much for one person to handle. But caregivers, because of their own complex feelings toward their parents, often place unreasonable demands on themselves. They go overboard in their zeal, insist on carrying the entire responsibility single-handedly, and discourage anyone else from sharing it. Brothers, sisters, and other relatives, initially willing and eager to help, will eventually back away when their offers are repeatedly rebuffed, at the same time resenting being rejected and shut out of the older people's lives. The caregivers may then complain bitterly to anyone who will listen about their heavy burdens and the selfishness of their families.

"I'm everyone's slave, Doctor," complained Sally Horgan, explaining during her physical examination why she was overworked and rundown. "After I've cleaned and marketed for my own family, I have to go over and do the same thing at Mother's apartment. And Mother's lonely—she needs company—so I have to visit a little, too. It makes her feel better. I fix her a little supper and then I have to go home and cook for all of us. I'm usually too tired to eat."

"You're an only child, then, Mrs. Horgan?" asked the doctor.

"No, Doctor. I have a brother and sister."

"They live far away?"

"No, Doctor—they're right here in Maplewood."

"Can't they help you out a little with your mother?"

"They always leave everything to me."

"Do you ever ask them to help?"

"They never offer."

"Do you ever ask them?"

"No, Doctor, I guess I don't."

The one in charge who does not ask for help, or rejects help when it is offered, ends up alone. The burdens become heavier as time goes on, and eventually the caregiver is likely to become the family martyr.

Friend or Enemy?

The caregiver may be seen as the most valued member of the family or the most hated. Brothers and sisters are often genuinely grateful to the one who performs a job they are unable or unwilling to do, and are often eager to do whatever they can to make the caregiver's life easier. The caregivers are often equally appreciative and report that the additional help they are given makes their responsibilities bearable. "There must be ESP in our family," one sister claims. "Whenever everything's about to get too much for me—almost before I know it myself—my brother and his wife take over for a few days. I'm always surprised, after all these years, that they keep on appearing just when I need them most." A sister in California tells her friends, "I always fly home to Philadelphia every summer to be with Father for a month. My brother and his family take care of him the entire year—they deserve a break. And anyhow I'm glad to know that I can spend some real time with Father every year."

The one in charge may be hated instead of loved by the rest of the family, for using the position to keep everyone apart. Aging parents can become pawns in family power struggles. They may be used to settle old debts and rivalries between siblings. A sister, always jealous of her brother, may deny him the thing he wants most: the chance to be close to their parents and share their final years with them. "Mary acts as if Father is her private property, as if *she's* the only one who cares about him," he might complain—justifiably—and then use every opportunity to draw his father over to *his* side. Poor Father, caught in the crossfire, is doubly threatened—by his own old age and by his own children.

> *The one in charge may be hated instead of loved by the rest of the family, for using the position to keep everyone apart. Aging parents can become pawns in family power struggles.*

The Caregiver under Fire

In many families, trouble may come from the most unexpected quarter: from the very child who seems the most remote from the parents, the least concerned, and the most willing to let everyone else take over. When plans have been put into action and seem to be working smoothly, an absent son or daughter may suddenly appear on the scene and imply to an elderly mother, "If I'd been around [or, if I'd been consulted], I'd never have let them do this to you." Mother, who may have been adapting pretty well to a new situation carefully worked out with the rest of the family, is likely to take several giant steps backward.

Social workers and other professionals concerned with the future adjustment of an older client know the value of including as many family members as possible in long-term care planning. A brother or sister may disapprove of a plan, not because the plan itself is ill-advised, but because someone else thought of it first: "Bill would have approved of the nursing home if he'd selected it," or "Mary and John would have liked Mother's homemaker if they'd hired her."

Snipers and critics may not make real trouble, but they can be constant irritants. Rather than acknowledge how much responsibility the caregiver does shoulder, his or her siblings (and other relatives) may be quick to point out any omissions and mistakes. Aware that they aren't doing much for their parents themselves, they find it comforting to snipe at him or her.

Older sister to younger sister: "Mother was so disappointed when you didn't visit on Thursday, Kim. She was in tears when I called." Kim visited Mother every day of the week—she just happened to miss that Thursday.

Younger brother to older sister: "How could you have let Dad gain so much weight since I was here at Christmas? Have you completely forgotten about his blood pressure?" Dad had lived with the older sister for 4 years. She watched his diet carefully, cooking special salt-free, low-cholesterol dishes. But Dad cheated, and she couldn't watch him every minute.

Younger sister to middle sister: "Aren't you ever going to get a new coat for Mother? She's been wearing that old rag for years. It makes me cry to see her looking so shabby." The middle sister did all of Mother's shopping. She bought food, shoes, curtains, nightgowns, dresses, cosmetics, and drugs. She just hadn't had time yet to look for a coat.

Caregivers must also defend themselves against well-intentioned relatives and onlookers, ready with unsolicited advice or criticism.

Caregivers must also defend themselves against well-intentioned relatives and onlookers, ready with unsolicited advice or criticism. Your mother's friends may gently but sadly intensify your own anxieties and conflicts through casual comments about how much worse she looks or how depressed she seems. They may ask if you *really* have confidence in her doctor, and remind you that she's alone too much, doesn't eat enough, and doesn't get out enough. You may already know everything they tell you and be doing the best you can, but these reminders usually carry the implication that you aren't doing enough, and that they could do much better.

A Permanent Split or a Closer Bond?

"We've not seen each other since Mother died," a gray-haired woman answered sadly when asked about her older sister. "I guess we're not on speaking terms."

The wounds that are given and received during a parent's illness or period of dependency are sometimes so deep and painful that they can never be healed. Relationships between brothers and sisters can sometimes be permanently broken off. Often those wounds are only the final blows ending a relationship that has been distant or seething for years. The sister who has given up too great a part of her life caring for an elderly parent may, even when she is free of her burdens, never forgive her siblings for not sharing enough of the work. A daughter burdened with remorse that she had never done enough for her father may, after his death, need to withdraw from the ones who did care for him. Siblings may resent the martyred caregiver who stood between them and their dying mother, making it impossible for them ever to resolve their feelings about her or to share her final days. Two brothers in Arthur Miller's play *The Price* voice their irreconcilable feelings toward each other while trying to dispose of their dead father's possessions:

Victor: You came for the old handshake, didn't you? The okay? And you end up with the respect, the career, the money and, best of all, the thing that nobody else can tell you so you can believe it—that you're one hell of a guy and never harmed anybody in your life! Well, you won't get that, not till I get mine!

Walter: And you? You never had any hatred for me? Never a wish to see me destroyed? To destroy me, to destroy me with this saintly self-sacrifice, this mockery of sacrifice?

The split may be less dramatic, resulting more from apathy and attrition than from resentment. When the parent and the parental home go, the unifying force in the family often goes too, and there is no longer the same need for siblings to keep in touch with each other. One child may try to take over that central role. If the family had always gathered at Mother's for New Year's, sister Ellie may try to preserve this tradition. But her New Year's celebration may be a conscious effort on her part rather than the spontaneous gathering it had always been when Mother was alive. Sister Ellie may succeed and establish a new family pattern, preserving it for the next generation. But she may fail, and the new tradition may never take hold. Next year, brother Jack may say casually, "You won't mind if we're not there for New Year's, will you? We've got a chance to go south for the week. We'd never have accepted if Mother were still alive. But it doesn't make much difference now, does it?" This will be the first defection, and others are likely to follow. Despite Ellie's efforts, brothers and sisters and cousins and nieces and nephews will, in the future, probably meet each other only at weddings—or more likely, only at funerals.

Money—The Root of Many Evils

Money and material possessions—abundance as well as lack—very often provide the real underlying source of family dissension.

Money and material possessions— abundance as well as lack—very often provide the real underlying source of family dissension. Brothers and sisters have been competing over inheritances since the beginning of time. They are still doing it today, especially when their elderly parents have sizable estates to leave behind. The recent public airing of the dispute between the 81-year-old son of 104-year-old Brooke Astor and her grandchildren is a case in point.

But even when a family has little money and only a few material possessions, these can still assume great symbolic worth. The struggle to win them may be out of proportion to their value. "Mother's leaving me the silver candlesticks because I'm the oldest," or "I should get the candlesticks because I've done the most for Mother." "Doing" for Mother therefore is expected to pay off. But will this kind of "doing" really pay off for her?

Money can cause trouble when there is none. If Mother is barely scraping along on her small pension and Social Security checks, and her children are in a better financial position, who is going to contribute how much? Should they all contribute equal amounts? Or should the contributions be from each child according to his or her financial situation? Or from each child according to his or her emotional need? Will the contribution be given out of generosity or guilt? Will the gifts have strings attached? Will Mother have to subordinate her own wishes to the wishes of the person who writes the biggest check?

Money is therefore power: "I give Mother the most; therefore, I have the right to decide what plans we should make for her." Does money ever buy that right? Many brothers and sisters say no.

Money can also be a substitute. A son who says, "I send my father a monthly check" may feel he has thereby discharged his total filial responsibility. Does his monthly check balance out equally with his brother's weekly visit or his sister's daily phone call? They may feel that their contributions have greater value and that no amount of money is a substitute for care and concern. Finally, money can be a contest. Competitive brothers and sisters who have money themselves may lavish luxuries on their elderly mother or father, not because either parent needs these gifts or even wants them, but to demonstrate which child has achieved the greatest worldly success.

Jason Neville was a successful man who prized success in others. His three children competed with each other throughout childhood to win his approval, and each one became successful as an adult. They constantly reminded their father of their success by sending him lavish gifts as he grew older and was often in financial straits.

When he was partially disabled by a stroke, they made arrangements for him to enter an expensive nursing home. The day he moved in, his daughter sent him an expensive bathrobe, his younger son provided a new radio, and his older son hired a limousine and driver to take the old man to the nursing home.

Eighty-seven-year-old Mr. Neville arrived in style—and alone. It was a full week before any one of his three children thought it necessary to visit in person to see how their father was adjusting to his new situation.

What About Your Own Family?

If you are involved with an ailing mother whose needs take up a lot of your time, your husband (or wife) and your children may give you great support, or resentment. Your family may share your problems, or add to them. Your conflicting loyalties may sometimes be unbearable.

Husbands, Wives, and In-Laws

Husbands and wives react in a number of different ways when their in-laws need help. A husband may have no particular animosity toward his mother-in-law herself, but he may be jealous of anything or anyone who makes demands on his wife's time or concern. A wife who actively disliked her father-in-law from the beginning may be able to keep her feelings under wraps until he becomes helpless and needs something from her that she is unable to give. A mother may have made it clear through the years that she never approved of her daughter's husband. Can he be blamed for keeping his distance when she is old, or for resenting the amount of time his wife spends with her?

Your family may share your problems, or add to them. Your conflicting loyalties may sometimes be unbearable.

Your husband's (or wife's) relationship with his own family also helps to determine how he behaves with yours. If he has always had a strong bond with his own parents, he may develop a positive one with his parents-in-law. A troubled relationship from the past, however, can affect his behavior in one of two opposite ways: he may, because of his conflicting feelings, be so emotionally tied to one or both of his parents that he has nothing left to spare for yours, or he may feel forced to separate from *all* parents—yours as well as his own—as if implying, "A plague on both your houses!"

Perhaps he came from an unloving family and hoped that your parents would make up for all that he missed in his childhood. He may come to resent them if they too let him down, fail to measure up to his expectations, and never become the parents he always wanted.

A son-in-law, as an outsider, may quickly size up the way his wife is treated by her family, and he may not like what he sees. She may have made her peace through the years and accepted the fact that her sister has always been the favorite, but her husband may never accept this. His feelings toward his wife's parents, therefore, may be determined by *their* feelings toward *her*. How can he feel close to people who do not appreciate the person he values? A daughter-in-law, wife of the least favored son, may never forgive her parents-in-law because they have been so blind and have never recognized her husband's superior worth. She may retaliate in two ways when they are old: either by withdrawing and trying to pull her husband with her, thereby adding to his problems, or by devoting herself overzealously to their needs. Her interest may be less in the welfare of the older people than in her continual desire to show up their favorite child.

The wife of the favorite son (or the husband of the favorite daughter) faces a different situation. She may have always known that her in-laws never considered her worthy of their son. She may always have to share him with them, or wage a constant and usually losing battle to win him away. When they are old and need to depend on him, she may sabotage his efforts to help them.

How Do Your Children Feel?

An endless variety of relationships may occur between aging parents and children-in-law: supportive, affectionate, caring, hostile, or antagonistic. An equal variety is possible between grandparents and grandchildren.

Even though many people like to cherish the rocking chair and "Whistler's Mother" images of grandparents, this image was probably more appropriate in the past. Grandparents these days, far from being white-haired and frail, are often vigorous men and women in their 40s, 50s, and 60s, still pursuing their own careers and interests. Many are actually relieved to be free of child care responsibilities and are not too eager to take on babysitting and domestic duties again. They may not even be comfortable in the role of grandparent and feel that it has been thrust on them too soon. Some may be pulled in a different direction, concerned about the welfare of their own parents, now great-grandparents, in their 70s, 80s, and 90s. But even when grandparents are older, they may not behave according to the ideal image.

The relationships that have developed over the years between the oldest and the youngest generations may determine how a

grandchild will feel and behave toward a grandparent who is beginning to decline and needs help. Occasionally, children see one particular grandparent as the person most important to them—more
important than their parents. The relationship can be simpler, less
pressured, less emotionally involved, and less conflicted than that
between parent and child. A daughter may admit, "Mother's always
driven me crazy, but Timmy won't hear a word against his grandma.
He thinks she's great, and she is—to him!"

A granddaughter may depend on a loving grandfather, trust him,
turn to him when she feels ill-used by the world, and see him as a
source of comfort, understanding, and knowledge. He may have time
to play with her when everyone else is too busy, time to tell stories,
to make things, to go fishing, sightseeing, or hiking. Grandfather, in
turn, may thrive on this relationship, knowing he is still important in
someone's eyes, delighting in the audience he has for his old stories
that no one wants to listen to anymore. A sense of family history can
be passed on from grandparent to grandchild, often skipping the
middle generation. When such grandparents grow old and feeble,
their grandchildren often share the family concern and try to do all
they can to be supportive. Older grandchildren may even share
caregiving responsibilities, including chauffeuring, visiting, housekeeping, and even nursing duties. When several generations join
together to help and comfort the oldest one, they usually comfort
each other at the same time.

That closeness does not always develop. Your mother may never
have been the ideal grandmother (or the ideal mother either), and
when she needs help, your children may not cooperate willingly.
They may resent giving up their own interests and activities: "Why
do we always have to go to Grandma's on Sunday?" or "Just because
of Grandpa we have to miss out on our camping trip!" Some grandparents are seen as stern or punitive figures, always disapproving
of something: language, lifestyle, dress, manners, or friends. The
younger generation, in turn, sees the older one as interfering, old-
fashioned, bigoted, or even physically distasteful: "I don't want
to kiss Grandpa—he smells," or "All Grandma talks about is constipation."

Such problems can be intensified, even reinforced daily, when a
grandparent lives in the same house with growing children. There is
little opportunity to relieve tension or let off steam. You may hear

yourself saying again and again, "Shhh, Grandma's sleeping," or "Turn that boom box down—you know Grandpa hates rap music." Your older children may ask resentfully, "How can I bring my friends home when Grandma's always there bugging everyone?" and solve their problems by staying away from home as much as possible.

Young children may feel jealous or abandoned when their mothers and fathers have to be out of the house all the time "taking care of poor old Grandma" if she is still living in her own home. Occasionally, children may become fearful, anxious, and bewildered when a sick older person lives in the same house with them. They may wonder what is really going on: "How sick is Grandpa?" and "Is he going to die?" One granddaughter, now grown up, remembers all the years her grandfather lived with her and her family; she also remembers standing at his door every morning on her way to school, listening carefully to make sure she could hear him breathing before she left the house.

The Games Older People Play

Your behavior toward your parents when they are elderly is determined by many factors in your personal history and your current life. But your behavior toward your parents is also determined by *their* behavior.

Older people are just as capable of playing games as younger people; in fact, they may become even more skillful over the years. Some children learn how to play the same games and win, but usually their parents come out on top because of long years of practice.

> Older people are just as capable of playing games as younger people; in fact, they may become even more skillful over the years.

Manipulation

A mother who has always played games with her family will know from long experience exactly how to manipulate her children to get what she wants from them when she is old. She may know she can go only so far with one but that the tolerance of another is limitless. She may vary her strategy accordingly with each one.

"She's a brave old girl," a son will say admiringly of his crippled mother. "She's going through hell, but she always manages to sound bright and chipper when I call."

"And how often do you call?" his sister may snap back bitterly. "I talk to her every day, and the minute she hears my voice, she sounds like the end of the world is here. I have to drop whatever I'm doing and rush over there to see what's wrong."

Denial of Infirmities

By pretending that they have no problems and refusing to admit that anything so terrible is going on, some disabled older people force their children into the same game.

"Everyone tells me I ought to go into a home," says Millie Farkas pleasantly.

"What do I need with a home? I'm doing fine here in my nice old apartment. I've got good children—we're a close family—they're happy to give a little help to their old mother once in a while."

Mrs. Farkas doesn't stop to define "a little help" or "once in a while." If she did, she'd have to revise her statement. She's not doing fine, and her children know she's not. Jack stops by on his way to work most days to see that Ma has breakfast and doesn't burn herself making coffee. Francie usually comes in at lunchtime, brings groceries, and cleans up a little while she's there. Grandson Billy brings dinner over every evening before he goes to night school; his mother, Laurie, has cooked it. When Mrs. Farkas is ill, her three children take turns sleeping at her house. By denying her incapacities, she has made the lives of three adult families revolve around her needs.

Exaggeration of Infirmities

The rules of this game require older people to exploit their age, insist that they cannot manage, play for sympathy, and demand attention. Some elderly players use their physical infirmities to control everyone. Loud music, late parties, and family arguments must be ended quickly if Grandpa has palpitations or if Grandma has one of her dizzy spells. When no one is looking, Grandpa doesn't hobble quite as painfully and can climb the stairs pretty well. Grandma can read the fine print of the TV schedule to find her favorite program, even though she tells everyone, "My eyes are gone."

Eighty-one-year-old Grandpa Allen, living with his son, used his age as an excuse to avoid any activity he disliked. He would have liked to help his daughter-in-law around the house, but his legs weren't strong enough anymore. (He had always hated any form of housework.) "Make my excuses to the minister," he would say to the family on Sunday. "Tell him I can't manage to get to church anymore." (He had always hated church.) "Make my excuses to Aunt Cissie. Tell her those family gatherings of hers are too much for an old man." (He had always hated family gatherings and Aunt Cissie.)

But when his oldest friend moved back to town and suggested they go fishing, Grandpa packed his gear efficiently, rose at dawn one day, and was off. His daughter-in-law stood at the window watching him leave and muttering to herself, "Okay, Grandpa—but don't play your games with me anymore."

Self-Belittlement

The elderly themselves can contribute to society's generally negative attitude toward old age. An older woman may deliberately draw everyone's attention to the miseries that old age has inflicted on her. "Look at these crippled hands!" or "Have you ever seen so many wrinkles?" or "I was beautiful once— would you ever believe it now?" She may reject herself before anyone else rejects her, answering all invitations, "Who wants an old woman like me along?" or "I'd only spoil your fun." The younger generation is then expected to respond, "Now, Mother, *of course* we want you to come, don't we, children?" The elderly may use self-belittlement to gain sympathy and manipulate their children, but also to quiet their own anxieties about their deterioration.

Some older people use money as others use love, or the withdrawal of love, to control their families.

The Money Game

Some older people use money as others use love, or the withdrawal of love, to control their families. They may try to buy attention, implying that certain behavior will be rewarded and other behavior will be penalized. Threats and promises that have price tags attached can keep entire families in line, bowing to the wishes of one frail old parent.

When old people play games with their children, it sometimes seems as if they always win. But their gamesmanship often backfires. It may create such resentment in their families that, when they really need help, everyone's judgment is so distorted that no one can function at all.

Can Old Patterns Be Reversed?

Family history can never be rewritten. Brothers and sisters cannot return to earlier days to heal old wounds. Husbands and wives cannot start married life all over again, this time loving their in-laws. The lifetime personalities of older people cannot be turned around, nor can their old relationships with their various children. But attitudes and perspectives can be shifted slightly—problems approached in different ways may become easier to deal with.

Lack of communication often produces deadlocks. Families may not realize that they are not communicating with each other—they may feel they are communicating too much. But sniping, complaining, or recriminating is not communication. How can it be, when everyone is talking and no one is listening?

Learning to listen is one step toward gaining new insights. Willingness to try new approaches is another. There may be a certain amount of trial and error. The new approaches may not work at all, or it may take time before they work smoothly. You may feel uncomfortable with the new relationships that emerge; they may seem forced, artificial, unnatural. You may, from time to time, slip back into old patterns. But after a while, the strains should begin to lessen; in addition, by working together for the first time, you may all come up with solutions that never occurred to any one of you when you were searching alone. (Chapter 11 shows in more detail how families can improve their communications with each other and get off the merry-go-round.)

Bob Morris: "I Wasn't a Doting Son Like My Brother"

Unlike me, my brother is a dutiful family man. Not only does he have children of his own and a wonderful marriage, he also has a very successful business. He's all about the family. And so, between us, you have one very amusing and fun-oriented younger brother—me—and an older brother, who is the family anchor. We are very close. And he can be very witty. But his primary impulse was and always is to put family first. So, as you can imagine, when it comes time to tend to aging parents, this causes tremendous conflicted feelings. Who's the better person, the better son? In terms of giving yourself over to your parents, what is enough?

I think he wanted me to do more, but he also understands me. And he understands that, like my father, I am the fun-loving person who could give to my parents in ways that weren't necessarily traditional. I just wasn't a doting son like my brother. He would always be making holiday dinners and having my parents up for the weekend to his country house in Westchester. They spent a lot of time with him when they got older, and it was a wonderful thing. I was present for them too; I just wasn't as giving and doting. I didn't constantly have them over for holidays. I didn't have that kind of home. I didn't lavish them with expensive presents. I didn't have that kind of income. I gave in other ways. And an advantage to having a son like me who doesn't have a family of his own—or even a spouse for most of the years when they were in decline—is that my schedule was more open. I could run out to see them more easily. I wasn't torn about where I had to spend my holidays because I didn't have to worry about my own spouse and family.

Like on Mother's Day, when my brother and sister-in-law would go to see her parents or entertain them along with her siblings, I always tended to my parents. One time, in my mother's last years, I went out to Long Island, intending to take them to a nice brunch. But my father was in a terrible mood—and I realized it was because he didn't want to be missing his baseball game on TV. So I told him he was excused and took my mother alone. I had just come back from England, where I had been writing a story about manners for a magazine. I'd been to a society wedding and had had lunch at the

House of Parliament. I had stories to tell her, and she was all ears. I showed her how the English use their forks and knives and how to butter a roll properly. I talked. She listened. Unlike my father, she was perfectly delighted just to be the audience. Later, she said it was the best Mother's Day she'd ever had. I think it was for me, too. I loved amusing her. And word got back to my brother that she had fun. It always made me feel so good that I could do that. He worked so hard at giving so much. My more modest attempts were equally appreciated.

The biggest conflict that arose between us occurred the week before my mother died. This was in 2002. She had been ailing and incapacitated after years of battling a blood disease called polycythemia vera. She was only 73, but she could have been 98. It was awful.

I had spent the summer in a rental cottage near my parents' home on Long Island, so I was around a lot for them. But at the end of the summer I was going to go on a Scotch-drinking tour around Scotland. It was with a bunch of fancy people, you know, going out for black-tie dinners and tasting Scotch for a week, a nice opportunity. The problem was that a few days before I was supposed to leave, my mother had taken a fall and was in the hospital. It wasn't lethal, and she wasn't supposed to be hospitalized for long. And she, along with my father and brother, told me to go to Scotland, enjoy myself. But when I got there, she really started to deteriorate in the hospital.

And, because the time difference made it tricky to call home—and I had no access to e-mail either—I didn't check in much. I didn't know the story. Toward the end of the week my brother left a message on my hotel's voice mail in Glasgow with words to the effect: "I don't know what's going on with you. I don't know why you haven't called. Maybe you just don't want to have your trip ruined with information from home. But as you know, Mom is still in the hospital, and she is not doing well at all. She may not even survive the week the way things are going. I don't know what you're thinking. But if you don't get back here soon to see her, and she's gone when you show up, I imagine you are going to be screwed up and in therapy for the rest of your life."

Now I knew what I was doing in Scotland. But even as I was thinking about my poor mother every day when I was there, I wanted to have my trip. And frankly, I felt that I had said my goodbye to her before I left. As I always did, I had sung to her at her bedtime while playing her piano, tucked her in, and kissed her goodbye. I remember that last night—she sang along with me in a weak, croaking voice I hardly recognized. She was almost gone by then. But on the other hand, she could have lived another year. What did I know? So why should I ruin my Scotland trip with phone calls and worries about her unless she was really dying in that hospital? I think my brother wanted those calls from me so I could show him that I was overwhelmed with worry. He needed me to go to the trouble of making the gesture of concern by calling daily. To be honest, I knew it would be best for her to pass on by then. But I couldn't say that to anyone. And I realize now that, more than anything, he was upset and needed someone to talk to about my mother's frightening and sudden decline. My father could only give my brother so much. I was his sibling and his soul mate when it came to worrying about our parents. And I was markedly absent at his time of need. In the end, I did come back early from Scotland. I cut my trip short, paid an additional 500 bucks to get myself home at the last minute. When I got to the hospital, she was obviously at the end phase of her life. That's another story.

4

What Have They Got to Gain and to Lose?

Eighty-five-year old Frank Barrett gained a lot and lost a lot in the 15 years after his retirement as a high school principal. For 10 of those years he lived with his wife Rhoda, having moved from their home of 30 years into a more efficient and accessible apartment near their married son and his family. Living comfortably on their retirement incomes, they were content with their situation and happy to be pursuing activities not permitted earlier in their lives. Not infrequently they would tell themselves and others that this was one of the best times of their lives—until Rhoda was diagnosed with cancer and died 5 years later. Even so, Frank continued living his own life with support from his family and friends, who shared his period of mourning. Several days a week he tutored teenagers with learning difficulties. He visited his friends, although their numbers were dwindling, and he enjoyed sports and the theater. He spoke to his children several times a week by phone, ate dinner with them frequently, and even babysat for his grandchildren occasionally.

But shortly after Frank's 85th birthday his children began to feel uneasy; they noticed little things at first. One day his daughter arrived and found the water running and overflowing the bathtub. Later that week she noticed that her father had burns on his arm. He seemed increasingly confused and often forgot what day of the week it was, which meal he had just eaten, and what his children had told him yesterday. He began to be irritable when they corrected or contradicted him and defensive when they questioned him. The day he fell and broke his hip, his children had already come to the realization that something needed to be done.

F RANK BARRETT'S STORY IS BEING REPLAYED BY NUM-bers of older people all over the United States and elsewhere and will be rerun even more frequently in the future with the aging of the baby boom generation. Your parents and older relatives may be living out similar scenarios right now.

Their problems, like Frank Barrett's, although disturbing to everyone in the family, may be relatively simple and straightforward. You may know exactly what kinds of solutions to look for, even though these solutions are often difficult to find. But things are not always so clear. Perhaps, instead, you are quite confused about what's happening to your parents. Perhaps you cannot put your finger on any single difficulty, even though you are aware that *something* is wrong. They may seem weaker, more tired, less alert—or withdrawn, full of self-pity and complaints, dissatisfied with everything and everyone. But even though you know that things are not right, you may not have the slightest idea how to make them better. How can you find answers if you don't even understand the questions?

Just as you may find it helpful to consider all the various emotions involved in your relationship with your parents in order to answer the question "How do you really feel about them?" it can be equally important to consider all the various changes in their personal world in order to answer the question "What's really happening to them?" You may never have stopped to wonder how the changes associated with growing old have affected their overall lives.

The Gains

Some of these changes are positive. A more optimistic view of aging is taking hold today, in part propelled by the impending waves of aging baby boomers. Extensive research findings also point to the benefits of late life for older Americans, and terms such as "positive aging" and "successful aging" are now familiar. They cite an extended life span for many who for the most part enjoy relatively good health, financial security, satisfying family lives and friendships, challenging volunteer work, and extended careers. As Frank Barrett and his wife discovered, freedom from the responsibilities of earlier adulthood was definitely a plus for them.

Creativity in Later Life

The gains in later life can be significant. Not the least are the increased opportunities to pursue creative activities and savor life. Noted gerontologist and psychiatrist, Dr. Gene Cohen of George Washington University, in his book *The Creative Age*, points to studies of aging that show that the potential for creative expression in later life is the rule rather than the exception, in spite of pervasive negative stereotypes to the contrary. He notes that creativity in later life spans a wide spectrum, from the work of authors and artists to the everyday pursuits of ordinary people. For many luminaries, such as Pablo Picasso and Sigmund Freud, creativity was undiminished in later life, and perhaps even enhanced. But non-luminaries such as Frank Barrett can also display enhanced creativity, in Frank's case by tapping in his long experience as a classroom teacher and a principal to find satisfaction tutoring troubled youngsters. The unique and dynamic combination of creativity and life experience is conducive to inner growth in later life, and some believe it leads to better physical and mental health as well.

> *The gains in later life can be significant. Not the least are the increased opportunities to pursue creative activities and savor life.*

Creativity in later life has biological underpinnings. Neurons, the nerve cells of higher intellectual functioning in the brain, do change with aging, but also continue to show adaptive capacity. To quote Dr. Cohen:

> We know that (in late life) the brain remains active—our "wiring" remains flexible—and that it responds positively to challenge, creating new connections that strengthen our capacity to respond to new ideas and generate them. We know that creative stimulation enhances our health, both biologically and emotionally, and that

some mental functions actually improve with age and experience. We know that even in the face of illness or disability, creative expression has the power to transform our lives with new opportunities and experiences of healing. (p. 66)

An Adaptable Majority Despite the Stereotypes

Despite popular belief, most older people adjust quite well to the changes in their lives. Your parents may be in this adaptable majority. Old age by itself is not a problem. It is the final stage in the cycle of living. Like every stage, it has its share of pleasure and pain, but unfortunate misconceptions and stereotypes prevail, perhaps accounting for the existence of "ageism" in many places and the prejudices against old age and old people held by many Americans. But the facts of aging, once they are known, can quickly prove these assumptions false. In the area of health, to take one example, although problems do mushroom during the later years, they are not nearly as universally incapacitating as many people suppose. Most men and women over 65 are healthy enough to carry on their normal activities—only 20% are not, and most of these are over age 75. Only about 5% of older adults are in institutions, nursing homes, or homes for the aged at any one time. Our elderly population averages fewer than 15 days a year in bed because of ill health, and even after age 65, illness and disability do not have to become chronic, but can frequently be cured or at least arrested.

The Losses

If any one word can sum up the varied catalogue of problems that do appear in old age, it is the word loss.

Still, if any one word can sum up the varied catalogue of problems that do appear in old age, it is the word *loss*. A 70-year-old woman may have had very little during a long and deprived life, but it's amazing how much she still has to lose as the years go by. Loss seems like a simple concept, but it often works in mysterious ways.

Children are usually quick to recognize obvious losses and to respond sympathetically to them. When Dad is widowed, everyone expects him to mourn. If Mom's arthritis seriously cripples her, it's easy to see why her daily life is so difficult. But loss is not always so glaringly apparent. When a 79-year-old woman considers it a tragedy that she cannot drive anymore, her family may be quite impatient with her. "What's she making such a big deal about? Can't she understand we'll take her anyplace she needs to go? Why does she act as if the world's come to an end?" They may not even begin to realize that *her* world *has* come to an end because she has lost what she valued most: her ability to go her own way and her independence. When aging Michael Parker's canary died, he could not be comforted. "It's only a bird," his children kept repeating in disbelief. "He wasn't this bad when Mother and Aunt Ellen died." They were right that their father had been able to recover more easily from greater losses in the past, but they did not realize that his canary's loss may have been one loss too many. While he mourned for his pet, he may also have been mourning for Mother *and* Aunt Ellen *and* his childhood friends *and* his fishing companion *and* his eyesight *and* his good digestion—*and* his teeth.

Loss comes in so many different forms. It can be a single blow: the death of a spouse or a sudden stroke. Or losses may be multiple: loss of work, combined with loss of social status, combined with loss of health, combined with loss of favorite activities. Your parents' ability to adapt to loss—whether single, double, or multiple—is perhaps the key that determines whether they experience a satisfying old age, an unhappy one, or a totally dependent one.

It's a High-Risk Period

Despite the generally positive attitudes held by those who are experiencing old age firsthand, there is no denying that the later years contain a considerable number of negative possibilities. More members of the older population suffer from chronic illness and disability than younger groups. Physical decline is often the underlying cause of other familiar problems associated with aging: mental illness, decrease in intellectual functioning, slowed reactions, and reductions in the gratifications and satisfactions of living. Even when older adults are in relatively good health, they have greater physical vulnerability, and that vulnerability may in turn affect many other aspects of their lives. The old definition of later life as a time when "stairs become steeper, print becomes smaller, lights become dimmer, and people are always mumbling" is no longer a laughing matter for many older people, but stark reality.

If the potential losses of old age were merely physical, they might be easier to deal with, but in our complex modern society, physical problems are usually interwoven with emotional and social ones. Throughout history we have been searching for the fountain of youth, but never with greater frenzy than in the period following World War II:

> Crabbed age and youth
> Cannot live together:
> Youth is full of pleasance,
> Age is full of care.

If these words were true in the sixteenth century when Shakespeare wrote them, how much truer they seem to ring today at the start of the twenty-first century. The emphasis on being young, looking young, acting young, and feeling young has grown more intense. Your parents have been told so often by the media and the fashion industry that they are out of step with the world that it's not surprising when they seem to believe it, too.

The spotlight is shifting now and is no longer directed exclusively on youth, partly because baby boomers, the generation that ushered in the youth culture after World War II, are now rapidly aging. But there are still forces in our culture today to persuade older people that society's needs can be met only by the young and the middle-aged. Despite the fact that Congress abolished mandatory retirement in 1986, many older people are still made to feel that their usefulness is determined by the calendar and the clock rather than by their ability to function and produce efficiently. Some, however, retire with grace, ease, and perhaps relief.

Some people's parents are able to adjust without much trouble to the losses they suffer. Other parents cannot do the job alone. Whether they are helped by you or by someone else, it may be useful now to review the major areas of loss that can accompany old age, sometimes singly, but more often in combination. Your parents may be experiencing one or more of those losses at this very moment.

Declining Functioning and Physical Health

The "Normal" Changes

If some genius in the medical profession were to discover a cure for chronic and disabling diseases, he or she would, of course, be removing some of the greatest problems that beset older people and would deserve worldwide gratitude and honor. But the process of aging would still keep right on, because some physical changes are inevitable. Fortunately or unfortunately, there is no built-in chronological timetable determining when these changes will take place and how rapidly, and how much damage they will do.

...some physical changes are inevitable. Fortunately or unfortunately, there is no built-in chronological timetable determining when these changes will take place and how rapidly, and how much damage they will do.

Your father may show them early and your mother much later, or vice versa. There is tremendous individual variation, and no two people are likely to follow the same schedule. Some seem to show hardly any deterioration at all.

Each organ system of the body is made up of millions of cells, and each system loses cells with advancing age (although, as noted earlier, brain neurons are more resilient). We can even watch this process taking place, since it is visible in the progressive wrinkling, drying, and sagging of the skin. Additional visible evidence is provided by diminishing height. Some older people actually lose stature because of the flattening of one or more vertebrae, which leads to a forward bending of the upper spine.

Each of the sense organs suffers some loss. Although only one of out six adults over the age of 65 reports serious vision problems, most experience vision changes. The lens of the eye loses elasticity, making it difficult to focus clearly, and we have all seen older people trying, with difficulty, to recover from the glare of a brightly lit room after they have come in from the dark. An older person's eyes may take eight or nine times longer to adapt to glare than a younger person's. The ear suffers its own nerve and bone changes, and hearing loss is noticed first by many older people, particularly in the higher frequencies. Sensitivity of the taste buds becomes duller, making it difficult to discriminate among foods. Sensory changes are often particularly difficult for the elderly to cope with emotionally, since these losses can so radically affect the pleasures of their daily living.

The aging process can also affect the nervous system and reduce sensitivity and perceptual abilities. You may have noticed a cut on your mother's hand or a large bruise on her leg and been surprised, or even irritated, that she seemed unaware of it. Frank Barrett's children reacted that way to the burns on their father's arm. Reduction in the pain response—its exact site unknown, but lying somewhere in the brain—may make it harder for older people to perceive pain within themselves. Other familiar signals transmitted by the nervous system that formerly alerted them to the part of their body in trouble may no longer come through loud and clear. A doctor may tell you that your mother has "walking pneumonia" or has suffered a mild heart attack that went unnoticed some time back. You can't blame her for not taking care of herself. Blame her nervous system for sending out inadequate signals.

The body must adapt to other reductions: the excretory function of the kidneys diminishes, the speed of the conduction of nerve impulses slows, and there is a decrease in heart output, which does not necessarily imply that the heart is diseased. Decrease in muscle tissue may produce a decrease in strength, and lung capacity may be reduced because the muscles no longer work efficiently. Digestive functions also slow down, including the flow of saliva and gastric juices, the motion of the stomach, and the contractions of the intestines—factors leading to constipation.

There is also *a decline in muscle strength,* and since so many everyday acts depend on physical strength and coordination, older people may find simple, everyday activities affected: walking, sitting down, dressing, and performing household tasks. When the declines in vision, hearing, and reaction time are taken into account, it is not surprising that the older adults are more fearful of accidents and more cautious than younger people.

Perhaps the most devastating reduction of all is *the depletion of the back-up reserves* that determine the human body's ability to fight off or recuperate quickly from disease. Your father may take a week to recover from the same virus that you and your children threw off in 24 hours. How much longer, therefore, and more precarious is the recuperation period from a more serious illness!

The aging process that affects us all would seem inevitable and irreversible, and indeed it is, for many conditions. Yet, what was yesterday a normal change associated with aging is today a treatable or untreatable disease, and tomorrow may be a curable condition. It is obvious that people are living longer and are in better physical shape than ever before. The need for continuing research is pressing, because, as the survival rate into the later decades increases, so do many chronic mental and physical disabilities.

What was yesterday a normal change associated with aging is today a treatable or untreatable disease, and tomorrow may be a curable condition.

There Are Compensations and Sometimes Improvements

Losses, even severe ones, are not always unbearable, and older people are often able to compensate for them. Your parents may have found this out for themselves already and may have discovered how to adapt. Keep in mind that they have survived many challenges over the years and are stronger as a result. Look at those with impaired vision who turn to large-print reading matter and "talking" books, those with impaired hearing who learn to ask others to speak slowly and clearly to them, and those with arthritis who search out more sedentary occupations to replace their more active ones. Some people with mild memory loss learn to keep a pad and pencil handy to jot down everything that needs to be remembered.

Normal memory loss, however, should not be confused with the symptoms of dementia, in particular, Alzheimer's disease. Psychologists have found that while memory may decline with age, judgment often significantly improves, and the ability to comprehend what is seen also improves with experience. When a rapid response is required, older people may not react as quickly as younger ones; they do not seem to be able to process as much information per time unit. But this slowdown is normal and is not a sign of mental impairment.

Some brain syndromes are not necessarily signs of irreversible and hopeless mental disorders. Reversible brain syndromes showing a variety of symptoms—confusion, disorientation, stupor, delirium, or hallucination—may result from any one of a number of causes, including malnutrition, anemia, congestive heart failure, misuse of medications, and infection. If diagnosed quickly enough, before too much damage is done, reversible brain syndromes can be treated successfully.

Modern scientists have provided a variety of inventions to compensate for the losses of old age. For example, cataract surgery followed by lens replacement has been very successful in restoring vision. For those with irreversible vision loss, efforts continue to improve and refine optical devices, and hearing aids are available for those with hearing impairments. Unfortunately, sensory-impaired older adults, who number at least one out of every four people over the age of 65, frequently reject these aids. Some are too impatient to learn to use these devices, which require training, and some are too vain to wear them.

Orthopedic surgery has been increasingly successful during the past 20 years, with total joint replacements now available to offset the devastating effects of crippling arthritis. Total hip and total knee replacements are now routine procedures, while replacement of other joints—ankle, wrist, shoulder—is under continuing study and evaluation. The number of prosthetic appliances is endless, including cane, walker, and wheelchair. Other important aids for persons with disabilities have been developed by architects, engineers, and other specialists. These include barrier-free environmental designs, ramps, motorized wheelchairs, kneeling buses, wide doorways, low wall telephones, and even the use of easily visible bright colors to provide cues for those with impaired vision. Thanks to the Americans with Disabilities Act passed in the 1990s and society's growing awareness of the challenges faced by persons with disabilities, the physical environment has become much more accessible to this population, young and old.

> It is important to keep in mind that many physical problems affecting aging bodies can be treated; some are even reversible.

Many Physical Problems Are Preventable and Treatable

It is important to keep in mind that many physical problems affecting aging bodies can be treated; some are even reversible. Disease and illness must be separated from the inevitable changes associated with aging, although undoubtedly those changes make the older adults more vulnerable and less resilient. Medical science is making great advances, and it is gratifying to know that some conditions once considered part of the inevitable process of aging can now be safely classified as diseases; therefore, they are potentially responsive to treatment, now or in the future.

For example:

- Diabetes is a disease in which the body does not produce or properly use insulin, the hormone that is needed to convert sugar, starches, and other food into energy needed for daily life. It is now considered to be of epidemic proportion, affecting 7% of the American population, including 20% of those over the age of sixty. Yet, as many as one third of those with diabetes are unaware that they have a disease that can be treated and its destructive effects on the organs of the body prevented with proper medical care. Type II diabetes, common in older adults can be prevented in some cases with control of weight and exercise.

- Arteriosclerosis, commonly referred to as "hardening of the arteries," was until recently considered part of the aging process because doctors found it more frequently in older people. It also seemed to become progressively more severe in particular individuals as the years went by. Today, however, it is seen as a complex metabolic disturbance and, thanks to advances in the management of hypertension and diabetes, is subject to treatment and alleviation.

- Osteoporosis, a disease in which the bones become more fragile and likely to break, was also once thought of as an inevitable part of the aging process. However, now this condition to some extent can be treated medically. We also know that women who exercise regularly and who have consumed adequate amounts of calcium and continue to do so are less prone to osteoporosis.

A few words of caution are necessary, however. If the condition has been present in various organs in an unrecognized form for a long period, irreversible damage may have occurred. Furthermore, diseases in the elderly are often of multiple origins, and it can be difficult to recognize and treat each one. But it is somewhat reassuring to know that chronic disease, while not curable, may be controllable. An abundance of information about diseases and conditions that are common in later life can be found online (see Appendix A for selected websites).

While the number of treatable conditions associated with aging has been expanding, unfortunately this is not the case with the number of geriatricians—medical doctors who specialize in treating older adults. This dilemma was reported on the front page of the *New York Times* on October 18, 2006. In 2005, the article noted, there was one geriatrician for every 5000 Americans over the age of 65, and the situation is only going to get worse since geriatrics is a specialty of little interest to medical students; furthermore, only nine medical schools out of 145 have departments of geriatrics.

Why Some Function Better Than Others

Except in severe situations, the physical losses of older adults should not be considered insurmountable problems. They become problems when they interfere with an individual's ability to function, to live a somewhat "normal life, and to carry on familiar routines.

Many younger people go through life afflicted with one ailment or another, but rarely need to stop their activities, except briefly. As a matter of fact, some mature and middle-aged people seem to carry their own special physical ailments as marks of distinction. Haven't you heard them announce almost with pride, "My allergies are terrible this month," or "My back's acting up again," or "I've got one of my migraines"? It's the same with older adults. Most should be able to function at least adequately and many do, but some do not. The irreversible processes of aging or the associated diseases may well be compensated for by one elderly person, while his neighbor, similarly afflicted, may be just barely getting along. Watch the progress of two patients recovering from the same long illness. One takes his medicine, follows the doctor's orders, and seeks out rehabilitation, while his roommate gives up and retires into semi-invalidism without making even a halfhearted try.

Arthritis may have turned your friend's father into a physically impaired shut-in who hesitates to leave the house. Why is it that

Except in severe situations, the physical losses of older adults should not be considered insurmountable problems.

your own father, no less arthritic, moving a little more slowly than before and possibly needing a cane, still travels in the same circles he has always enjoyed? Your mother may refer to herself as "half-blind" and consider herself seriously incapacitated, while your colleague's mother, with equally deficient vision, tells the world that she's lucky her sight is holding up so well—and believes it, too.

To the despair of their children, some older adults are unable to make satisfactory adjustments and seem unwilling to try; they almost perversely reject other people's suggestions. Listen to the conversations at the next social gathering you attend—cocktail party, sewing club, lodge meeting—it's almost predictable that you'll hear the same old familiar refrains: "Mother's a diabetic, but she won't stick to her diet," or "John's mom won't consider a cataract operation," or "Father's got a walker, but he's never tried to use it," or " 'We bought Ginny's dad a hearing aid, but he's never worn it once."

Certain losses may be more difficult to bear for individual, personal reasons. A vain woman may be able to compensate for impaired hearing, but may be totally devastated by her wrinkled skin—something that another woman might accept as a natural, although unwelcome, fact of life. Your parents' feelings, attitudes, psychological makeup, and personalities are often the factors determining whether or not physical losses are seen as overwhelming problems.

Reduced Social Contacts

Just as cell loss inevitably takes place in your parents' bodies, almost as inevitably do social losses occur in their world, particularly in the later years. Patterns of living, working, communicating, and socializing that built up over all the earlier stages of their lives often break down completely or at least are harder to maintain. The universe of the very old tends to become a smaller, more confined place, less crowded with the familiar faces of friends, relatives, and co-workers. As people die, husbands are left without wives and wives without husbands.

There are always exceptions: because of some unusual event or accomplishment of their own, or the rise to prominence of a son or daughter, men and women in their 80s and beyond may find their horizons expanding and discover new faces, new experiences, and even new geographical locations. But for many, their social world is a shrinking planet. The situation may be less confining for today's better educated, health-conscious middle-aged, who will be tomorrow's old. Their social world may be a different one, with wider horizons.

Here again, as with physical loss, the variation among older adults is tremendous—and mysterious. For some, the social losses can be devastating. For others, the impact is not unbearable—they may have always been self-sufficient. Severe physical impairment and financial privation can produce the greatest social hardships, but your parents' ability to accept their social losses depends (as it did with their physical losses) on a number of factors: their own personalities, developed over a lifetime; the stability of their marriage or other relationships; their relationship with their children and other family members; their roots in their community; the plans made in earlier years for their retirement period; and their own attitudes toward old age and even death.

Changes in Human Relationships

Physical problems are difficult enough to cope with, but the social problems that result from severe physical decline can be the source of additional trauma. If your father has been immobilized by arthritis or paralyzed by a stroke, if he is confined to bed or just confined to the house, if he can no longer board a bus or take a walk by himself, or if he cannot go out with you in your car, then his world will become no larger than his own apartment or house. It may even be no larger than his own room, if he is bedridden. Then, in addition to the physical pain he is suffering, he will also suffer the pain of loneliness. Your mother, if she is alive and healthy, will inevitably share some of this isolation. Because of *his* incapacity, *her* life will also become more limited. Visits by a steady stream of relatives and friends can help to bring the world to the housebound. A few concerned neighbors who drop in regularly can help alleviate loneliness. For the less fortunate, with no relatives or friends nearby, social isolation can be relieved only by planned visits from staff and volunteers from social service agencies and faith-

> *Physical problems are difficult enough to cope with, but the social problems that result from severe physical decline can be the source of additional trauma.*

based organizations and even occasional impromptu contacts with mail carriers, delivery people, and neighborhood children. The role played by pets in alleviating loneliness cannot be underestimated.

Social isolation can also increase when older persons can no longer communicate easily with the world around them because of impaired vision or hearing. Here again, the more physically active partner suffers some of the same isolation. When familiar social patterns, formerly shared by both husband and wife, are lost for one, they are often lost for both.

But social isolation does not only come from physical causes. It can also come from the death of close family members—husband, sister, brother—or friends. Even more tragic for the elderly is when death strikes younger generations: children, nieces, nephews, or grandchildren. When those ties that have been so close for so long have been broken, how can they ever be replaced? Many old people do form new friendships, but some very old people live long enough to see the disappearance of their entire generation and every close relative and friend they have known.

Changes in the Environment

Loneliness may also result from changes in familiar patterns. Ours is a mobile society; friends and children (even loving and devoted ones) may move far away for jobs or a preferred style of living. Thousands of miles may separate parents from children and friends from friends, although relationships can still remain close, even when they are no longer conducted face-to-face. The telephone, e-mail, the tape recorder, and the video camera can keep contacts amazingly alive. Friendly neighborhoods change, too. They become more built-up, less cared for, less residential. Familiar faces disappear from the streets and are replaced by unfamiliar ones. Favorite stores, where shopping was a comfortable, even a sociable process, change hands, and new stores carrying new merchandise can cause bewilderment in elderly customers. Mr. Malatsky's little delicatessen on the corner may have been replaced by a new modern supermarket, but for your elderly mother, nothing will replace Mr. Malatsky. Many children try arguing, shouting, or pleading, in vain attempts to dislodge elderly parents or a widowed father or mother from an apartment or a house situated in a neighborhood that has become rundown and unsafe. "It was good enough for your father and me for 40 years. It was good enough for you as a boy. It's good enough for me now," is a typical response, and nothing short of abduction or a crowbar will budge the speaker. Because they risk being mugged, robbed, or beaten if they are alone on the streets, some older people fear going out at all. They become shut-ins or limit their outings to certain "safe" times of day. To the despair of their children, elderly parents often cling to familiar walls, even though an alien country lies right outside their front door.

Fewer Familiar Roles

Older adults cannot escape undergoing some changes in their customary roles, and for some, these changes are experienced as a loss. In the course of a lifetime, people assume a multitude of roles. Some of these roles might be parent, breadwinner, homemaker, spouse, church member, or athlete—even black sheep. But then, as individuals age in our society, they lose or voluntarily give up a number of their earlier roles—in extreme cases, all of them. Here again, there is variation. Some roles are given up easily; others are more painful to lose. Most older people no longer fulfill a parenting role unless they live with their children and grandchildren, and even then, they may take on few parenting responsibilities. With retirement, the breadwinning role is given up. Eking out a small income by working as a babysitter or a security guard does not replace the prestige of the role of breadwinner.

In other times and other societies, older adults who no longer were able to perform their former roles could turn to auxiliary ones and continue to be, as well as feel, useful and needed in their communities. Among the polar Eskimos, old couples helped in summer to store the winter's supply of bird meat; old women too feeble to travel stayed indoors doing household chores and repairing clothing. They tanned leather, chewing it to make it soft. Elderly men made seal spears and nets. There is a shortage of meaningful auxiliary roles for the elderly in our society. "Older persons are our great unutilized source of labor," writes Malcolm Cowley in *The View from 80*. "A growing weakness in American society is that it regards the old as consumers but not producers, as mouths but not hands."

The one role left for many older people is the role of householder. "My own place," whether a house or an apartment, can symbolize the last rampart, and it can become crucially important to defend it. That may be one reason why older people so often refuse to leave familiar neighborhoods and are far less likely to move than younger Americans. The presence of a home health aide is sometimes viewed as an incursion on this last rampart, and even the final role of house-holder is removed when older adults need to enter a nursing home or an assisted living facility. Here they can only fill a dependent role: the role of patient or resident is rarely satisfying.

Many older people do make successful adjustments to their role loss. Some actually thrive on being relieved of burdensome demands and find greater contentment in the final years than in the previous ones. "I'm an old lady and glad of it!" insisted one active grand-mother on her 80th birthday. "I don't have to prove anything to anyone anymore. No more competing, no more pretending—I can just be myself now." There are those still working at first or second careers and actively involved as volunteers. There are some who find it painful to lose the parent role, but derive compensatory satisfac-tion—sometimes even greater satisfaction—from the role of grand-parent. Some older people maintain their sexual identities, their male and female roles, through a continuing active sexual life. But even taking these successful examples into account, loss of an important role can be a painful blow to the self-regard and emotional well-being of some older people.

Financial Insecurity

One of the most heartening developments in recent years is the great improvement in the financial picture of older people. There has been a dramatic decline in poverty among the elderly. In 1959, 33.2% of men and women over 65 lived below the poverty line. In 2000, this percentage was only 10.5%. Social Security, Medicare, and past improvements in pension systems are largely responsible for this welcome change. Despite this progress, 3.5 million men and women over the age of 65 still live below the poverty line, and another 2.3

million rank as "near-poor," with incomes just above poverty level, making a total of 5.8 million poor or near-poor older people.

Even though there is greater financial security for older adults these days than in the past, this should not suggest that most of those over 65 are affluent. Many have to live on diminished resources, while the threat of medical expenses and long-term nursing home care are ever-present, haunting concerns. For those who live on fixed incomes, the fear of inflation is not an irrational anxiety. Increased energy costs are a case in point.

In other times and places, older adults could expect that the struggles and labors of their earlier years would be rewarded in their later years by comfort and security. "I shall cherish your old age with plenty of venison and you shall live easy," was the customary assurance of an Iroquois son to his father. Even poor Job, afflicted for so long by trial and tribulation, could relax when he became old!

> So the Lord blessed the latter end of Job more than his beginning: for he had fourteen thousand sheep, and six thousand camels, and a thousand yoke of oxen and a thousand she asses.
> Job 42:12–17 (King James Version)

There are many growing old in America today who cannot expect such comfort and security ahead. Too many learn that to grow old is to grow poor.

There is a misguided assumption that older people need less money to live on. Whether the old need to spend as much on clothing, travel, entertainment, or furniture as the young is open to argument, but there is no argument about the fact that the old have greater medical expenses. For example, those over 65 spend, on average, three times as much for prescribed medicine alone as those under 65. The Medicare and Medicaid programs administered under the Social Security Act cover many health costs, but there are significant loopholes in both programs, including the recently enacted Medicare part D to "cover" the costs of prescription drugs.

There is a misguided assumption that older people need less money to live on.

Earlier in this chapter, we mentioned that some people seem able to compensate better than others for the variety of losses experienced in old age. It is not always easy to explain these different reactions, but in light of diminished finances, they are more understandable. An older person living on a small Social Security check and a small pension may desperately need orthopedic appliances to compensate for progressive arthritis, but simply may not have the financial ability to purchase them. If compensatory devices are not provided under Medicare, they might as well not exist. Financial limitations are among the most severe obstacles blocking elderly people from compensating for the problems of aging.

Financial insecurity and money problems do not vanish for those living above poverty level. Fear of reduced income may realistically haunt even middle-income elderly couples and individuals who have substantial assets, a car, an unmortgaged house, and many personal possessions collected over a lifetime. When regular salaries and incomes stop coming in, healthy 70-year-olds with thousands of dollars' worth of assets are not unrealistic when they worry, "When this is gone, what will happen to me?"

Increased Dependency

The combination of some or all of the losses described in the previous sections—loss of physical health, familiar roles, social contacts, and financial security—can precipitate another loss that has particular meaning in our society: the loss of independence, a highly regarded personal asset. The loss of independence can be a stunning blow to an older person's self-esteem.

... loss of physical health, familiar roles, social contacts, and financial security— can precipitate another loss that has particular meaning in our society: the loss of independence, a highly regarded personal asset.

Independence, of course, is a misnomer regardless of one's age and capabilities. We are all dependent on others to greater or lesser degrees, but within societal bounds, we have control over our personal lives. The increased dependency forced on disabled older persons can pose severe problems for them and for family members who care for them. Not infrequently it can trigger a troubling depression, or the older person who is disabled may overreact to his or her needs and become too dependent and too demanding. We've all heard relatives commenting helplessly from time to time, "We try to do everything Mother wants, but it never seems to be enough!"

Conversely, there are those with disabilities who try vehemently to deny their dependency by insisting, in the face of all handicaps, "I can manage perfectly well," and refusing the willing offers of help essential to maintaining health. They may try to mask the magnitude of their disabilities by "showing who's boss" and ruling their relatives, wives, and children, curtailing everyone else's freedom. Maintaining a semblance of independence can be admirable, but when carried too far, it can lead to trouble.

Some older people fear losing their independence when they are financially insecure. You may be financially able, willing, and eager to provide additional funds for your parents. You may even insist on doing so. But when forced to accept money from their children, many older people feel that in return they are surrendering control over their lives. The extra income may prove to be at best only a mixed blessing. Your monthly check may be a sweet and loving gesture on your part, but it may be received as somewhat bitter medicine by your parents, who had grown accustomed through their lives to earning their own money, paying their own way, and feeding and educating their families—and taking care of *you*.

If the day finally comes when an older person finds it impossible to manage on his or her own, financially or physically, and must accept institutional living, the greatest sacrifice for this person may be control over the activities of daily life. Institutionalization, by its very nature, seems to symbolize that ultimate loss, and this probably explains why so many older people prefer inadequate, isolated living conditions to the protective care of even the best institutions.

Escalating Mental Health Problems

Each of the areas of loss examined in this chapter has psychological ramifications. Mental health problems resulting from losses in later life, as well as those triggered by other threats, real or imaginary, are often the most difficult to handle. In dealing with your own parents, you may have already discovered that their psychological problems place the heaviest demands on your own emotional resources. Physical incapacity can present enough problems, but the picture grows more complex when psychological problems are added.

Psychological problems can be very perplexing for the children of older people, especially when the emotions of both generations become intertwined. It is not unusual for a family to report that an elderly relative has undergone a real personality change: "He's not the same person he used to be," or "I just don't know my mother anymore." Surprisingly enough, some personality changes are for the better, although many, admittedly, are for the worse. As your parents begin to age, mental health problems may appear for the first time, developing in direct response to physical and social losses. But these difficulties may also be continuations of lifelong emotional problems that were successfully held in check at earlier times, but become intensified in old age. They may also be related to reversible or irreversible organic brain conditions.

What Are the Mental Health Problems?

They include a familiar list—depression, anxiety, alcoholism, cognitive impairment, and sometimes severe psychotic reactions. There's nothing really new or special in this list. These are the psychological problems of all ages—the young as well as the old—but statistics reveal that some appear with greater frequency in the population 65 and over. There is a higher incidence of depression among older adults as well as a higher incidence of organic brain disorders that produce their own special symptoms, including disorientation, loss of memory, and confusion.

"Normal" Reactions to Loss

Before you jump to the conclusion that your parent has a serious mental health problem, it is important to keep in mind that it is normal to react to loss with strong emotions.

The emotions your parents feel in their old age are no different from childhood emotions, young adult emotions, and middle-aged emotions. The infant faces loss when giving up

Before you jump to the conclusion that your parent has a serious mental health problem, it is important to keep in mind that it is normal to react to loss with strong emotions.

the close, dependent relationship with his or her mother; the adolescent when breaking away from parental authority; the middle-aged adult when facing the loss of youth. The older adult reacts with the very same emotions to the physiological and social losses accompanying old age as well as to the indignities and neglect imposed by society. Since losses appear with greater variety and frequency in old age than in any other stage of life, anxiety and depression, fear, anger, and guilt can be anticipated. They are normal, even appropriate, emotions.

- *Mourning.* You would certainly be surprised if an older person who had suffered a severe loss did *not* seem to be sad or angry—if he or she did *not* grieve. More damage can be caused when the mourning process is circumvented. "We shouldn't leave Mother alone today because she'll only sit and think about Dad"—this may be an understandable, well-meant, loving reaction from concerned children shortly after a father's funeral. Yet, perhaps that's just the very thing Mother *needs* to do for a while before she's ready to do anything else. Mourning plays an essential part in making a healthy adjustment to the loss of a beloved person. It helps those who mourn to work through their grief and redirect their energies to new interests in life. There is no timetable for mourning, nor should one be imposed. For some, a period of mourning may last more than a year.
- *Anxiety and fear* play equally useful roles. There's nothing abnormal about an older person's fears for his future—he or she has every right to be afraid, within reason. If your father's eyesight is failing, it is perfectly realistic for him to wonder how he will manage for himself and to feel a diffuse sense of foreboding. It's also realistic for someone who has already had one heart attack to be concerned about his or her health or even to fear approaching death.
- *Anger* is also to be expected as a normal emotional reaction to loss. When you've suffered an injury or an insult, what's wrong with being angry? After all, anger is an emotion of retribution, a way of striking back at whatever has caused an injury. Just as a young boy might get angry at the hammer with which he has hurt his own finger, an older person may get angry at the gods or fate or whatever he believes may have

caused a particular loss. Your father may even direct his anger at you, for lack of a better target, and feel guilty as a result. There's no need to be alarmed when your parents exhibit fear, anxiety, grief, or anger. They are not pleasant emotions—no one claims they are—but they may be necessary, even therapeutic, at certain periods. Your parents should not have to feel guilty if they show those emotions, nor should you feel guilty yourself. There is room for those feelings in the total context of life.

Older people, like younger ones, develop special behavior patterns that help them to ward off anxiety, depression, or a fear of uncontrollable rage. These behavior patterns are important to their own sense of survival. They may be within a "normal range," although you may, on occasion, find them bewildering, frustrating, or even infuriating. It is important to note that these patterns of behavior are seen in people of all ages, although the old may rely on some of them more than the young.

- *Reminiscing* is one of the most potentially effective behavior patterns employed by older adults, yet it is often misunderstood by their families. As death approaches, many older people spend much time going through a life review. Remembrance of things past can be a painful process, but it can also be comforting. It can provide meaningful significance to the final years and help to reduce fear and anxiety. Living in the past is often mistakenly seen as a symptom of brain damage: "What's the matter with Father? He can remember the name of his first-grade teacher, but he can't remember his neighbor's name or whether he's had lunch or not!" At best, the tendency to live in the past is viewed as unnecessary nostalgia—an unfortunate disengagement from the present—or as self-preoccupation. You may despair that your parents seize every opportunity to discuss their past life with you or with anyone else who will listen, but it may be an indication of health rather than a sign of deterioration. If this does not seem to be merely meaningless repetition but rather something that gives them pleasure or possibly even rejuvenates them, it should be encouraged, not stifled.
- *Preparatory Mourning.* Some older people, while not seriously depressed, do not bounce back from a period of mourning

and are never again ready to contemplate new directions. Mourning can become a lifestyle, best described as *preparatory mourning.* It can be seen as a protective pattern of behavior and is often reflected in a morbid interest in death, fascination with obituaries, and a preoccupation with funerals—even those of strangers. All of us know people who, even in the prime of life, turn first to the death notices in the daily paper. Some older people find this their favorite section. One testy 70-year-old used to horrify his grandchildren at the breakfast table by chuckling cheerfully as he scanned the obituary page of the newspaper every morning, often saying, "Well, I see another old friend of mine has made headlines today."

- *Denial.* "Old Mr. Jones is really showing his age these days, isn't he?" commented Mr. Smith to his daughter. Mr. Smith himself is 80 years old, bent with arthritis, walking with a cane, and increasingly hard of hearing. He is able to notice the signs of aging in others, but not in himself. His own old age and impending death are not conscious realities to him. He uses *denial*—a common defense—to avoid facing his own advancing years and the accompanying painful feelings. Denial, used in moderation, can be helpful in maintaining a sense of stability and equilibrium. If it is carried too far, however, it can become hazardous.

Denial, used in moderation, can be helpful in maintaining a sense of stability and equilibrium.

The elderly may deny pain and physical symptoms until they are beyond help; they may deny dependency, deafness, blindness, and confusion, thereby jeopardizing their safety. Denial need not be limited to physical symptoms or sensory losses; it may involve other losses as well. A 75-year-old widow seemed to take the drastic reduction in her finances after her husband's death with remarkable good will, or so her children thought—until they discovered that she had simply denied her financial problems and continued to spend her dwindling capital and use her charge accounts as if there had been no change in her circumstances. Denial is not uncommon, nor is it dangerous in itself. Only if it interferes with reality and prevents sound decisions can it legitimately be considered a serious problem.

- *Mistrustful Behavior.* You may sense that your father is becoming increasingly suspicious as he grows older. That is quite possible. *Mistrustful behavior* is not uncommon in older (or younger) people. Some forms of this behavior arise when people project their own unconscious and uneasy feelings elsewhere—away from themselves. Mistrustfulness, which has no visible roots, can be bewildering and upsetting to families, and it may, if carried to extremes, be considered a mental illness. Some mistrustful behavior can be more easily understood and clearly grounded in reality. It may be realistic and self-protective. A frail old man can be at the mercy of other people who are stronger. He may become a prime target for abuse and exploitation. Caution and suspicion may be the only weapons he has with which to protect himself. Sometimes the elderly are not mistrustful enough!

  Other forms of mistrustful behavior, although unwarranted, are rooted somewhere in reality and stem from the anxiety that aging men and women feel as independence slips away from them. Once able to care for themselves independently, but now increasingly dependent on someone else, they begin to wonder if that "someone" is really doing right by them. They feel they must watch out for their own interests or "someone" will take advantage of them: cheat them, rob them, or even hurt them. You may find it quite painful when that suspected "someone" turns out to be you. The concerned child who is trying hardest to help may accidentally become the target for mistrust and the focus of the anger that can accompany it.

- *Stubbornness and avoidance of change* are two particularly successful and related adaptive patterns of behavior used by some older adults. Both are likely to be extremely frustrating to children, close friends, and other relatives. "I can't budge him!" is a familiar cry from a long-suffering son or daughter trying in vain to help an aging father. "He won't listen," "won't move," "won't see a doctor," "won't watch his diet." Stubbornness is also used as a magical solution to fight the forces that disrupt life, and it's remarkable how strongly a failing, 100-lb old woman is able to resist the combined weight of hundreds of pounds of concerned relatives. So many changes and losses are forced on older people as the years go by that they may often try to control their lives in such a way that they can avoid change whenever possible. To that end, a whole way of life may be developed. When your parents insist on remaining in a familiar house, apartment, or neighborhood, even though they agree with you that the neighborhood has changed, the house is too big for them, and the apartment is too isolated, they are obviously avoiding change, although you may see this as stubbornness.

A pattern of avoidance can also operate more subtly. It can explain fear of travel—or fear of even leaving the house—or refusal to consider new activities, meet new people, or try new doctors or new medicines, even though they know the old ones are not doing them much good. Avoidance of change and stubbornness can be used by some older adults as a kind of protective armor that wards off the changes well-meaning children or relatives would like to impose.

Mrs. Gross became a quasi–shut-in. She went out only for occasional emergencies. Her children made superhuman efforts to dislodge her, urging her to "come to dinner," or "come to the movies," or "come for a drive." "It's for your own good," they insisted. But she turned down all invitations. She was, however, very sociable, always delighted to have visitors and to serve light meals very hospitably. Mrs. Gross did not ask her children for help and was contented with her life.

- *Worship of Independence.* Closely connected with avoidance of change is a passionate, although often inappropriate, *worship of independence.* Many older people see independence as another weapon with which to protect themselves from outside interference. To the horror of family, friends, and social agencies, aging men and women may reject safe and protective surroundings and endure drab furnished rooms, inadequate nourishment, and irregular health care in order to preserve that treasured state. It is painful to accept the fact that when independence is weighed against protected living in a child's home, independence often wins. But painful as that is, relatives should understand that when such a value is given to independence, its loss could trigger a devastating emotional reaction.

Serious Mental Health Problems

Behavior patterns and feelings, "normal" when kept within limits, become serious when they go out of bounds and interfere with your parents' overall ability to function and adversely affect their physical health. Someone who is still in deep mourning after more than a year and showing no signs of recovery may be suffering from a severe depressive reaction. Someone who gets angry for an inordinate amount of time and, even worse, engages in verbal, even physical, violence—is certainly showing a serious emotional problem. Grief, anger, and anxiety—all normal emotions—can lead to severe difficulties that may require psychiatric attention when they are unremitting and intense. It is important to note that psychological problems among older adults are not always expressed in extreme emotional states or difficult behavior. Organ systems depleted by cellular loss and tissue change can show physiological breakdown as a result of psychological stress. Anxiety, in particular, has been shown to be related to cardiovascular difficulties.

> *Behavior patterns and feelings, "normal" when kept within limits, become serious when they go out of bounds and interfere with your parents' overall ability to function and adversely affect their physical health.*

Other severe problems, such as Alzheimer's disease, may develop independently of these intense reactions to loss and stress. To a significant degree, however, these reactions play an important role in the mental disturbances of older persons. Here are several of the more common ones.

- *Clinical Depression.* As a mental disorder, depression is quite different from mourning a loss and the temporary moods almost everyone experiences from time to time, moods we describe by saying, "I feel so depressed today." The symptoms of clinical depression go beyond "blue" feelings and are not always obvious. Prolonged periods of insomnia, fatigue, lack of appetite, agitation, and various psychosomatic ailments may all be indications of a serious depression, although the correct diagnosis

  > *The symptoms of clinical depression go beyond "blue" feelings and are not always obvious.*

is often overlooked. Depression by itself can affect cognitive and physical functioning.

So-called depressive reactions in later life often can be related to earlier experiences. A person who lost a great deal as a child, for example, may suffer periods of depression repeatedly throughout the life cycle. Depression, mild or severe, may return when there is a reminder of early childhood trauma, such as the loss or rejection of a parent, illness, or deprivation. The onslaughts of aging can be such grim reminders of earlier losses that they can trigger acute depressive states. Depression can also be an extension of unresolved mourning. Extreme depression is one of the causes of the high rate of suicide among older adults.

Depression can mask other feelings, such as severe guilt, shame, or unacceptable anger. If a person cannot accept these feelings, he or she may turn them inward, bringing on an apparent state of depression. Loss normally produces some depression and anger, but those who feel in any way responsible for the loss may also suffer painful feelings of guilt and shame. That is especially true when death comes to someone who has been very dependent, very troublesome, or very unloving. The partner who survives may feel very guilty. (The same kind of depression may afflict grown children when a difficult, troublesome parent dies.)

In recent years, significant progress has been made in the treatment of depression, through both medications and psychotherapy. While there are now more than 20 antidepressant medications, not all are as effective in older adults as in younger ones, and care must exercised in their prescription. Their potentially harmful interactions with other medications must also be taken into consideration. Chapter 12 speaks more to this point and the skill and experience of the prescribing physician. Too often, however, older adults regard depression as an inevitable part of aging, and they do not seek treatment. The stigma of mental illness also makes some older people reluctant to seek treatment.

- *Alcoholism.* Various studies have shown that a drink or two a day is beneficial to the health of older adults. As reported in the September 2006 issue of the American Geriatrics Society, it was found among older women that being a nondrinker of alcohol was associated with a greater risk of death and poor health, and that moderate alcohol intake may carry health benefits in terms of survival and quality of life. This said, there is a growing problem among older adults with abuse of alcohol and other substances. Some older adults may be coping with lifelong addiction problems that may be exacerbated by the stresses of aging and increased life burdens. Some may start drinking heavily for the first time to mask depression and anxiety. Those who were light or moderate drinkers earlier in life may find their tolerance for alcohol diminishing as their bodies age: they can feel the effects with less alcohol. Alcohol metabolizes more slowly in older bodies, so blood alcohol levels remain higher for a longer time after drinking, increasing the risk of falls and accidents for many hours.

Closely related to the problem of alcoholism and substance abuse is the misuse of medications, which is discussed in detail in Chapter 12. Here it should be underscored that consumption of alcohol, even a small amount, in combination with the various prescribed and over-the-counter medications that many older adults take, can result in serious health problems.

A problem with alcohol consumption can occur without anyone noticing it at first. Some of the symptoms might be shrugged off as the common signs of aging or illness. The warning signs can include memory loss, difficulty in concentrating, sadness, falls, bruises, burns, incontinence, poor hygiene, and a lack of interest in activities, family, and friends. These red flags can signal other conditions as well and call for medical attention.

A problem with alcohol consumption can occur without anyone noticing it at first.

- *Psychotic Reactions.* Some people may see, hear, or think things that have no basis in reality. Anxious, depressed, and angry feelings can precede such psychotic reactions, which can result from severe impairment of the sense organs and the brain. Loss of hearing can affect mental stability; some with hearing impairments may turn to their own inner world for sensory clues. Unable to hear what is going on around them, they invent explanations. Furthermore, cognitive impairment can interfere with an older person's ability to process information from the real world, thereby setting off or compounding a psychotic reaction. Paranoid states are a type of psychotic disorder involving delusional thinking and false beliefs of persecution and victimization.

- *Alzheimer's Disease.* Last but not least among the mental disorders suffered by older adults are the dementias, the best known and most prevalent of which is Alzheimer's disease (AD). Estimates suggest that 5%–10% of people over 65 are affected by AD, a devastating condition in which there is marked deterioration of intellectual performance. As with other age-related disorders, AD occurs with far greater frequency among the very old, involving up to one half of the over-85 population.

The specific problems experienced by persons with AD include gradual loss of memory, problem-solving ability, and other aspects of abstract thinking. Other related symptoms include disorientation in time and space; personality changes; difficulty in communicating, word-finding, and learning; decreased attention span; and impaired judgment. In the early stages of dementia, people with AD might have trouble remembering familiar names and places and forget what they did earlier in the day. The symptoms can begin as almost imperceptible personality and behavior changes. They may also resemble those of other psychological conditions discussed previously. As the disease progresses, however, the changes become more marked and interfere with the person's daily life, requiring a caregiver's attention. When severe symptoms appear, including incomprehensible speech and lost of bladder and bowel control, 24-hour/day care is required. In addition, the severe impact of advanced dementia on intellectual functioning and personality, resulting, for example, in the inability of the older adult to recognize even loved ones, can be particularly difficult for family members.

There is no known cure or treatment for the symptoms of AD, although research has increased dramatically in recent years, and much more is now known about the pathological changes that occur in the brain. Reliable means have been developed to determine the presence of the disease with 85%–90% accuracy. These include a thorough medical examination as well as psychiatric and neurological evaluations to rule out other conditions that can mimic AD. Indeed, as noted, the symptoms of dementia may be due to other conditions, some of which are treatable. Included here are depressive reactions, malnutrition, drug toxicity, and anemia. Therefore, when the symptoms of dementia occur, medical, neurological, and/or psychiatric evaluations are needed not only to establish or exclude a diagnosis of AD but also to treat reversible conditions that cause similar symptoms.

> When the symptoms of dementia occur, medical, neurological, and/or psychiatric evaluations are needed to establish or exclude a diagnosis of AD and to treat reversible conditions that cause similar symptoms.

The good news for families of persons with AD is the dramatic growth in recent years of public awareness of the condition, its devastating effects on the family, and the extraordinary demands it places on the long-term care system. Contributing to this public awareness and growing concern has been the advocacy of the Alzheimer's Association, an organization founded in 1980 by families of persons with dementia. Today this organization has chapters throughout the United States that provide essential information and counseling for families as well as support groups. Its web site address is www.alz.org.

There is little question that one of the greatest losses that can be experienced by elderly persons is the ability to function intellectually and keep in touch with the world around them. Just as devastating for some older persons is the loss of sight, the loss of hearing, or the loss of home, money, or independence. For family members, the losses brought about by Alzheimer's disease are probably the most devastating and most feared. The total dependency of the persons in advanced stages of the disease and the changes in personality place great physical and emotional burdens on the family. Chapter 9 addresses the steps families can take to address this daunting challenge.

The Gains Versus the Losses and Your Role

No one can deny that a broad array of losses may be incurred in old age—losses that often multiply and interact. Much space has been devoted to the discussion of these losses to deepen your understanding if and when your parent experiences difficulties. It is essential to be aware of them. Equally essential to keep in mind, though, is that a significant number of older people do *not* suffer from conditions such as dementia; many can function fairly independently despite the various challenges they may face, and they could function better if they were aware of *what can be done* when those challenges arise. The family is an important resource in seeing that *something is done.*

For some of us, aging is a downer; for others, it is uplifting. Short of devastating illnesses, such as AD, there is much to gain in later life. The stories of those who are enjoying these gains could fill the pages of this book. Old age is full of endless possibilities—long-suffering acceptance, dreary monotony, grim misery, and high tragedy—as well as deep satisfaction, unexpected gratification, serenity, and even fun, and surprisingly, *creativity.*

A person who is growing old may perceive the glass as half-full or half-empty. The research repeatedly documents the decisive role that family members play in keeping the "glass half-filled." For many disabled and ill older adults, hands-on caregiving or care management—although needed and deeply appreciated—is not what they value most from their children. Most important are understanding, empathy, socialization, entertainment, and inclusion as an integral part of family life.

Bob Morris on His Father's Suicide Attempt and on Bringing Happiness into His Life

My father had a fantastic year after my mom died. He jumped right into dating, and was running around and really was happy. He was like a Palm Beach snowbird on speed. He just was running around from bridge games to dinners to movies and dating.

My brother and I just stood back, thrilled to watch him go: "Go, Dad, go." You know, he didn't need a lot of phone calls for consolation in the months after mom's death, and there was very little talk of her passing. We even gave him a big 80th birthday party 6 months after she died. Secretly, I think, my father and I were relieved not to have the sadness of her suffering in our lives anymore.

But then, once he had his great year after mom died, finding new love and everything, he was aware that he had a shortness of breath having to do with his heart—hypercardiomyopathy, a weak heart, with thickened musculature causing an arrhythmia, an irregular beat. And there was a breathlessness that started to disturb him enough that he went to see his heart specialist in the city. When he got word from this specialist that there was nothing to be done and that he would find himself losing energy as his heart continued to fail, my father lost heart—no pun intended. He lost all hope of having a pacemaker or some other kind of restorative procedure to reverse his situation. A chief expert on his heart condition had told him, "I'm sorry—really, there's nothing we can do." And that's a terrible thing to say to somebody.

So Dad, who had so vigorously dated, played bridge, and was always on the run for some kind of fun all of a sudden went into a state of despair. He canceled a trip to Vermont for the summer with his lady friend, who went on without him. He didn't feel he could keep up with her and didn't want to cramp her style. She was younger and far more vigorous.

And then he took six Ambien, which was not enough to kill him, but it did knock him out for a day. He left a very long suicide note with instructions as to where certain money accounts were and where to place his obituary, including the *Fort Lauderdale Sun-Sentinel* and the *Palm Beach Post,* but *in season*—which would have meant January, not July. He had everything carefully laid out in this suicide letter, but very few words were spent describing his emotions. He simply wrote, "I hope you will forgive me for leaving you at this time." He actually thought six Ambien would let him off the hook with life. But of course, he ended up in the emergency room instead. I don't even think they had to pump his stomach.

Later, he told us he had chosen that moment for his suicide attempt—at the end of a July weekend—because he felt it would be the most convenient for all of us. "I knew you'd all be getting home from your weekends out of the city," he told us. Or something like that.

The next day he was in the hospital, getting an intake interview by the staff psychiatrist, and I was watching him answering questions as if he were on a talk show. But then reality set in. And in the days that followed, he was, of course, terribly depressed. Can you imagine having tried to kill yourself, and failed, and not even being glad that you've been saved and are still alive? I was in conflict. I wanted so much to let him know that I might want to do the same thing if I were in his shoes—just cut all the years of misery short and have a nice exit after a nice life without the prolonged decline he was facing. But I also knew that wasn't fair to the people who love me. You have to want to live, right? You have to tell someone life is worth living, don't you?

On the other hand, maybe there's something to be said for honesty, for not masking the bad feelings with the Zoloft he started taking. Maybe it's more helpful to allow or even encourage an aging parent to have all the terrible feelings he wants to have. Do you try to motivate him to cheer up when he has no reason to cheer up? Instead of trying to cheer him up and look for solutions, maybe all we had to do was hold his hand and say, "Look, Dad, I know you're really scared. I know you're really frustrated and depressed. You have every reason to feel that way, and I'm not here to tell you to cheer up. Let's talk about this if you want to. Or let's not."

My father was not a friend of psychotherapy in any way and wasn't emotionally conversant or articulate with his feelings. But, once he realized that he wasn't going to be getting better anymore— and that he saw a debilitating year or two ahead and realized that he'd just lose all his energy, according to his doctor—he wanted out. So he tried and failed. I appreciated that. "The only thing I don't like," I told him only half-jokingly, "is that your death would have cast a pall over my stage show about you that's coming up in the fall. And what about your granddaughter's Bat Mitzvah? Wait until after that; give it a few months more, and we can talk about your wish to leave us. Is that fair?" I didn't want him to think I didn't understand his wish to die.

In the year after his failed suicide attempt, in addition to lifting his spirits by visiting him at his assisted living place in Great Neck, playing ukulele and piano for him, taking him for drives, and doing whatever I could—I really let him vent about the uselessness of living. I egged him on. And it seemed like it was good for him. Instead of saying "Oh, come on, Dad, things aren't that bad," I'd tell him he was right, he should have died, and it couldn't be worse. I got the feeling that he wanted us to know that he was right in trying to kill himself. He loved being right. And so I think that that was what motivated me to say, "It is a mess. You're right—it would have been better if you had gone. But since you're still here, let's just sing this Cole Porter song, okay?"

I was on the side of happiness, not the bigger picture of happiness, but happiness in the moment. The ice cream floats I could make for him. The gossip items I could read him from the tabloids. The stories of my life that made him proud of me. The stories of his life that he was always more than happy to tell me. Singing. Joking. I felt that I could be most effective by facilitating happiness.

5

Marriage, Widowhood, Remarriage, and Sex

Like my father, I've learned that the love we have in our youth is superficial compared to the love that an old man has for his old wife. "My old gray-haired wife," my father used to call my mother. And I can still remember her saying as she passed the food around the table on their 50th anniversary, "I thank God for giving me this old man to take care of."

—Interview with philosopher Will Durant,
New York Times, November 6, 1975

WILL DURANT WAS CELEBRATING HIS 90TH BIRTHDAY on the day of this interview. He himself had been married to his wife, Ariel, for more than 62 years. The public responds with delight to such stories of marital longevity and contentment. Pictures in magazines and newspapers of a white-haired couple cutting the cake on their golden anniversary are sure to arouse pleasant emotions. No words are necessary—those pictures evoke images of love, tenderness, fidelity, companionship, and mutual support. In some cases, these images are true. In others, they are not. For better or for worse, old

For better or for worse, old age affects not only each husband and wife individually but also their life together—their partnership.

age affects not only each husband and wife individually but also their life together—their partnership.

The institution of marriage and other intimate partnerships has been examined, probed, and analyzed by scholars, professionals, and the clergy. Much attention has been focused on marital problems in the early and middle years, but little of that scrutiny has been turned on marriage in the later years. Part of this neglect in the past may have been because of the lower life expectancy. Few marriages continued intact with both partners alive in their 70s and 80s.

But there are many of these durable marriages today. There will be even more in the future. In 2006, 52% of men and 48% of women were married. This marriage gap between men and women does widen with age. For those over the age of 65, 72% of men and only 40% of women were married. The numbers of homosexual partners are increasing among older adults as well.

Marital Adjustment in the Retirement Years

After 30 or 40 years of life together, it would seem that two people would have come to know each other as intimately as possible and, assuming that the marriage has been a relatively stable one, there would be few surprises left. But there may be plenty of surprises in the post-retirement period, the greatest one probably being that the partners might not know each other quite so well after all.

In the middle years—particularly if there are children in the family, but even when there are not—husbands and wives usually function independently of each other much of the time, even in the closest of relationships. When they both work, each one goes off every day to a separate place. Even if they share all household tasks equally, they are physically in each other's presence only in the evenings, on weekends, and on holidays. When the husband is the sole breadwinner and his wife cares for the home and children, there are also many hours of separation. The two may thoroughly enjoy the time they do spend together, yearn for more, steal occasional weekends away, and resent the stresses of life that prevent them from being together more often. But the fact remains that their hours together are limited.

In the post-retirement years, their hours together are limitless. Unless they have prepared themselves in advance with activities and routines to share or interests that will take them in different directions for some time at least, they may face each other 24 hours a day, 7 days a week, including Saturdays, Sundays, and holidays. Like children on rainy afternoons, they may say, "There's no place to go. There's nothing to do."

When both husband and wife have had careers, each one at some point past 60 may have to develop a new, different (sometimes even more rewarding) lifestyle for the retirement years. But the housewife and mother whose children are launched by the time she is in her early 50s or younger usually faces her midlife crisis—sometimes known as "empty-nest syndrome"—much earlier. She may face menopause at the same time. Her husband, still in his mid-50s and probably still in mid-career, may remind her, with understanding and compassion (or possibly with irritation and exasperation), that she has always wanted to "eat dinner at a civilized time," or go back to school, sell real estate, volunteer at the hospital, spend time at a club, or go into politics. He may even wonder how she can be depressed when she finally has the time to do all the things she always complained she had no time for. She may go ahead and do any one of these things, or instead devote herself to domestic routines, gardening, or close involvement with children or grandchildren. During the next 10 or 15 years, while her husband is still actively involved in his own work, she may establish a very satisfactory way of life for herself. But suddenly one day, after the gold watch has been presented and the farewell dinner for her husband is over, she may find that she suddenly has a constant companion sharing or possibly interfering with that new way of life.

She may watch her husband go through some of the same confusion and uncertainty she herself faced years before, and she may say to him, as he said to her long ago (also with understanding or exasperation), "You always wanted to go fishing," or do more carpentry; take up golf, painting, or sculpture; learn a foreign language; or work in a settlement house. Many men—sometimes joined by their wives—do develop new interests by enrolling in adult education classes or university course. But often the same activities that, in their working days, seemed to promise relaxation and satisfaction now lose their appeal for the retirees and appear more as idle puttering and meaningless time-filling.

The breadwinner often feels that by losing his job he also loses his valued role and therefore his prestige, purpose, and self-respect. He may feel aimless, rejected, cast aside, excluded, and forgotten, and often reacts with depression, anger, or resentment. If he directs those emotions toward the person who is closest to him—his wife—a great strain will be placed on their marriage. You may notice that your parents disagree and bicker as never before. Some newly retired men age dramatically in the first years of inactivity or go through a period of depression—fertile ground, according to some experts, for premature disease and deterioration.

> *After all those years of knowing how to spend weekends and holidays together, a retired couple may seem virtual strangers to each other on weekdays.*

After all those years of knowing how to spend weekends and holidays together, a retired couple may seem virtual strangers to each other on weekdays. "Is that what you eat for lunch?" a husband asks his wife as she spoons out cottage cheese. Married for nearly 40 years, he may not have the slightest idea of what goes on in his house for 8 hours every weekday. "I never knew your father was such a busybody," your mother may sigh to you. "He's into everything I do. He's forever asking me what I'm doing and why I'm doing it, and then telling me how to do it better. I don't have a minute's privacy. Who does he think has been taking care of this house all these years, I'd like to know?" She may complain on a regular basis that he intrudes on her kaffeeklatsches with her friends, insists on buying the groceries, and monitors all her conversations. "The next time he says to me, 'What in God's name do you and Flora have to yak about every day?' I'm going to throw the phone at him."

You may find yourself drawn into their disagreements and be tempted to take sides, either with the parent you are most closely attached to or with the one who seems to be most ill-used. If your father is withdrawn and apathetic, you may criticize him for giving your mother so little pleasure: "He's burying her alive! He doesn't want to do anything himself, and he won't let her do anything either." Or you may take his side against her: "Why can't she let him alone? He's worked hard all his life. Doesn't he deserve a little peace now?"

Instead of taking sides with either, you may be critical of both of them and quick to tell them all the mistakes they are making and what they ought to do instead. You may even come up with a variety of wonderful ideas that appeal to you tremendously, but might not give them the slightest satisfaction. If, instead of pushing your own solutions, you are able to show some concern, patience, interest, and understanding, they will probably, in time, work out their *own* solutions—in their *own* way.

Some couples, confused and disturbed by their unaccustomed incompatibility, turn not to their children but to friends, ministers, doctors, and other professionals. "Imagine me—at 67—going to a marriage counselor!" a retired salesman said sheepishly, at the same time admitting that he and his wife really needed someone to help them smooth out the fraying edges of their 44-year marriage. Not infrequently, couples, finding life in the later stages as difficult as in the earlier stages, are turning to professional help. Marriage counselors report what many couples find out for themselves in time: if a marriage has strong bonds and a firm foundation, it is likely to weather the post-retirement crisis and come out intact. Any marriage that has lasted more than 40 years has undoubtedly weathered its share of crises in the past, but at the same time, one cannot overlook the fact that the rate of divorce among older couples, including those who have been married for many years, is increasing.

Fortunately, many men and women prepare themselves by thinking through alternative patterns for the future and developing compromises that will satisfy both partners in a marriage. Increasing numbers are postponing retirement into their 70s and even 80s, and embarking on second careers and volunteer activities. (Not to be minimized is an older couple's need for additional income.) Such advance preparation is usually the best insurance against the apathy, depression, anger, and interpersonal conflict that lie in wait for many couples.

In Sickness and in Health—for Richer, for Poorer

In addition to adjusting to the changes in daily life produced by retirement itself, many older couples may also have to adjust at some point to each other's failing health and the dwindling of their joint financial assets. The famous words spoken at wedding ceremonies are really put to the test when husbands and wives live on together into their 70s, 80s, and 90s. Poverty and ill health may come separately or in combination, since the more frequent or chronic the physical disability, the more money must be spent on medical expenses.

Reasonable, well-thought-out plans for retirement can be disrupted overnight by the sudden illness of one partner or by the gradual decline of one or both.

Reasonable, well-thought-out plans for retirement can be disrupted overnight by the sudden illness of one partner or by the gradual decline of one or both. Your mother and father may have developed an enjoyable pattern of living, pursuing some activities independently and sharing others, but what if your father has a stroke, a heart attack, or crippling arthritis? He may need constant care. The new life the two have made together may come to an end, yet another pattern has to be developed. Your mother may be ready and able to care for your father, but at the same time, whether she admits it or not, she may resent being so tied down. The strain may affect their relationship with each other.

Illness can also reverse long-standing behavior patterns. A wife who has always been dependent and submissive may find herself forced to take control when her invalid husband can no longer run the show. If a domineering wife is incapacitated, she may, for the first time in her married life, have to turn to her more passive husband, expecting him to manage everything *and* take care of her. Frequently, those formerly submissive spouses rather enjoy their new-found power and flourish, despite the burdens they have to assume. They may even turn the tables completely, becoming dictatorial and autocratic, to the amazement of their children, friends, and relatives.

Dwindling financial resources, inadequate pensions, Social Security checks that cannot keep up with the nation's rising inflation rate, and heavy medical expenses: all can strain marital relationships, particularly in marriages where money—or the lack of it—has always been a source of conflict. An elderly couple may have to give up their home because of increased rents, higher taxes, or rising maintenance costs, and cramped quarters may contribute to irritation. If they are able to stay where they have always lived, there may be no money at all for entertainment, relief from monotony, or occasional escapes from each other. Medical expenses may erode their food budget, and their health, emotional as well as physical, may deteriorate from inadequate nutrition.

Couples who were always in great conflict when life was easier may be drawn closer together by the harsh problems of ill health or poverty. Their days are devoted to fighting off the enemy at their gates, concentrating their energies, husbanding their resources, and caring for each other with greater determination than ever.

As they get older and physically less active, some couples become even more closely involved with each other, zealously watching over each other's health, protecting each other from excitement, and sparing each other exertion. At the pace they establish for themselves they may read, walk, market, do housework, watch TV, listen to music, garden, and take their medicine—always together. Relatives and friends may report with admiration, sometimes mixed with irritation, "They don't really need anyone else. They're only interested in each other," or "They think alike, they talk alike, they even look alike."

If the wife in such couples ages more rapidly or is more seriously incapacitated than her husband, he may try to assume full responsibility for her care. The wife may respond in the same way to her invalid husband. These relationships can become so totally interdependent that in time they can tolerate no separation at all. Not infrequently, the death of one spouse is followed within a short time by the death of the other, who may have seemed in comparatively good health. One doctor reports that he was obliged to place a 94-year-old man in intensive care after a severe stroke, even though his 89-year-old wife begged to be allowed to take care of him at home. Two days after her husband was hospitalized, she died of a heart attack.

The family may be understandably concerned when a very old relative insists on nursing her bedridden husband. Everyone may try to persuade her to institutionalize him or hire a nurse, saying, "You've got a right to live, too." But that may be the only way she wants to live. One 77-year-old wife, persuaded against her will by her children to place her paralyzed husband in an excellent nursing home, agonized constantly that he was not getting the right care: "They don't shave him the way he likes," or "They always forget the pillow he needs under his legs," or "He'll starve with that slop they feed him." She could not enjoy a minute of her new freedom. "But, Ma," her children kept saying, "he's better off in the home. You would have killed yourself if you'd gone on any longer." She had only one answer: "I should have died trying."

Discord in the "Golden Years"

Your parents may not have such an exclusive relationship. Instead of turning to each other, they may turn to you, trying to involve you and their other children in their conflicts. Hearing them fighting or complaining about each other may make you very uncomfortable. You may remember that they fought all the time you were growing up, but somehow you may have expected all this to stop as they grew old together. The answer to the question "How can they still be fighting, at their age?" is "Why should they stop now?"

> For forty-seven years they had been married. How deep back the stubborn gnarled roots of the quarrel reach, no one could say—but only now, when tending to the needs of others no longer shackled them together, the roots swelled up visible, split the earth between them, and the tearing shook even to the children, long since grown.
> —Tillie Olsen, *Tell Me a Riddle*

There is no reason to expect tempers and personality clashes to fade away with the years. Occasional conflict is to be expected in any close relationship. It can provide a catharsis, a release. Conflict may even arise for the first time in the later years, as couples struggle to cope with the stresses and difficulties caused by their aging. When there is a strong bond between husband and wife at any age, periodic quarrels can serve to cement rather than destroy a relationship. But some couples—perhaps your parents—make quarreling a way of life.

There is no reason to expect tempers and personality clashes to fade away with the years.

Young children are often terribly upset when their parents fight, particularly if they carry on directly in front of the children. Even if the parents try to keep their conflicts private, a child can be just as upset knowing that something terrible is going on in the house. Years later, the child may be upset all over again when the parents attack each other and may need to withdraw for his or her own protection. "I'm nearly 50, but I still get that old sick feeling in the pit of my stomach when I hear Mom and Dad fighting," a daughter admitted to her mother's doctor, trying to explain why she visited her parents so rarely.

A successful writer claims that he invariably falls asleep at the theater when the scene onstage involves a marital battle. As a child, he had always used sleep to escape hearing the thing he hated most: his parents fighting. They are in their 80s now and still at war. Their son visits them, although infrequently, and after he visits, he usually goes home and sleeps.

Some partners in stressful marriages that have held together during the middle years "for the sake of the children" feel free to break up when the family is launched. Couples separate, divorce, and start afresh with new partners at 50, 60, or even beyond 70. This pattern is expected to continue. Some couples feel that it's never too late to separate. In Marian Thurm's short story "Sounds," an elderly mother says to her daughter, "It's over, thank God," as her husband in his early 70s drives off to meet his young bride-to-be. "It went on forever, didn't it, like a bad movie you can barely manage to sit through, but it's finally over."

Margaret Mead, the famed anthropologist, would not have been surprised at the rising divorce rate among older couples. She claimed that we have an antiquated idea about marriage lasting forever. When life expectancy was 45 and couples vowed, "Till death do us part," death parted them pretty quickly. In Mead's opinion, that's why marriage lasted forever: everyone was dead. Since couples now stay alive much longer, there is more time for them to outgrow each other or to develop "irreconcilable differences," or to find new and more stimulating relationships.

By contrast, other seemingly shaky pairs, while using their children as the rationale for staying together, remain intact permanently because of their dependence on each other. Despite constant threats through the years to separate, they never follow through, to the surprise of their children, who report, "We grew up expecting our parents to get divorced—we almost still expect it now—but they're still together and still at each other's throats."

The Vaughans' marriage had always been a battleground. No one had heard Philip Vaughan refer to his wife by name for years—only as "that woman." Even when they grew older, their conflicts continued, and they frequently spent long periods refusing to speak to each other. In their later years, they often communicated with each other by making long-distance calls to their daughter, Edna, who had moved far away from her parents. "Tell your father to see a doctor about that cough of his," Mrs. Vaughan would say to her daughter, who could hear her father coughing in the background. Edna, in New Hampshire, would then speak to her father when he got on the phone in Iowa and urge him to see a doctor. In reply, her father would shout, "Tell 'that woman' to stop worrying about my health all the time."

At least the Vaughans, despite their bickering, managed to keep a close watch over each other's physical well-being, but other couples may remain so wrapped up in their conflict that they no longer communicate about anything else. Each one may keep quiet about a disturbing physical symptom, refusing to admit to the other that something hurts somewhere. Thus, they may keep their fears to themselves until it is too late.

Children, friends, and relatives even go so far as to recommend divorce or separation to an elderly couple who battle on a daily basis. An outsider may not realize that, along with all the anger, there are also strong bonds holding the two old people together, and that beneath the conflict, they may be deeply attached to each other.

Seventy-nine-year-old Mavis Wood had been threatening to leave her husband, who was a year older, for most of the six decades of their marriage. In her mid-70s, she was confined to a wheelchair and was dependent on his help, so her threats were somewhat idle. When a double room became available in a nearby nursing home, their children, tired of being drawn into their conflicts, urged their parents to move in. Harry Wood was reluctant for one reason only: "She'll leave me when she has someone else to take care of her." But he was persuaded, and the two moved in, carrying their conflicts with them. Now they involved the nursing home staff as well as their children.

After some time, the staff, tired of the situation and convinced that the two would be better off separated, offered to move Mrs. Wood to another room. When the move was made, she was delighted: "You never believed I'd ever leave him, did you? Well, I did!" she gloated to everyone. Her children and the staff were relieved during the peaceful period that followed, but their relief was short-lived. Within 4 days, Mrs. Wood was back in her old room with her husband once again, ready and eager to resume their old, combative relationship.

Widowhood

A marriage may remain intact, in harmony or in conflict, for 40, 50, or 60 years, but sooner or later, it will inevitably be broken by death. Unless they die together in a plane crash or another disaster, one partner will have to face life without the other for some period.

Of all the losses that must be faced in old age, the loss of a partner is often the most cruel and disruptive of all. In most cases, the wife will survive her husband. According to current statistics, women can expect to live 7 years longer than men. Since women tend to marry men older rather than younger than themselves, the likelihood that they will survive their husbands is even greater In 2003, 43% of women over the age of 65 were widows, but only 14% of men over the age of 65 were widowers.

Of all the losses that must be faced in old age, the loss of a partner is often the most cruel and disruptive of all.

In addition to the grief and upheaval caused by the loss of their husbands, many elderly widows living alone (along with other elderly single women) face financial privation. In 2005, nearly 20% of older adults over the age of 85 (the majority of them women) had incomes below poverty level.

Because most wives are aware of the strong possibility that they will outlive their husbands, some go through a kind of "preparatory widowhood" in the later years, talking to their children about what lies ahead, thinking through specific plans, working out budgets, or concentrating their efforts on protecting their husbands' health and well-being. Even if they prefer not to think about the future, they cannot avoid the fleeting thought "Am I next?" as more and more of their friends become widows. Husbands, by contrast, are generally not prepared for the possibility that, despite the statistics, they may be the ones who survive, and many give little or no thought to the idea that one day they, too, could be alone. Widowers may be even more shocked and helpless than widows in the initial stages.

But prepared or not—even if death follows a long period of illness, even if it is expected, almost hoped for—the loss of a partner is almost always a devastating occurrence followed by some period of grief and disruption. Mourning usually involves a number of emotional reactions—numbness, apathy, longing, sorrow, remorse, and guilt—as well as physical symptoms of weight loss, insomnia, irritability, and fatigue. But there is great variation, depending on the individual, in the intensity and duration of the emotional and physical reactions. It may be hard for you to predict in advance just how your own mother or father will react.

When a surviving husband has always been particularly dependent on his wife (or vice versa), it is understandable that he will feel utterly lost without her. But dependency in marriage is often a very subtle process. You may have always thought that your father was a very independent, self-sufficient, dominant type, who ran everyone's life. Why should he seem so shattered by your mother's death? It is worth remembering that the most independent of husbands may, underneath, be very emotionally tied to their wives and dependent on them, although heaven forbid they should ever admit it! You may not believe that your father could ever feel dependent on anyone—he may not even believe it about himself. The realization may only dawn on him the day he is widowed, and his reaction may shock everyone.

On the other hand, you may have always underestimated the strength of your surviving parent. Although your mother may have seemed docile and passive, inner reserves you never saw before may surface when your father dies. You may have a sneaking suspicion after a while that she actually seems somewhat relieved, which may seem quite surprising and inappropriate under the circumstances. But once the funeral is over and the mourning period is past, some widows and widowers experience an unexpected sense of freedom rising above their feelings of loss. If a husband has been domineering, a kind of parental figure, his wife may be quite relieved to be free of his control. She may need some time before she can reactivate her rusty old self-sufficiency, but she may surprise everyone, including herself, with her ability to think and act as an independent person.

A similar sense of freedom may be felt by widows and widowers who have spent long years caring for physically or emotionally dependent spouses. A husband who felt duty-bound to care for his invalid wife, who never could bring himself to gain his freedom by institutionalizing her, will be freed by her death—and not through any deliberate act of his own. He may then find he still has time to make use of his new freedom, although for many it comes too late.

If relief seems to be an unexpected emotion, you may be just as surprised if one of your parents reacts to the loss of the other with calm tranquility. Some widows and widowers, after a short time, reflect this quality in the midst of sadness. They seem able to pick up their lives and carry on, even start afresh.

Disruption Is to Be Expected

Widowhood for elderly men and women almost invariably involves disruption, which may last longer than the grief itself. An elderly widow is no longer anyone's wife, anyone's companion, or anyone's sex partner (for the time at least). She has no one to care for or to run a house for, except herself. With no one to cook for, she may not bother to cook at all and may become further weakened by malnutrition. She may have to change her lifestyle completely because of reduced income. If her husband has always been the handyman, finance officer, and business executive in the marriage, she will have to grapple with these unfamiliar roles. Widowers face similar disruptions in habitual patterns of daily life.

If the couple's social life has always been carried on together, that, too, will be disrupted temporarily—or permanently. Widows and widowers often report that they don't "fit in" anymore, that they are no longer as comfortable or as welcome in their old social niches, although widowers are more likely than widows to be sought out and included by friends. A widow often senses (rightly or wrongly) that her old friends are uncomfortable with her grief, that they feel depressed around her, or that she has become a fifth wheel in couple-oriented activities. Widows are more likely than widowers to discover that if they do not drive or can no longer afford accustomed forms of

> *Widowhood for elderly men and women almost invariably involves disruption, which may last longer than the grief itself.*

entertainment, their social life begins to fade away. Older widows have one compensation denied to younger ones: since it is unusual to be widowed early, young widows often feel out of step with their married contemporaries, while older widows, because of their numbers, can often find kindred spirits among their contemporaries. A steady diet of female companionship may not be completely satisfying for most, but for some widows, it beats loneliness.

Loneliness itself is not a simple feeling and can mean different things to different people. When your widowed mother tells you that she is lonely, you may not understand exactly *how* she is lonely. Helen Lopata, in *Widowhood in an American City*, reported that the widows she interviewed defined their loneliness in a variety of ways: some were lonely because they missed everything about their dead husbands; others were lonely for companionship, for someone to organize their days around, for escorts, for someone to love or to be loved by, for someone to share activities with. Widows and widowers have to learn how to live with their own individual variety of loneliness.

In recent years, subjects that formerly were not discussed openly have been dissected minutely in the press and on TV and radio talk shows—even in television dramas, movies, and theater. Old taboos have disappeared. Buzzwords abound and are used—and misused—broadly and authoritatively. There is a danger of nonprofessionals becoming parlor psychiatrists after exposure to a barrage of pop psychology. The public has been bombarded with a similar battery of material on aging and widowhood. Friends and relatives may flaunt their newfound expertise, even when they are not asked for advice.

> "Just yesterday, I heard Dr. Simonov say on TV that mourning should only last a year. Phil's been dead 2 years. You better start making a new life for yourself"—words of a so-called friend to a widow.

If your parents do not conform to patterns of mourning that you have heard experts put forth, this does not mean that there is necessarily anything wrong with them. Experts discuss overall patterns—there's always room for individual differences. Your mother may hear a different drummer and follow a different star.

If your parents do not conform to patterns of mourning that you have heard experts put forth, this does not mean that there is necessarily anything wrong with them.

Statistics may indeed show that widows and widowers make bearable adjustments within the first year or so. But your father may need to follow his own timetable.

Unless she is totally dependent on others because of ill health or prolonged depression, your widowed mother (or father) is likely to adjust eventually to the disruption in her life and develop a new pattern that may go on for many years. Things will never be the same for her again. Life will certainly be different; it will probably be bearable; and it may—in some cases—even be better.

When Mourning Goes Out-of-Bounds

While shock, pain, and depression are not only normal emotions during the mourning period, but actually necessary ones that make it possible for survivors to work through their grief and eventually resume life again, some widows and widowers never recover.

Prolonged mourning was more obvious in the past, when the process was more ritualized. Some widows refused to give up their "widow's weeds" and lived on, shrouded in black, never letting themselves or the world forget their loss. Although less visible, prolonged mourning is not unknown today.

While experts agree that the survivor of a marriage is more susceptible to physical and mental illness in the early days of widowhood—a higher rate of suicide is reported in this period—they also report that the intensity of these emotions and of physical symptoms normally eases with time. Those who remain in a state of perpetual grief may have conflicting feelings about their dead partners or may have been known to have depressive episodes in the past. What seems to their families to be a state of perpetual mourning may actually be a state of severe depression set off, but not caused by, the bereavement itself. Simple remedies that help to ease normal grief will not work. Some form of professional help may be needed.

Queen Victoria gave the world a classic example of prolonged mourning. Victoria, as Queen of England, was one of the most powerful figures of her time. No one could possibly say she did not have enough to keep her busy. Yet in 1861, after the death of her husband, Prince Albert, she retired, at the age of 42, into seclusion at Windsor Castle. For 3 years, she never appeared in public, and she did not open Parliament again—an annual duty for British monarchs—until 1866. Even though she lived another 40 years after her husband's death, she never let her country forget her loss. The poet Rudyard Kipling suffered permanent royal disfavor when he dared refer to his queen as "the widow at Windsor."

The Death of a Parent: the Effect on You

The previous discussion has focused on your parent's reactions to losing his or her partner, but your own personal ones cannot be ignored. When your father dies, you may feel some responsibility to help his widow (your mother or your stepmother) recover from her loss. But you may have a hard time behaving in a cool, level-headed way yourself, because her loss is yours as well. She has lost a husband, it's true, but you've lost a father. If your father is widowed, he mourns for a wife, while you mourn for a mother. When sympathy goes in two directions, when the older generation is able to acknowledge that the younger one is suffering too, it is easier for everyone. But that does not always happen. A mother may complain to everyone, "Carol carries on so! You'd think she'd lost a husband. Can't she think what it's like for me?" But Carol may tell a different story: "Mother acts as if she's the only one who misses Dad. Doesn't she remember that I loved him, too?"

Even if both generations recognize each other's grief, they may mourn in different ways. Your mother may turn to religion after your father's death, taking her comfort in ritual and prayer, visiting the cemetery, lighting candles, wearing black. None of these rituals may be at all helpful to you—they may even seem distasteful. Many families are in disagreement about the entire mourning process, starting with the funeral itself. Some members may want a lavish ceremony and a constant stream of condolences, and find comfort when the world seems to share and witness their grief. Others can mourn only in privacy. If you find no comfort in the rituals that comfort your mother, there is no reason why you should be forced to do everything her way—but no reason, either, to prevent her from taking comfort where she finds it.

You may be so shattered by your own grief after your mother's death that you find it painful at first to talk about her at all, even to mention her name. Your father may need to talk about her all the time. For your own sanity, you may need to withdraw a little and let others do the listening.

A particularly painful situation occurs when a son or daughter has had
a stronger bond with the parent who
has died and greater conflict with the
surviving one. If you had an especially
close feeling for your father, his death
may be devastating to you, and you
may find it almost impossible to com-
fort your mother. You may even resent her for still being alive while
he is dead, and also for never—in your opinion—treating him well
enough or appreciating him enough during his lifetime.

A particularly painful situation occurs when a son or daughter has had a stronger bond with the parent who has died and greater conflict with the surviving one.

Although it has always been customary to speak well of the dead,
children are frequently amazed at the way the surviving parent
manages to remember the dead one. Widows and widowers often
seem to find comfort in idealizing relationships that were actually far
from satisfying and are quite skillful at rewriting their own marital
histories. Relatives may listen in disbelief as a widow describes her
dead husband as "the gentlest soul on earth," when everyone knows
he was tyrannical and demanding. A widowed father may remember
his wife as "selfless and saintlike" after her death, when in reality she
had been self-centered and hot tempered.

What You Can Do to Help

Your involvement when one of your parents is widowed depends on
your mutual relationship, your desire to help, how many other
people are available, and where you live. Obviously, if you live far
away, you will not be able to do much more than return for the
funeral (or possibly during a final illness) and help out with the
arrangements and initial problems. You may be able to continue to
help from a distance by keeping in touch by phone and visiting more
frequently, especially in the early period.

It is important to keep in mind that mourners go through many
different stages on their way to recovery, and some of those stages
may be difficult to deal with. Your mother may be full of self-pity at
one time and consumed by anger at another. She may withdraw from
you and your siblings this week, and accuse you of neglecting her
next week. Those stages may be surprising and burdensome, but they
are likely to pass.

The mourning process does not necessarily proceed in a straight line—improving steadily from the deepest distress to reasonable normalcy. The mourner may well take one step back for every two steps forward. Innocent, seemingly insignificant reminders may precipitate setbacks—a song, a picture, a bit of "your father's favorite cake," the smell of "your mother's favorite flower." Anniversaries—and not only the obvious annual ones—may trigger temporary relapses. One daughter was puzzled because her father always seemed lower in spirits at the end of the week than at the beginning. Eventually it dawned on her that her father dreaded Thursdays because he became a widower on a Thursday.

Mourning usually takes time, and since older people are likely to move more slowly in all situations, they cannot be rushed through their grief or accept changes before they are ready. "We can't let Mother stay here alone. Everything here reminds her of Dad. We'll have to sell the house" may seem like a logical conclusion, but Mother may be worse off and her recovery permanently jeopardized if her home is sold out from under her and she is bundled off to a strange environment. Familiar surroundings and familiar faces are very comforting, although temporary changes of scene can be helpful.

When elderly widows or widowers are initially helpless and bewildered because of their grief, children may be tempted to rush in with impetuous invitations. "Come live with us—you can't live alone here," may seem like a kind solution at the moment, but unless it has been considered carefully from all angles in advance, it may turn out to be far from kind for anyone. Your mother, persuaded to become dependent on you before she has given herself a chance to test her self-reliance, may forfeit her independence forever, while you and your family may come to resent the unnecessary and uncomfortable adjustments you have to make in your own lives.

Older persons themselves, in an attempt to escape their grief, may be the ones who rush into impetuous decisions. They may ask or demand to live with you. A widow may decide to sell her house and move into a one-room apartment or a hotel. Once the move is made, she may regret it. A widower, thinking he cannot face a winter alone in a cold climate, may pick himself up with little notice and move to a warm place where he knows no one. You may be able to forestall radical moves that could boomerang in the future by agreeing with the idea in principle, but suggesting alternative approaches. "I can see why you don't want to stay here alone, Dad, but why sell the house? Why not rent it this winter and see how you like living in Arizona? If you don't like it there, you'll always have a place to come back to."

Even if a widowed mother does not seem to need anything from her children, it is usually helpful for her to know they can be depended on. Dependability and availability are important; so are sympathetic listening and genuine concern. It is equally important to help widowed parents build up their self-confidence and to encourage them to take their first independent steps. Your first instinctive reaction to your widowed mother may be to protect her in every way. "Don't worry about a thing, Ma, we'll take care of everything" may be a well-intentioned offer, but may only make her more dependent than ever. A more effective approach would be to reassure her that she is perfectly capable of taking care of herself, but that you're ready to back her up when she needs you.

Even if a widowed mother does not seem to need anything from her children, it is usually helpful for her to know they can be depended on.

On occasion, widowed parents who no longer have partners to share their lives focus all their attention—and their demands—on one particular child. A daughter may be expected by her father to take the place of her dead mother, or a son to replace his dead father. (Children themselves sometimes try to assume these roles, and are hurt and angry when their attempts are rejected and their parents prefer to be self-reliant.) The only way to prevent those expectations from taking hold is to set firm boundaries from the beginning: "No, Mother, I can't spend Saturdays working in the garden with you like Dad used to do. You know I coach Jim's Little League team on Saturdays. But we'll be over to see you after church on Sunday as usual." Or: "No, Father, I can't get over to see you every day. You know how much I have to do at home. But don't forget you're spending the weekend with us." The situation is more difficult to handle when the requests are less specific. It is harder to set boundaries when your mother wants you to be responsive to her emotional needs, just as your father always was. It is equally hard to reply to broad, nonspecifc complaints, such as, "I feel blue," "My life's so empty," "Why am I living?" Trying to counteract these statements with encouraging, upbeat sermons is likely to be a waste of breath.

Here again, a concrete, specific reply given with an understanding tone may be more helpful: "I know you're lonely and it's hard for you, but Aunt Flo's coming back next week and we've all got tickets for the ice show. How about going out to dinner first?"

Remarriage

Older men and women, widowed or divorced, may remarry, even in their 80s. It will be impossible for anyone to predict after your father dies just *what* your mother will do. You can't be sure and neither can she. A categorical *never* can be said only in cases where individual survivors are seriously incapacitated. Widows and widowers often swear during the mourning period that they will never marry again. Their children usually believe them, often finding the mere idea inconceivable. You may share this view. Yet your widowed mother may surprise herself—and you, too.

The chances of remarriage are obviously greater for older widowers than for widows, because single women over 75 outnumber men of the same age 3 to 1. The field, therefore, is wide open for the widower, and his selection is not limited to women in his own age group. His new wife could be 10, 20, 30, or 40 years younger than he is. Women, because of social mores, are less likely to marry men who are much younger. Winston Churchill's mother, Jennie, was a famous exception. After she was widowed, she had two more husbands, both younger than her own sons. Such exceptions seem to be on the increase today.

Some older widows and widowers are unable to contemplate marrying again because they feel it is somehow improper, undignified, or frowned on by society. Their children frequently agree and voice even greater opposition, adding a new concern of their own: money. When a father remarries, who will inherit from him? His children or his widow? If he marries a younger woman, he may have children with her. Who will be his heirs? His first set of children or his second? Or will the inheritance be less for everyone because it has to be shared? Prenuptial agreements are sometimes made by an elderly pair to reassure the children on both sides that their "rightful" inheritances will not be lost.

You may approve in principle of the idea of remarriage for older people, but find it appalling when your own father remarries. Your reasons for thinking it is ill-advised, in his particular situation, may seem to be valid. His new wife may

You may approve in principle of the idea of remarriage for older people, but find it appalling when your own father remarries.

be after his money; she may be from a different background or have different interests or less education. Her health may be poor, and you may be concerned that he will have to take care of her or possibly that you will have to take care of both of them. But actually, if you are completely honest with yourself, you may admit that these are not your real reasons for opposing his marriage. You may be against it because you feel it is disloyal to your mother. It may be too painful for you to think of another woman taking your mother's place in your father's life, using her things, sleeping in her bed. You may be jealous that your father prefers another woman and is not content to depend on you. Finally, you also may feel that remarriage at his age makes him look ridiculous—and therefore makes you look ridiculous, too.

But unless elderly men or women are seriously disturbed and not responsible for their actions, their children might be better advised to consider the consequences of opposing a remarriage. A son who seriously opposes his mother's marriage is telling her that she is better off living with her loneliness than with someone *he* considers inappropriate. Is she really better off? Can he be sure?

Although you initially opposed the idea, once your widowed parent has remarried it may become easier for you to accept. The closeness you once had may be gone, however. The new remoteness you feel may be obvious if you refer to the woman your father has married as "my father's wife" rather than as "my stepmother." Many children are never reconciled and continue to feel hurt and resentful because a father treats his new wife better than he ever treated them or their mother, or because a mother seems to show more affection to her new husband than she ever showed to their father.

Although remarriage after the death of a spouse, particularly soon after, may appear to children and close friends as disloyalty to the memory of the dead man or woman, it actually may be the reverse. Some experts claim that when there has been a good, solid, mutually gratifying relationship in a marriage, there will inevitably be pain and grief after one partner dies, but the survivor will eventually be freer to start life again and even to contemplate marriage again. A widow or a widower whose former married life has been gratifying may want "more of the same" and hope to continue, in a new marriage, patterns enjoyed in the old one.

When the marriage has been difficult, conflicted, and unsatisfying, with elements of dependency, anger, and resentment, the death of one partner will not wipe out those emotions for the survivor. The grief that follows may be intense and as conflicted as the marriage itself. Those conflicts may prevent the survivor from making a new life or a commitment to marriage again. Even though the marriage was generally happy, a widow may reject remarriage if her husband was ill for a long time before his death and she carried the major burden of his nursing care. Or conversely, if her widowhood came suddenly, with no warning, she may say, "I never will go through that again," when the subject of remarriage comes up.

A woman (or man) remarries late in life for a variety of reasons: for companionship, for financial security, to share common interests, to have someone who cares about her or someone she can care about, or to satisfy sexual needs.

Elderly widows and widowers, even those who have all these needs, may decide not to remarry for many reasons: fear of making a mistake, family opposition, lack of desire to resume marital responsibilities, and lack of opportunity. But they may find alternative ways to satisfy their needs. Just as young people are turning to more unconventional lifestyles, so may their grandparents: group marriages, shared living arrangements, communes, and homosexual or lesbian relationships. Their financial situation frequently makes marriage economically unwise, and to protect their assets, they may decide to live together without legal ties.

Such unconventional living arrangements, difficult enough for the elderly themselves to accept, may be hair-raising for their sons and daughters, who may already be having a hard time accepting the unusual lifestyles of their children. Consider the discomfort of the conservative middle-aged man who is forced by current mores to refer to "the girl my son is living with" or "the boy who shares my daughter's apartment" at a social gathering. How much greater his discomfort will be if, in addition, he has to include "my father's girlfriend" or "my mother's boyfriend"! He may prefer to withdraw from both generations.

Sex after 65—Myth Versus Reality

Many children like to ignore the fact that sex plays a part in their parents' lives at any age. That possibility can be ignored even more easily when their parents are old because of the prevailing

Many children like to ignore the fact that sex plays a part in their parents' lives at any age

assumptions that sex is not possible, necessary, or nice in the later years, and furthermore, that it can be hazardous to the health! You yourself may never have given a conscious thought to your parents' sex life or discussed your own with them, and may accept the belief, passed on through the centuries, that while the other appetites last indefinitely and must be satisfied, sexual appetites die young.

> You cannot call it love, for at your age
> The hey-day in the blood is tame . . .

said Hamlet to his mother, Queen Gertrude. He could not understand why she married with such "indecent haste" after his father's death, and denied that a woman of her age could be motivated by love or passion. Yet Gertrude's age was probably less than 45. It's easy enough to smile at Hamlet's naïveté, to point out that knowledge of human biology was very limited in Shakespeare's time, and to say that things are different in the twenty-first century. But popular attitudes, supported by some members of the medical profession, are not so radically different today, despite the advances in scientific knowledge. Beliefs about sex and the later years continue to be distorted by old myths and false assumptions. Many young people, for example, still believe that a woman's libido vanishes after menopause and that impotence lies in wait for middle-aged men.

Plenty of aging men and women, of course, know from personal experience that these myths are false. Their own continuing sexual activity is all the proof they need. But plenty of others still buy into outmoded ideas about sex. If they feel any sexual drives or suffer any sexual difficulties, they often worry that something is the matter with them, and they may hesitate to seek advice about their anxieties for fear of looking foolish. In addition, they are constantly reminded by the media that to be old is to be undesirable—another way of saying *sexless*.

Any example of passion and sexual potency still surviving in the later years is considered unusual or "abnormal" enough to be newsworthy: the marriage of a 79-year-old man and a 30-year-old woman, fatherhood at 80, an affair between an older woman and a younger man, or a crime of passion. Such stories should make people question their old assumptions, but public response is most likely to be, "Oh, yes, but these are the exceptions."

Studies of human sexuality have shown that sexual activity among the elderly is far from unusual. Nearly 50 years ago, Alfred Kinsey's first studies showed that while the frequency of intercourse declines steadily among men through the years, the majority of men continue some pattern of sexual activity. A number of men are sexually inactive at 70, but a greater number still have intercourse with some regularity at the same age or older. (Kinsey's sample included one 70-year-old man whose ejaculations were still averaging more than seven a week, and a man of 88 who had intercourse with his 90-year-old wife anywhere from once a week to once a month.) Kinsey also reported that the sexual capacities of women show little change with aging.

Present-day researchers confirm Kinsey's earlier findings. Their studies show that men and women can, and often do, remain sexually active at 60, 70, 80, and beyond, and furthermore, that older couples who maintain sexually gratifying lives are usually continuing the pattern of a lifetime. Sex may be less frequent, possibly less intense, but just as meaningful in their old age as it was when they were young, and perhaps even more satisfying. Similarly, single men and women—widowed, divorced, separated, or never married—who have always been sexually active are likely to seek out sexual relationships when they are old, although partners are increasingly difficult to find as the years go by. (Kinsey found that among previously married women, masturbation became more important with age, possibly as the only available sexual outlet.) Far from dying out with age, sexual feelings, if they have been strong and satisfied through the years, may be intensified when an elderly man or woman is alone and lonely.

Sexual patterns of behavior may start early and continue late, but may only be considered socially acceptable in the earlier years. A young man who sows wild oats at 20 may be admired and envied, but he would be branded a roué at 50 and a "dirty old man" at 70 for the same behavior. "Mother, you were flirting with the butcher!" a daughter may say reprovingly, but the white-haired old woman may merely shrug off the reproof: "I can't change old habits at my age."

Eyebrows are usually raised when an elderly man marries a younger woman. People are quick to assume that she married him for his money, for security, for social position, or because she needs a father, and that he needs someone to take care of him. But their assumptions may easily be wrong.

> Friends and relatives were happy when 82-year-old Phil Richter married his 50-year-old housekeeper a short time after he was widowed. "How nice for him," they said. "He was so lonely. Now he'll have companionship at least." They were quite upset some time later to learn that the marriage had not worked out and that the newlyweds had separated. Rumors circulated that the trouble was caused by sexual incompatibility. "Of course," everyone quickly assumed, "she was too young for him. She still needed a physical relationship. Poor old man—how sad—he probably couldn't satisfy her."
>
> Those closest to old Mr. Richter knew that the situation was reversed. The younger woman had always found sex distasteful and was glad to marry for companionship, convinced that nothing more would be expected of her. Mr. Richter had other ideas. He had maintained a high level of sexual activity all his life, not only with his wife, until she died, but with a series of mistresses as well. Now in his 80s and widowed, he needed companionship, but he needed a sexual partner, too, and expected to find it in the younger woman he married.

Age, therefore, is not a barrier to healthy, ongoing sexual activity. The barriers come rather from physical disability, mental disturbance, long-standing sexual maladjustments, and—more frequently—lack of an appealing or willing sexual partner.

The Elderly May Be Misinformed, Too

Scientific research has broken down many of the myths that have surrounded the subject of sex and the elderly, but many older people still do not fully understand the changes taking place in their own bodies as they age. Temporary setbacks in their sexual performance may quickly revive the old myths. Their anxiety may then make temporary setbacks permanent. A woman may know intellectually that her libido will not be affected after menopause even though her ovaries stop functioning, but she may not be aware of other possible changes: thinning of the vaginal walls and a decrease in elasticity and lubrication, resulting in painful intercourse. Those conditions can usually be treated, but unless she gets good medical advice, she may decide by herself that her sex life is over.

A man may be concerned that his sexual potency will be gone after prostate surgery or may worry merely because his reactions are slower, and because it takes him longer to achieve an erection and an orgasm. He may be concerned that he is becoming impotent, and his anxiety may make the impotence a reality—a self-fulfilling prophecy. Many problems, not necessarily related to age, can cause periods of impotence in younger as well as older men, such as certain medications, drinking, fatigue, worry, fear of failure, or boredom. Careful physicians are often able to pinpoint the problems, suggest ways to overcome them, and reassure elderly patients that impotence is not necessarily permanent. But sexual failure seems so shameful to many men that they are reluctant to admit the problem. If they decide to consult a doctor, they are often told, "Don't worry about it—it's to be expected at your age!"

Modern medical thinking has exploded another old myth: that sex is hazardous to the health of older people. Many doctors are convinced that the opposite is true, even for the elderly with heart conditions and arthritis, and that sexual activity can actually be therapeutic in reducing tension, heightening morale, and maintaining a sense of well-being. Nursing home rules once required the segregation of the sexes, or permitted only married couples to share a room. But today, some of the more concerned institutions, realizing the importance of sex to the adjustment of elderly residents, are making it possible for unmarried couples to have privacy together. This practice, while producing great happiness for the residents concerned, often produces consternation among their children.

Modern medical thinking has exploded another old myth: that sex is hazardous to the health of older people.

What Will the Children Say?

Sir Laurence Olivier, in a 1992 interview in the *New York Times*, discussed the play, *The Seagull,* and its author, the late British playwright Ben Travers:

> Travers is well into his 90's. It's a very naughty play indeed. He discovered sex very late in life. He was thrilled by it and quite ashamed of the play. He put it in a drawer. He didn't want to shock his children, all of whom were over 60. We persuaded him that they would be able to take it.

Perhaps Ben Travers's children were able to "take it," but children are not always so open-minded. They may accept a widowed father's remarriage to the elderly woman who was their mother's best friend, or a mother's remarriage to a kindly old man everyone loves. If sex is considered at all in these marriages, everyone may like to assume that the elderly couples maintain separate bedrooms or at least separate beds.

But what if you cannot make any such comfortable assumptions in your own father's situation—or your mother's? What if the behavior of one or the other makes it perfectly clear that a sexual relationship is going on? A special set of feelings may be aroused, and suddenly, although you firmly believe that sex is normal and appropriate for other people's fathers and mothers, it may now seem highly inappropriate for your own. You may try to prevent what you feel is an "unwise" marriage or break up a relationship that does not seem "right." You and others in the family may insist that "he is making a fool of himself" or that "she doesn't know what she's doing." You may even consider that your elderly parent is becoming mentally impaired. It is dangerous to jump to such conclusions. Although other people who have seriously deteriorated mentally or physically may lose the defenses they once had that inhibited inappropriate sexual acts, you may have a hard time deciding if your father's behavior is *truly* inappropriate or if it just *seems* inappropriate to you and simply makes you uncomfortable or ashamed. Perhaps you want your father's or your mother's affections to be exclusively yours and are jealous when someone else comes between you. Perhaps you cannot bear to see your once very proper parent, who cautioned you against sexual display, exhibiting open sexuality.

When children feel ashamed or jealous of an elderly parent's sexual relationship that is appropriate and gratifying to the parent, it is the children's problem, not the parent's. The children may deal with their problem by learning to accept the relationship or by staying away from it as much as possible. Worrying, "What will the children say?" may make older men and women hesitant to remarry and may also prevent them from establishing new relationships, forcing them to settle instead for unnecessary loneliness and sexual abstinence.

Whether closely embroiled or not, adult children are affected by the ups and downs of their parents' marriage in late life, by the death of one partner and the challenges presented by the surviving spouse, and by the sexual partnerships the surviving spouse may enter into—even remarriage. But if you are accepting of your possibly mixed feelings about these changes in your parent's life and concern about your relationship, you will find great comfort and pleasure in this new phase in your mother or father's life.

Bob Morris on His Father's Pleasures as a Widower

Three months after my mother died, I was planning to spend the day with my dad in Florida. I had gone down to see him. And he suddenly wasn't so available, because a woman called him up—who wanted to take him to a bridge game. I went down to his parking lot to say hello to this very put-together 85-year-old in her little silver Lexus. And she looked at me, and she said, "Joe—he looks just like you!" And then she drove him away. And I thought, "Wow!" I wasn't sure what that relationship was, but it was a taste of what was to come.

Six months after my mother was gone, my father handed me a personals page that he had ripped out of a free Jewish weekly in Great Neck, and he had some ads circled. And he said: "I wonder if you can help me out. Would you call these women for me? I can't figure out how to do it. It says you can't do it from a cell phone—I only have a cell phone. Here are these women's ads—call them up for me."

I said, "This is ridiculous. You've got so many friends; you've got your kids—what are you doing? What is this need to be in love all about?" He said, "It worked so beautifully with your mother for 50 years—I would love to do it again." What could I say to that?

And so the dates started coming in, and I found myself in the position of trying to monitor the situation. He was 80 years old at the time. I was concerned about a couple of things. So on this superficial level, I didn't want him to end up with somebody who would be an embarrassment because my father was a very open-minded guy, who did not have the screening system most of us have to tell you if someone is a little trashy. I mean, if my father could have found a Jewish Dolly Parton, he would be with her, you know? On a superficial level, I was worried about just what he was going to fish up from the widow pond.

But the other thing that I found myself feeling was, "I don't want him to find somebody who might ruin our relationship," which was decent in his last years. It took so long. And it wasn't, really, until I was in my 40s that I started to realize what a privilege it is to have a father, and to have such a good guy around to enjoy. And so it would have made it sad for me if there was this high-strung, nervous, egomaniacal, difficult new woman . . . keeping company with him all the time. I know—it probably sounds ridiculous, but I wanted to be friends with him.

Then I started worrying that all his bad habits would make it harder for him to find a nice woman on the dating trail, like the fact that he had a habit of using a toothpick at the dinner table. And I warned him not to talk about Mom very much on first dates because who wants to hear about the love of someone's life on the first date? He couldn't be trusted to wear the right shirt that wouldn't show his V-neck T-shirt underneath. His car was an absolute pigsty. Sometime he would fly off the handle in discussions about politics, alienating everyone around him.

But, generally, he took to the dating life beautifully. And he was very lucky. He rented in Palm Beach, which is such a great area—full of seniors. And then, ultimately, he finally did have a big romance—after casting about for 8, 9 months—he did finally find somebody who proved herself to be right for him. And then that lasted right up until he got really sick, weak, and infirm. Love and the pursuit of love made those 2 years after my mother's death so active for him.

The story I love to tell is when I sold my father's car to somebody after he passed away, I thought I had cleaned out the whole thing—filling 12 contractor bags with his junk. But I missed one thing, a little compartment over the rearview mirror. The man who was looking to buy the car was an accountant, very prim and correct. He was sitting behind the steering wheel, and he reached up to open this little compartment overhead, and out of it fell a condom. My father couldn't have been younger than 79 when he had stored that up there with high hopes for a good night. He had a condom at the ready, just in case. I thought it was very optimistic. He was an optimistic person.

6

Facing the Final Crisis

"He is certainly of an age to die." The sadness of the old; their banishment...I too made use of this cliché and that when I was referring to my mother. I did not understand that one might sincerely weep for a relative, a grandfather aged seventy or more. If I met a woman of fifty overcome with sadness because she had just lost her mother, I thought her neurotic: we are all mortal; at eighty you are old enough to be one of the dead....But it is not true...the knowledge that because of her age my mother's life must soon come to an end did not lessen the horrible surprise.
— Simone de Beauvoir, *A Very Easy Death*

THE DEATH OF AN ELDERLY MOTHER OR FATHER INEVItably touches the children who are left behind, whether they are just grown up, middle-aged, or nearing old age themselves. Even if it is expected because of a hopeless illness, even if it is welcomed as an end to suffering, even if there is remoteness or estrangement between the generations, the death of a parent cannot be a casual event.

Any review of life in the later years must therefore include a consideration of death. Death becomes more and more of a reality with every passing year. Its closeness touches not only those who are about to die but also those who love them and will survive them.

According to the laws of nature, the younger generation will survive the older one. But the process is not necessarily without pain. A son expects to survive his father, but also expects to mourn him and to feel some amount of sadness, regret, and loneliness. He may also realistically expect to feel a certain sense of relief when the burden of caring for an invalid is lifted, particularly if the invalid has been difficult or demanding, or has suffered. Many children respond in just these ways when their parents die. Others surprise themselves and wonder why they respond with more painful emotions—inconsolable grief, anger, fear, guilt, and a sense of abandonment—when someone who has been old, sick, and helpless—and no longer able to enjoy life—finally dies.

Painful reactions should not be so surprising. Parents are crucial figures in our lives when we are children. If they live on into their 70s, 80s, and 90s, they may continue as integral parts of our adult lives, too; we and they may even grow old together. When a mother dies at 85, her children at 50 or 60 may learn for the first time the meaning of life without her. Each one of us has only one mother or father to lose, and when either or both die, some part of us dies with them.

When a mother dies at 85, her children at 50 or 60 may learn for the first time the meaning of life without her.

Our personal being is in some way, to a greater or lesser extent, diminished. A strong force linking us to our past is gone. As our parents' lives end, an eventful chapter in our own life history ends, too. It may not have been a particularly good chapter for us, but it is finished and can never be revised or rewritten. There will never be an opportunity again for reconciliation, for explanation, for understanding, or for saying things left unsaid for years: "I'm grateful," "I'm sorry," "I love you."

Psychologist Clark E. Moustakas, in *Loneliness*, describes the thoughts of a son watching his dying mother:

> This was my mother; and the word "mother" brings on a flow of feeling and past experiences and years of living together, loving together, and hating, too. The fighting and conflicts do not seem important anymore, the arguments and intense pains and emotions that clouded the relationship have evaporated. This was my mother, and I realize the uniqueness of our relationship. It was not an impersonal fact of

someone having cancer and dying, but it was a basic relationship that can never be repeated, a piece of eternity, never to be the same anymore.

There is also the story, fact or fiction, about a 60-year-old man who, when asked to indicate on an insurance form whether he was married, widowed, or divorced, wrote in the appropriate space "orphan." While this word did not describe his marital state, it did describe the state of his feelings. Many of us have a similar feeling, if only for a fleeting moment, and the old fear of abandonment is remembered from childhood. As long as our parents live, we are always somebody's child, no matter how old we are. Whenever they die, we are orphans for life.

Most of us are unprepared for this feeling. If we sense it in advance, we are likely to laugh at it and at ourselves for being ridiculous. We certainly are not likely to discuss it with our parents who are close to death, yet undoubtedly they must know something about it—after all, they have probably been orphaned, too.

The Conspiracy of Silence

As a matter of fact, we are likely to talk to them about very little that relates to their death, and more likely to stop them from bringing up the subject. Families with deep religious faith may be able to deal with death more directly, to talk about it and what comes after, but the subject of death has been generally taboo in modern society. Freud discussed that taboo in his essay "Obscure Thoughts on War and Death":

> . . . we were of course prepared to maintain that death was the necessary outcome of life, that everyone owes nature a death and must expect to pay the debt—in short, that death was natural, undeniable and unavoidable. In reality, however, we were accustomed to behave as if it were otherwise. We showed an unmistakable tendency to put death on one side, to eliminate it from life.

For some, not only the subject but also the word is taboo. Euphemisms are used instead: "passed on," "gone," "departed," "lost," "at rest." Not wanting to be reminded of the inevitable, people find it safer to avoid the topic; if they talk about it at all, they tend to do so in general, impersonal terms, with no names attached. A wall of silence, therefore, can grow up between those who are about to die and those who care about them most. That silence can deprive both of help, comfort, and support, just when they are needed most. In *I Knock at the Door*, Sean O'Casey writes of a dying old man:

> And here he was now reclining in a big horse-hair covered armchair, shrinking from something that everyone thought of, but no one ever mentioned.

The same taboo that makes it difficult for us to discuss death with the dying makes us uncomfortable with mourners. "What can I say?" you may have asked every time you sat down to write a condolence note or went to visit friends in mourning. A few conventional, stilted words of sympathy—and then on to safer, more pleasant topics. The subject uppermost in everyone's mind is the subject that is hardest to bring up. Children, uninhibited as yet by social taboos, often spontaneously break the conspiracy of silence and refer point-blank to the thing that terrifies them.

> When Peter and Eleanor Thorne returned with their two children after a 3-year assignment in Japan, their homecoming was a sad one. Eleanor's father, who had always lived with them, had died at 82 while they were all overseas. He had been extremely close to his daughter, son-in-law, and grandchildren, and they were all acutely aware of his absence when they came back to the house he had shared with them for so long.
>
> Friends who dropped in to welcome the family were also aware of the pain of the homecoming and were determined to be helpful. A succession of visitors came and went, each one full of bright chatter and careful to avoid any reference to the missing person. The Thornes were surprised at first when no one mentioned Grandpa—they would have liked to talk about him—but they decided it would put a damper on their friends' efforts to be cheerful, so they kept silent, too.
>
> At the end of the day, a small boy arrived with his parents, surveyed the piles of luggage scattered all over the house, spotted a giant duffel bag standing upright in the corner, studied it with fascination, and then, to the horror of his mother, asked in a shrill voice, "Is that where they keep the grandfather?" The silence was broken.

Humans have orbited in space, harnessed nuclear power, walked on the moon, and mapped the human genome, but death remains undiscovered territory, terrifying in its mystery. The motto observed by many is, "When terrified—hide." So they try to hide in silence, but that does not always provide real shelter. Without a word being spoken, our parents' aging forces us to acknowledge the fact that we are trying to ignore. Their increasing frailty, their whitening hair, their fading vision, and their advancing birthdays can be daily reminders of their mortality, and by extension, our own. No wonder many of us react with anger and impatience if, on top of those visible reminders, they want to talk about dying. They are likely to find themselves cut off before they have a chance to begin:

Father: I'm not going to be around forever.
Son: Nonsense! You'll outlive all of us! *[The subject is
          closed.]*

Mother.   When I'm gone . . .
Son: Oh, Mother, stop talking that way. *[The subject is
          closed.]*

Father: I've had a good life, but I . . .
Daughter: Don't act as if it's over. You've got years to go.
          [The subject is closed.]

These are all direct references to death, but some older people make more indirect allusions that sensitive sons and daughters are quick to catch and resent.

Bernard Hill's father always had his affairs in order. "His drawers are all neat and tidy," Bernard reported. "He's always reminding me where his papers are and which keys fit which locks. He used to be like this when we were kids before we went on a trip. He always seems packed for a trip these days and ready to go. Whenever I visit him, I feel like I ought to say goodbye. I hate it."

Every time there was a sale—sheets or underwear or stockings or towels—Meg Corwin always asked her mother whether she needed anything. Her mother invariably answered, "No, I have enough to last me." Meg always groaned when she heard this. "Why does she have to keep on reminding me all the time that she's going to die?"

Other adult children don't so much resent their parents' allusions to death as try to navigate the elaborate code system those allusions sometimes assume. As one middle-aged woman recalls:

> My father has been planning for his demise since he was 30, deciding who should keep track of his affairs and what should go to whom after he is gone. Now 86, he is completely obsessed with two things: the weather and money. He plots how to keep the government from getting "our inheritance" and badgers his broker every day, sometimes twice a day, about moving this or that stock into something else. When he calls me or my brother or sister, each of us hundreds of miles away, he always starts by telling us what's he heard on TV about our weather (as if we couldn't look out our own windows and know whether it's raining), and then he segues over to his latest postmortem financial plans. We don't talk meaningfully about his sadness about the end of his life or about his friends who are dropping like flies now. We don't talk about death at all, except in the cold and practical terms of estate planning. Sometimes, he'll slip in a funny old story about his irritating, social climbing sister, now gone, or my mother's five aunts, each completely loony and all long since deceased, and then his voice quavers and breaks. He misses them all. He misses his life, his youth, himself. He wants everything and everyone back, including the social climber, and he knows that's not possible. So it's back to stocks and bonds and the lake effect snow in Buffalo. All we seem to be able to do is listen to the things he can say and feel for things he can't.

Other adult children don't so much resent their parents' allusions to death as try to navigate the elaborate code system those allusions sometimes assume.

Some People Need to Talk about Death

If death were not so taboo, if it could be talked about more freely, those direct and indirect references might stimulate rather than abort discussion. The discussions would not be likely to go on indefinitely, or to monopolize all conversation. The elderly are not usually preoccupied with thoughts of death every minute. Thoughts and fears come and go. When they come, it can be comforting and reassuring to voice them occasionally. Not much response is required except listening and a few words: "I know," or "I understand," or "I remember, too."

Your father may be looking for a chance to talk to someone about himself—to reminisce about what his life has meant to him, what certain people have meant to him. He may wonder what he has meant to others—to you. He may want to talk about his accomplishments, mistakes, regrets—or perhaps his fears not only of death but also of the process of dying. He may hope to be reassured that he will not die alone or be in pain. He may also want reassurance that he will be remembered, that he will be able to leave some kind of legacy behind for future generations. He may want to discuss his will and the distribution of his material things, his feelings about funerals and burials. His concerns may be not only for himself but also for those he will leave behind, people he worries about: you, or your mother, or your brother, or a grandchild. He may not expect to find answers to all his questions, but talking about them can be therapeutic if only there is a willing listener.

Children frequently look back on lost opportunities after a parent has died and wonder why they did not listen more, both for their parent's benefit and for their own.

Children frequently look back on lost opportunities after a parent has died and wonder why they did not listen more, both for their parent's benefit and for their own. After his father died, John O'Brien said regretfully:

> I'd get pretty bored when Pop rambled on about the old days and what happened before I was born. But he always seemed to catch me when I was busy—I'll admit I hardly ever listened. But I wish I had. Who is there left now to tell me the name of the town in Ireland where my great-grandfather is buried? Who remembers Aunt Tessie's mother's maiden name? Why should I care about such silly, unimportant things? But I do. And he'll never know I do.

Direct and indirect references to death are often ignored, but sometimes the subject never comes up at all; there seems no way to open it. You may feel you would like to talk to your mother when you realize she is failing and may sense that it would help her to talk to someone, but both of you may be uncomfortable and uncertain how to begin. There may be awkwardness and reticence on each side. It's easy enough to say to her, "Listen—before you take off for California, is there anything we should go over together, anything you need me to do for you?" It's harder to speak so freely when she is not going to California, but is going to die. Much, therefore, is likely to be left unsaid by both of you.

> Do not go gentle into that good night,
> Old age should burn and rave at close of day;
> Rage, rage against the dying of the light.

So wrote the Welsh poet Dylan Thomas, opening one of the best-known contemporary poems about death. According to those who knew him, Thomas wrote those words for his dying father, but never could bring himself to read them to him because of the great reticence in their relationship. The poem has been read by countless strangers instead of by the one dying man for whom it was written.

It has been generally assumed that the older adults fear death less and face it with greater equanimity than the young. This may be true for many old people. They undoubtedly have had plenty of experience with death. Most of them are forced by their advancing age to acknowledge their own mortality, and their awareness is constantly reawakened as, one by one, close friends and relatives die. But even though they may fear death less, this does not mean that they are not afraid. Many are fearful until the end and never reconciled, continuing in Dylan Thomas's words, to "rage, rage against the dying of the light." Sons, daughters, and close relatives may go through parallel emotional stages before they, too, can accept irrevocable separation.

The conspiracy of silence has generally included not only the relatives of the dying but also the healing professions. Physicians, by training, are more concerned with fighting death than with helping their patients meet it more easily. Their professional life is dedicated to avoiding, preventing, or at least postponing death, and to developing life-preserving procedures: antibiotic therapy, chemotherapy, transfusions, infusions, transplants, and life-sustaining machines. By machine, lungs can now be kept breathing, hearts kept pumping, and kidneys kept functioning. In the past, human organs had no such miraculous support systems, and without them, greater numbers of people died, and died younger. The only possible benefit offered the dying then was that more of them died at home in a familiar atmosphere, with people who loved them nearby.

The patient dying in the hospital today is in an alien environment made more alien if he or she has to be surrounded by strange tubes, bright lights, machines, and monitors— with teams of experts and skilled technicians, all strangers, concentrating their efforts on preventing death. While so much necessary intensity is concentrated on physical needs, there is a danger that the dying patient, as a person, may be forgotten, his or her other needs brushed aside.

While so much necessary intensity is concentrated on physical needs, there is a danger that the dying patient, as a person, may be forgotten, his or her other needs brushed aside.

Intensive care procedures often save lives, and those whose lives have been saved are thankful, but some speak later about the sense of personal isolation they experienced. They could hear voices, but the voices did not usually talk to them; they were touched by gentle, capable hands, but the hands, busy with tubes and wires, usually transmitted impersonal messages. After surviving a critical illness, the recuperating patient is able to resume human contacts again, but many of the elderly remain isolated until death.

Care and Concern for the Dying

Fortunately, the conspiracy of silence is not as pervasive as it once was. Among certain groups of people, death is currently being discussed openly and examined freely. It is the subject of books, articles, seminars, institutes, workshops, and public lectures. Concern for those who are about to die is coming not only from physicians but also from psychiatrists, social workers, philosophers, scientists, and theologians. Popular books, magazine features, and TV programs are making the general public aware that more can be offered to the critically ill than medical procedures alone to make the process of dying easier and less painful.

Thanatology, the study of death, is a growing field of science, its name derived from *thanatos*, the Greek word for "death." Particular concern has been focused by the growing number of professionals in this new field on the emotional needs of those who are nearing death and on easing and improving the dying process—both for the dying person and for his or her loved ones. In some hospitals and nursing homes, staff members are given special training to make them more responsive to the needs of the dying and the feelings of the dying person's family.

Hospice Care

A more all-encompassing type of care is provided by hospice programs, established originally in England for the sole purpose of offering comfort to the dying and their families. Modern hospice care began in 1967 when St. Christopher's Hospice opened its doors in London. This approach to treating the terminally ill soon spread across the Atlantic, and the first hospice in the United States was established in 1974. Today there are more than 4000 hospice programs across the country.

Some hospices operate with a full team of physicians, nurses, psychiatrists, and social workers as well as home health aides and specially trained volunteers. Others are not so fully staffed, but all hospice workers are trained not to cure but to comfort the dying and to help sustain them and their families. The goal of hospice care is to alleviate pain and other symptoms caused by the illness itself or by the side effects of medication. Most hospice care is provided in the home by professionals and volunteers on a daily or occasional basis, according to the individual patient's needs, but some hospice services are located in hospitals and nursing homes. The location is not important, since the hospice is not a place, but rather a system of care that offers physical, emotional, and practical support to the terminally ill. It also recognizes and tries to ease the strains imposed on caregivers and family members, who have probably had to endure weeks, even months, of rigorous daily and nightly routines. Some hospice programs provide counseling for family members after the death of a relative they have cared for so constantly.

Hospice care is financed by different sources, including Medicare, Medicaid, most private insurance plans, managed care organizations, and the Department of Veterans Affairs. To receive Medicare coverage for its hospice services, an agency must be approved by Medicare. For all forms of coverage, a doctor must certify that a patient has less than 6 months to live if the disease runs its normal course. Families can pay for services out of pocket, and most hospices with the support of charitable contributions provide services without charge if the patient has limited financial resources. See Chapter 9 and Appendix A for more information.

Palliative Care

Whereas hospice services are specifically geared toward care in the last months of life, palliative care—which also has the goal of providing as much comfort as possible to a patient—may be deliv ered at any point in an illness and over an extended period. It is characterized by concern for symptom relief and promotion of general well-being and psychological, spiritual, and social comfort for the person with a life-threatening or life-limiting illness. The need to maintain quality of life has become increasingly important, not only in the dying stages, but also in the months and years before death.

Palliative care can also be provided in the hospital, nursing home, or at home, but currently Medicare and Medicaid do not offer a "palliative care" benefit. The services covered will depend on the patient's Medicare, Medicaid, or private insurance coverage, and it is important to determine what, if any, costs you will be asked to pay. (See Appendix A for organizations and web sites that can provide more information on hospice and palliative care.)

Telling the Truth to the Dying

Many of those who work closely with the dying are convinced that frankness and honesty about their physical condition is usually essential before patients and their families can begin to work through the stages of dying. A dying man has the same right to know, whether he dies at 40 or at 80. While that may be the best approach in most cases, there are always exceptions. It may be necessary to take a somewhat more cautious approach with an older person who is confused or mentally disturbed, and there will always be some older people—just as there are younger ones—who do not want to hear the truth, rejecting it and denying it when it is offered to them. There obviously can be more than one approach to death, and truth should not be forced on anyone; neither should it be denied to those who ask for it or are willing to receive it.

You may think, as many loving children do, that you are protecting your mother, whether she is at home or in a hospital or institution, when you urge her doctor not to tell her the facts about her physical condition. You may honestly believe it is kinder to lie to her. But how kind can it be to keep her completely in the dark about what's wrong with her? How can she understand why she feels so terrible? How can she explain her aches and pains? How can she accept her limitations? Nothing is more confusing to an older person—or a younger one—than to sense that something is seriously wrong and then to be told by everyone that it's nothing, just a minor problem that should go away soon. Yet relatives and doctors have been equally timid about being honest, not realizing that uncertainty, confusion, anxiety, and distrust are usually much more damaging than the simple truth.

When Lily Simmons, a nursing home patient, complained of abdominal pain at 82, her physician, in consultation with her family, decided not to tell her the diagnosis that had been made—carcinoma of the stomach—but told her instead that she had an allergic condition. That did not really satisfy Mrs. Simmons, a bright, alert woman, since it did not explain the severity of her pain or her sense of foreboding.

One day, as she was signing some insurance papers, she noticed that the diagnosis of her condition—carcinoma of the stomach—was filled in on the form. She went immediately to the nurse on the floor to ask the meaning of the word, and when she was told it meant cancer, she demanded that the nurse tell her the truth. At first, she was angry and resentful of both the doctors and her family, but eventually she understood their motivation and in time began to reconcile herself to her condition. Since her cancer progressed slowly because of her advanced age, she found herself once more taking an interest in the world around her and decided that there were things she could still enjoy before she died. Until the last months, which came several years later, she remained quite actively involved in life around her.

Although it is important that your mother understand the truth about her condition and its implications, it is not necessary to go into great detail or to keep referring to it continually. Once she knows what's going on, she can begin to prepare herself, ask questions, raise her fears, and receive reassurance. She may wonder how much pain and discomfort lie ahead and how these can be alleviated. It is not necessary, either, to tell her she is dying in so many words, because she may not be dying at the point the diagnosis is made. Her cancer may be inoperable and it may cause her death one day, or her heart condition may be serious and her next attack may kill her, but she may surprise everyone. There are all kinds of terminal illnesses, and many make slower progress in elderly bodies than in younger ones. Cancer may be detected in an 80-year-old man, but he may die of a massive stroke before his cancer has had a chance to do much damage.

Professionals are reluctant to pinpoint months and years. The dramatic "death sentences" so popular in drama and fiction—"You have 3 months to live" or "1 year at the most"—are less likely in real-life situations today. The future is unpredictable, even for the elderly. There is evidence to suggest that those who are about to die can sometimes, in some mysterious way, postpone their death to remain alive for some particular occasion or until some particular piece of work is finished. It is not uncommon to hear families report, "Mother was determined to live until Ned came home from Iraq," or "Father wanted to see Susan and Fred get married," or "He managed to stay alive until he finished his book." One indomitable grandmother kept herself alive by setting herself a series of goals. As soon as one was reached, she set a new one. By age 90, she was determined to see a great-grandchild. So far, none has been conceived.

Just as there are disease factors governing death, so social and psychological factors play important roles. Statisticians, demographers, and social psychologists have documented the existence of a phenomenon that they have termed the "death dip," in which the death rate among certain groups of people drops prior to a special occasion and rises shortly afterward. A study reported in the *British Medical Journal* suggested that, among the elderly, an approaching birthday can be a motivation for survival since research showed that fewer older people died in the 2 months before their birthday. An earlier study of more than 300 famous Americans, whose birthdays were of national significance, revealed the same pattern.

The death dip has also been noticed prior to less personal occasions, such as Thanksgiving and other holidays. In two separate studies of big cities with large Jewish populations, a death dip was documented among Jews in the period immediately preceding Yom Kippur, the most solemn day in the Jewish calendar.

Thomas Jefferson, at 83, and John Adams, at 91, both died on July 4, 1826, the 50th anniversary of their country's founding and of the signing of the Declaration of Independence, which they had both shared in drafting. The words of the doctor who was with him document the fact that Jefferson was aware of the significance of the date until the end.

> About seven o'clock of the evening of Thursday, he [Jefferson] awoke, and seeing me staying at his bedside exclaimed, "Oh, Doctor, are you still there?" in a voice, however, that was husky and indistinct. He then asked, "Is it the Fourth?" to which I replied, "It soon will be." These were the last words I heard him utter.
>
> —Merrill Peterson, *Thomas Jefferson and the New Nation*

A Time for Closeness

The conspiracy of silence about death, the awkwardness so many feel about it, their discomfort, often makes those most closely involved with the dying do just that—waste their energy covering up their feelings, the very feelings that could provide so much comfort and support. But sometimes there is little opportunity for this closeness. Babies in the past were born at home, with fathers and close relatives hovering nearby. The dying died in the same environment. Birth and death were events not to be experienced alone, but to be shared. In that intimate atmosphere, emotions could be shared, too—the painful as well as the joyous ones.

Birth and death in the past century, to a large extent, have moved out of the home into institutions. The moves were essential to provide the greatest protection for the new lives and the old ones. But in this highly efficient and highly sterile atmosphere, strangers may usher in life and usher it out, while those with the deepest personal ties can feel like trespassers. Fortunately, now the family has been reinstated in the process of birth. In most hospitals, fathers and even other close family members are allowed to be with mothers during delivery so that the ones most intimately involved can share the first minutes of life. It is increasingly recognized that the same kind of closeness could be allowed during the last minutes of life as well. Hospice care provided in the home makes this possible for many. But this is not always possible, as one middle-aged son discovered:

Fathers, and even other close family members, are allowed to be with mothers during delivery. . . . It is increasingly recognized that the same kind of closeness could be allowed during the last minutes of life as well.

Ellis Martin was very fond of his friend Tom's father and quite shaken when he heard the elderly man had an inoperable brain tumor. But Ellis learned a lot from watching his friend's family during this period. He described it this way: "When they learned that nothing more could be done for Tom's father in the hospital, they—his wife and his children—decided to bring him home to die—to the house by the lake that he had inherited from his own father. This was what he wanted, and they knew it. I thought it would be terribly hard to visit him, but it wasn't—even when he got much sicker. He lay there in his room, looking out over the lake that he had always loved, and he could hear his family in other parts of the house—his wife, his children, his grandchildren—preparing meals, playing games, talking to each other. He could hear laughter and music. They didn't hover over him, but they didn't leave him alone much either. Every once in a while, someone would stop by his room to talk a little, to read, or just to sit quietly with him. Even the littlest children came. I thought then, 'What a wonderful way to die, with your whole life around you—past, present, and future.' I hoped my father could die this way, too."

But Ellis's father didn't. He had a massive heart attack when he was 83, and the family had to have him hospitalized. They did everything they could to save him. "We were there with him, but there was no place for us. We were only allowed to see him for a few minutes at a time—never long enough to say much. We didn't know what to say anyhow. We were in the waiting room when somebody came out and told us he was dead. I wonder if he knew we weren't with him when he died—and that he was dying alone."

Should Life Be Prolonged?

That question has been asked over and over again. Many people would give the old familiar answers: "Life must go on," or "While there's life, there's hope." But is there hope for the hopeless? Must life go on in any condition? The right to die is a controversial issue, becoming even more pressing recently as more and more life-sustaining procedures have been able to keep alive men and women—old and young—who would have died 50 years ago. But there is a great difference between "being kept alive" and "living." It is possible through "heroic measures" to prolong life, but it is much more difficult to assess the value of the life that is being prolonged.

The controversy over the right to die continues to make front-page news with dramatic cases involving young and hopelessly ill people, so dramatically illustrated by the Terri Schiavo case. But the controversy has been ongoing, although less publicized, over the old and hopelessly ill. It is possible to prolong the life of a 75-year-old man who has been in a coma for months. It is possible to keep an elderly woman alive, even though a stroke has condemned her to a vegetative existence. It is possible to extend life for someone over 80 with one operation after another, each one causing additional suffering. But is life worth prolonging under these conditions?

Opinion today is divided about the right to die. Some deny that right, abiding by religious teachings and secular law or the belief that life itself must be valued, regardless of its condition. Others are convinced that life without meaning and dignity has little value. The controversy is not new. In sixteenth-century England, Sir Thomas More, sometimes called the "Father of Euthanasia," wrote in his *Utopia*:

> If the disease be not only incurable, but also full of continual pain and anguish, then the priests and magistrate exhort the man that . . . he will determine with himself no longer to cherish that pestilent and painful disease . . . . And in so doing they tell him he shall do wisely, seeing by his death he shall lose no happiness, but end his torture. . . . They that be thus convinced finish their lives willingly, either by fasting, or else they are released by an opiate in their sleep without any feeling of death. But cause none such to die against his will.

Euthanasia for the aged was not uncommon in certain primitive cultures. Some peoples, because of the rigors of their life—particularly in nomadic tribes—were forced to abandon their very old who were helpless and ill, leaving them alone to starve or freeze to death. Some Eskimo groups left their aged to die on ice floes. But other groups found euthanasia more humane than abandonment. As one Chukchee, a reindeer-herding nomad of Siberia, put it:

> Why should not the old woman die? Aged and feeble, weary of life and a burden to herself and to others, she no longer desired to encumber the earth, and claimed of him who owned nearest relationship the friendly stroke which should let out her scanty remnant of existence.
>
> —Leo Simmons, *The Role of the Aged in Primitive Societies*

Today even those who believe in the right to die are not unanimous in their feelings about it. There are the advocates of "active euthanasia," the ending of life for the hopelessly ill and disabled, and the advocates of "passive euthanasia," the withdrawal of all life-saving medications and interventions without which life cannot go on. Whatever the logic and reason in either approach, one crucial question remains unanswered: "If such decisions are to be made, who will make them?" Who will decide what condition is hopeless? Who will decide when life is no longer meaningful? Will it be the relatives of the dying—those with the closest emotional ties? Or will it be the doctors—those with the best medical judgment? Such power over life and death may be too great to be entrusted to any single person or group of people, who might use it irresponsibly or for personal gain.

Advance Directives

Many older people feel that they themselves are the only ones who should have the power over their own lives, and many are careful to let their feelings be known clearly in advance. Some discuss their desires with their families, exacting promises that no "heroic measures" be taken on their behalf. Others

Many older people feel that they themselves are the only ones who should have the power over their own lives, and many are careful to let their feelings be known clearly in advance.

feel safer when they put everything in writing; just as they specify certain funeral arrangements or bequeath their bodies for medical research, in the same way, they may leave written instructions about their desire to die with dignity or sign a "living will." One such document is addressed "To my family, my physician, my lawyer, my clergyman. To any medical facility in whose care I happen to be. To any individual who may become responsible for my health, welfare, or affairs." The document states:

> If the situation should arise in which there is no reasonable expectation of my recovery from physical or mental disability, I request that I be allowed to die and not be kept alive by artificial means or "heroic measures." I do not fear death itself as much as the indignities of deterioration, dependence and hopeless pain. I, therefore, ask that medication be mercifully administered to me to alleviate suffering even though this may hasten the moment of death.

Since the first living wills were distributed by the Euthanasia Educational Council in 1972, millions have been signed. These documents have legal status in 38 states and the District of Columbia. Similar legal documents, such as "end-of-life directives" and "medical power of attorney," are recognized as well. It is important that these directives are drawn up or at least reviewed by a knowledgable attorney and are available to the family (elder law attorneys and the Personal Papers Inventory are discussed in Chapter 7). It is also important to consult with your parent(s)—when they are well—about what their wishes are regarding "heroic measures." Presumably, you have made these provisions for yourself as well.

Now and then, older people are not content to put their trust in others, and they make their own decisions on when and how to die, choosing to end their lives by suicide. The public—as well as philosophers, scholars, and theologians—usually responds with shock to the act of suicide, which goes against most religious and moral teaching. In 1975, 78-year-old Dr. Henry P. Van Dusen, a world-famous theologian, and his wife committed suicide together. Ill for several years and knowing they would both soon become completely dependent on others, they felt there would be little meaning or dignity in the life ahead for them. In the letter they left behind, the Van Dusens wrote: "Nowadays it is difficult to die. We feel this way we are taking will become more usual and acceptable as the years pass. Of course, the thought of our children and our grandchildren makes us sad, but we still feel this is the best way and the right way to go." In commenting on their suicide in the *Saturday Review*, former editor Norman Cousins asked, "What moral or religious purpose is celebrated by the annihilation of the human spirit in the triumphant act of keeping the body alive? Why are so many people more readily appalled by an unnatural form of dying than by an unnatural form of living?"

When the Family Must Decide

The decision to prolong life in the case of a dying comatose patient falls on the shoulders of the closest family members without an advance directive that is recognized by the hospital staff. Ideally, family members can agree on steps to take in consultation with medical staff, and a feeding tube or respirator may be removed. In a hospital, there are instances in which the staff may disagree with a family's decision and insist on more aggressive treatment. But, increasingly, the comfort of the dying patient is taking precedent over aggressive treatment, and these types of confrontations—particularly if there is an advance directive—are avoided.

Family members can also disagree on whether to prolong life, as in the case of Terri Schiavo. There was no written advance directive in this case, and the dispute ended up in the courts, which ultimately supported the position taken by the husband. Short of becoming a legal dispute, family members—spouse, sons, and daughters—may find themselves embroiled in a highly emotional disagreement about the best steps to take on behalf of the dying patient. Some family members may not want to be responsible for prolonging the patient's suffering, others may not want to let the parent go, and others may have ethical concerns. This is an appropriate time to seek counseling from an objective third party—although, as spelled out in Chapter 11, the family may be able to reach consensus on their own.

But regardless of the decision reached by the family, to prolong life or not to prolong life, it is usually made with misgivings.

Bob Morris
on His Mother's Dying

She was a wreck. Ranting and raving in the hospital, completely uncomfortable in her failing body. Yet my brother just thought she could be fixed with the proper assessment from her doctors. But I looked at this—and this is truly the most conflicted thing I've ever felt in my life—and I thought, "Why are we keeping her alive? Why is she going through this? And, what would her life be like if we did get her out of this hospital?" She had to be lifted off and on her bed all day. She was falling all the time. Two weeks ago, I had picked her up off the bathroom floor in the doctor's office. She had soiled herself. It was the second time I'd been through that with her in a year. Can you imagine how she felt? And because I'm not afraid to sound self-involved here—imagine how I felt, too. All of us.

So I wandered around the hall in this hospital—where my un-moored mother was attached to tubes and actively struggling in her room and my brother was calling doctors and consulting with attending physicians to figure out how to help her, make her more comfortable, get her back on her feet. And all I saw was her babbling—fighting in her bed as if she were drowning. So I went over to a head nurse and asked her what she thought might be going on with my mother. And she said, "Well, you know, this is what I see when people are at the end. It may be near her time." Imagine—a nurse in the hospital who sees this thing all the time. Who would have a better perspective than hers?

And so I said to her, "So, from your point of view—having worked here for 20 years—this looks like the onset of dying? So what should we do?" And she said: "Well, if I were you, I would stop trying to prop her up with, you know, pumps and needles, and whatever you're doing, and consider increasing her morphine drip to give her more comfort from her pain. She'll drift off eventually. And that way, she can have a peaceful ending, and you'll all be here together to say a long, peaceful goodbye."

I thanked her. Then I went to my brother, and I said, "You know, you should speak to this head nurse. She thinks that Mom's condition is indicating that she's close to the end and we should remove the tubes and just make her comfortable and think about letting her go."

And my brother said to me, "Why? Because it's more convenient for you?" And I, of course, was devastated by this. This brother I loved so much once again was calling me on my selfishness. And I will admit again here that, by then, I was looking forward to my mother's passing. It was just too sad and too difficult, and was only getting worse every day.

I made him talk to the doctors. And it wasn't until the doctors talked him through it that my brother agreed that the process of letting her leave us could begin—removing the tubes and making her comfortable and increasing the morphine. Once that agreement had been made—once my brother was able to say, "Okay, you're right. We have to let her go"—once that happened, then we just became very united in seeing her out well.

I remember sitting with him outside the hospital once this decision had been made, and there were still going to be many hours ahead of us before she actually died. He was saying, "I can't believe this is the day that Mom is going to die." It was a Friday. We're Jewish, and we went and bought some candlesticks and candles and some really nice CDs to play in her room. Stuff my father would like to hear, too. I made sure that as many machines were turned off as possible to stop the beeping and humming, and we did whatever we could to have a peaceful vigil. We lit candles and listened to music and sang to her and talked to her for 8 hours, hoping she could hear us. We were exhausted by the time her breathing finally stopped.

Sadly, she struggled almost to the end. And so, in my brother's mind, even now, he believes that she was fighting death, and that she wasn't ready. But I don't know if she ever would have been ready for death. I will never really know. And my brother has come to terms with the fact that it's possible that we did the right thing.

Part II
Taking Steps

7

Stepping Forward—Helping When They Can Manage and Preparing for When They Can't

Marian Franklin—77, widowed, somewhat arthritic, and mildly diabetic—continued to live in her old neighborhood, which had gone dangerously downhill. Her children, comfortably settled in pleasant suburbs, were frantic. They worried when their mother went out alone and worried when she stayed home alone. They complained that she "exhausted" herself with volunteer work at her church and were upset every fall when she went apple picking at a friend's orchard. She kept telling them that she was fine, steadily refused their offers of help, and rejected their repeated invitations to make her home with one of them. She was reasonably content with her life.

Eventually, her children found the opportunity they needed when an elderly woman was brutally mugged in the lobby of Mrs. Franklin's building. All the tenants were fearful and understandably upset, including Mrs. Franklin herself, and her children were able to persuade her that she was unsafe in her apartment. Within a short time they helped her move out to live with her younger son in a room they redecorated especially for her. They were delighted that they were finally able to "give Mother a good life," but wondered why she didn't seem to enjoy it the way they expected she would. She was somewhat bewildered during the move, remained apathetic and uninvolved in her new surroundings, and seemed physically frail. Everyone was heartbroken when she died of pneumonia less than a year later. They all continued to believe that they could have prolonged her life if only they had insisted she make the move earlier.

I T COULD BE SAID THAT MRS. FRANKLIN WAS FORTUNATE. She had loving children, eager and able to help her as she grew older. Many older mothers and fathers would envy her. It could also be said that she was unfortunate, because those loving children were unable to understand the kind of help she needed. With the best of intentions, they weakened rather than supported her.

"Help" sounds like a simple four-letter word, like "love." But many steps are involved in the process, and being ready and willing to help is only the first. A second step is knowing the right kind of help to give, and when. Many well-meaning adult children take the first step easily, but are unable to take the second. Their best intentions can be undermined by lack of knowledge, lack of understanding, or total misunderstanding. In many instances, they jump to false conclusions about what is best. That's often because too little listening is done and too little attention paid to the desires and inclinations of older adults. Too little time is taken to understand them and to evaluate the adaptation they are making to old age and its accompanying losses. For their help to be truly effective, families have to arrive at a realistic assessment of what kind of help—and how much—an older person actually needs to get along.

What does old age mean, anyway? Although it's commonly used to describe the sector of the population 65 and over, that may cover a 30-year or longer time span in some lives. The over-65 population is a tremendously diverse group, and as individuals they go through many different stages. Your father may live one kind of life at 65, another at 75, another at 85, and still another at 95. The young are inclined to forget that the needs of older people are determined not by chronological age but by their ability to manage their lives. A term gaining in use is "functional age" to reflect the capabilities of older adults. As one daughter described her father, "he may be 85 years old, but he lives and behaves like a 70-year-old."

In the next chapters we shall consider the help and understanding likely to be supportive to the older adults at strategic points along the continuum of need, ranging from the totally independent to the totally dependent:

- Older people who can manage alone and know it
- Older people who can manage alone but think they can't
- Older people who can manage alone some of the time
- Older people who need around-the-clock care

Those in each of these categories have suffered, to varying degrees, the losses and stresses of aging. Many are able to handle the transitions in their lives successfully and find at least some compensation. Others give up without a struggle. Older adults are capable of an amazing range of adaptations, and their capacities can be strengthened by the effective support of their children—or weakened by their children's well-meaning interference. Although with some particularly determined parents, children have no effect at all!

"I'm Okay"—Those Who Can Manage and Know It

A surprising number of the older adults take old age in their stride. They are somewhat content with their lot, and would be justifiably offended if anyone were to suggest that they were not competent to handle their own daily routines of cooking, cleaning, dressing, and shopping. In addition, they feel perfectly able to take care of their own finances, entertainment, and health. Whether they are continuing to work or enjoying a quiet life of reading, watching TV, and seeing a few friends, they still consider themselves functioning members of society, perfectly capable of making their own decisions and deciding what is best for themselves—by themselves. A self-reliant octogenarian has a real sense of pride and personal dignity; he may even delight in flaunting his age and letting the world know he's not finished yet. The energetic older couple who insist on roughing it on camping vacations take pleasure in ignoring the anxious pleas of younger relatives that they vacation instead in a "safe and comfortable resort."

There are numbers of remarkable older people who even chart new courses for their lives and experience a kind of rebirth. Stories appear frequently in the press of 70- or 80-year-olds who have just completed the requirements for a high school diploma, a college degree, or a graduate degree. It is not unusual today for a retired businessman to start a new business venture at a time of life when many of his contemporaries are in wheelchairs. Those admirable examples are endlessly reassuring to the younger generation, who can say to themselves, "That's what I'll be like when I'm old." The world loves a "fabulous old guy" or a "spunky old gal."

Even though your parents don't want to be dependent, they probably like to know that you are dependable.

If your parents currently fall into that enviable group, the best approach to take is to give them quiet support. Let them know that you accept, even admire, the lifestyle they have chosen for themselves. Jumping in with unsolicited advice or offering unwanted help may only disrupt the valuable equilibrium they have established, or create bad feelings. A good rule to follow here would be to let it be known that you are willing to discuss things with them and that you are willing to help if they want you to help. Even though your parents don't want to be dependent, they probably like to know that you are dependable. Lewis Carroll made this point in *Alice's Adventures in Wonderland:*

> "You are old, Father William," the young man said,
> "And your hair has become very white;
> And yet you incessantly stand on your head—
> Do you think, at your age, it is right?"

Father William wasn't asking for anyone's help or permission to stand on his head. His feat was a bit unusual, but if he could still perform it, how could it possibly be considered wrong? If your parents have established a way of life they feel works for *them*, it would be foolish to try to impose a different lifestyle just because *you* feel it is more appropriate.

It is easy enough to take this live-and-let-live attitude when your parents adopt a socially acceptable mode of life in, say, a safe, comfortable retirement village that offers plenty of congenial companionship. But what if they adopt a way of life that stands *you* on your head? What if your father still pursues an active sex life and your mother talks about her dates and going dancing? What if you fear for their safety (as did Mrs. Franklin's children) or find their friends embarrassing? A laissez-faire philosophy may not be so easy then. But if your father's choices seem to be working for him, you may have to keep reminding yourself that it's his life and not yours. It does not matter that you would *prefer* him to live differently, nor what the neighbors say to your face or behind your back. If he is able to take command of his own destiny, however irritating his behavior, he deserves a willing go-ahead. If, however, a parent's accommodation does not work well—for example, your father's gambling is depleting his resources, or your mother ignores a dangerous physical symptom—then some interference may be necessary.

The Pseudo-Helpless—Those Who Can Manage but Think They Can't

In contrast to resolute, independent older adults, who insist on managing their own lives, another group of their contemporaries presents a totally different set of problems to their children.

Your mother may be in relatively good health, enjoying solid enough finances and fairly pleasant living conditions. She may be managing perfectly well. But the problem is that you can't convince her that she is doing fine. Unable to adapt to the decrements of aging, she shows increasing self-pity and inordinate anxiety, while demanding unreasonable amounts of time from you and your family. Sometimes this behavior is short-lived, following a time of crisis, but it may become chronic.

Some in later life who feel they cannot abide their old age by themselves often tyrannize their children. Chapter 3 described how one particular child may be chosen or may assume the role of "Mother's support," sometimes becoming a martyr to Mother's old age. Some of the pseudo-helpless like to claim that they can manage, but the minute the focus of attention is drawn away from them, they will cry for help. These older adults often have a sixth sense of the exact moment when the child they depend on is particularly involved elsewhere.

John Farnetti's mother managed quite well some of the time, but could turn helpless overnight, particularly when her only son and his family were about to leave on a trip, when a new baby was about to arrive, or when a particularly important business deal was pending. At every crisis in his life, John could always expect that the phone would ring (usually late at night) and he would hear his mother's voice saying faintly, "You're going to be very upset with me." This was the dreaded but familiar opener: the overture to a new crisis that would demand John's immediate attention. He was expected to put his personal affairs on a back burner while he made an emergency trip to another state to settle his mother's problem yet again. It must be admitted that John allowed his mother to run his life and his family's.

Older adults who behave this way do so for many reasons. One is simply a lack of knowledge about the normal aging process. Each minor physical symptom becomes exaggerated into a drama of fear and anxiety. Given greater understanding, they may be able to take their physical ups and downs with greater equanimity. In some cases, when logical explanations and reassurance are given by a child, a nurse, a doctor, or a social worker, anxiety can be allayed and episodes of panic prevented. For others, however, reassurance and understanding do no good at all. They make self-pity their way of life, exploiting their difficulties to gain an inappropriate amount of time and attention.

Eighty-year-old Carl Forbes was obsessed with his failing hearing and had been for years. His daughter, who had been helpful and sympathetic for a whole decade, was relieved when he finally agreed to a hearing aid, but she could not enjoy peace for long. Within the next few months, when his hearing improved, he began to complain of intestinal pain and sinus trouble. By moving on to new symptoms, he could regain the attention he lost when his hearing improved.

If life histories were to be taken of such pseudo-helpless older folks, they would probably reveal that these people had always been overly dependent. Old age merely provides a golden opportunity to exploit the pattern more openly. Their helpless behavior can also cloak a guilt-provoking twist of the knife, a ploy the parent may have used throughout life with various family members. Variations on the old tune—"I brought you up and now you leave me out in the cold"— are favorite types of guilt producers. Comments like that can incite tension headaches or irritable bowel syndrome in quite sturdy children! And they are probably meant to do just that. Admittedly, there are situations in which such bitter complaints are rooted in reality, and there are children who deserve them. But the words are just as frequently used as ammunition against the most devoted of children, who keep asking themselves, "What more can I do?"

When to Say No

Just as unreasonable demands on the part of young children, teenagers, and adult friends can and should be turned down, it's not wise to give in to unreasonable demands from your parents. The boundaries you have set for yourself—for what you can and cannot do—must set the agenda, not your parent's demands. If you have no boundaries, the resulting bitterness, tension, and resentment building up inside you may render you completely ineffective when your parents legitimately do need your help. Some children, who have never learned to say no firmly, find their only solution lies in cutting loose completely and disappearing from their parents' lives, a potentially guilt-producing act in itself. There is no reason to grit your teeth, penalize your children, or disrupt your work while trying to satisfy your mother's unreasonable demands. Your pulse will be steadier if you can learn to say no.

Once you've said it, you may be surprised that your answer is often accepted with relative equanimity and little argument. Your mother may be relieved to know where you stand and exactly what she can expect of you. She also may catch a supportive message that tells her, "We will not treat you like a baby, because you aren't a baby. You are not helpless; you're doing all right on your own." There may be initial bitterness, but if you can live through this period, the ground rules for living will be more firmly established for everyone.

> *The boundaries you have set for yourself—for what you can and cannot do—must set the agenda, not your parent's demands.*

"But I Can't Say No"

"My parents worked so hard all their lives, they deserve to be pampered and indulged," you may tell yourself. Still, it would be a good idea to think things through less sentimentally and consider the debilitating effect on your parents themselves if you allow them to become unnecessarily dependent on you. A greater gift to them might really be to resist behavior that helps them grow old prematurely.

What else might be getting in your way? Guilt, shame, anxiety, and anger—all those unresolved legacies of manipulative parents to their children—make it seem easier just to say yes. Then you don't have to deal with those unpleasant emotions directly. If you find it impossible to say no directly, it helps to run through the probable long-range effects on yourself and the rest of the family. Consider the consequences of saying yes.

> How can I say no when Mother suddenly announces she wants to spend the summer with us?
>
> If I say yes and let her come, we'll have to give up the camping trip to Camilla that we've been planning and saving for all year. Ruth won't be able to have her best friend spend August with us because there won't be enough beds. The dog will have to be boarded because Mother's allergic. And I'll have to give up coaching the softball team because Mother hates it if I'm out at her suppertime.

After looking at the results of giving in to Mother, a better question to ask yourself might be, "How can I say yes?"

> How can I say no when my father says he doesn't want to live alone in the big house anymore? But he won't give it up, and he wants us to give up our apartment and move in with him.
>
> If I say yes, it will mean that Jim will have to commute an hour longer to his job, the kids will have to change schools, I'll be tied down with extra housework, I'll have to give up my hospital work, and I'll have to cook two sets of meals because of Dad's low-fat diet.

How can you say yes?

> How can I say no to Mother when she begs to come to live with me? She's afraid to live alone, even though she's managing

quite well. If I say yes, we'll both go under. Mother is 85 and I'm nearly 60.

I'm having enough problems of my own. If she comes to live with me, I'll never be able to take care of both of us.

Saying no to Mother will be kinder to her and to yourself.

Saying no doesn't mean that the subject is closed and that the desires of the older generation are ignored. A different approach can be taken: "I'm sorry, Mother (or Father). I know things are hard for you now, but your idea just won't work. Let's try to figure out a different way that's better for all of us." By rejecting the unreasonable demands of the pseudo-helpless, the younger generation need not always be accused of callousness, selfishness, or indifference. The firm *no* can ultimately be the greatest blessing to both generations.

Prepare for the Day When They Can't Manage

Whether your parents can manage and know it, or can manage but *think* they can't, there is no guarantee that the situation will continue. The time to look into the future is while they are still living independently. It's also the time to explore what will happen if and when their independence runs out.

Some of the blows of old age are beyond all remedy, and no amount of thinking ahead can soften them. But many can be averted completely or made easier to bear. Advance planning is probably one of the most important and most neglected areas of help for older people. That is why so many of us are caught unprepared when a crisis occurs in our parents' lives.

Advance planning is probably one of the most important and most neglected areas of help for older people.

Ideally, planning should start in young adulthood, although few young people make any such moves other than entering a pension or savings plan. Certainly, planning should begin by the middle years. But it is never really too late to begin, and if your parents are in their 60s now, they are likely to have quite a future ahead of them—well into their 80s and older.

It's great to be able to boast with pride about a parent's independence, good health, and varied activities. It's wonderful to be able to say, as some 50-year old sons and daughters can, "Mother's 85, but she looks 65 and does everything for herself. Last year, she traveled to Europe alone." The strong possibility is that this 85-year-old woman will run into some type of difficulty before she's finished, unless a massive stroke, a fatal heart attack, or a plane crash makes it possible for her to die with her boots on.

Serious difficulties can lie ahead for even the most active parents, if for no other reason than because tragic gaps exist in the support our society provides. The sad results of insufficient forethought are seen over and over again in hospital emergency rooms or in substandard nursing homes where families literally have to "store" older relatives who can no longer manage. Such a crisis might have been avoided if they or their families had given any advance thought to what would happen to them. When problems occur because of lack of planning, the family usually feels the greatest sense of failure, but the older person who has not thought ahead should share the blame. Careful anticipation of future crises by all concerned can offset the shock, grief, disruption, and guilt that accompany them. When it comes to planning for old age, a stitch in time saves more than the proverbial nine—it can save whole families.

Let's Talk about It

Although it is easier said than done, the best way to initiate planning is in the context of respectful, relaxed discussion. Some parents bring up the subject spontaneously with their children or with one particular child whom they consider (sometimes mistakenly) to be the most level-headed or caring. They want to talk about what they will do if they become sick, if their money runs out, or when one of them dies. They may just want to talk and have someone listen, or they may ask for help, suggestions, and guidance. Some middle-aged children, however, are not receptive to these overtures because of their own anxieties about death and dying.

Other parents play their cards closer to the chest, remaining secretive about their resources and about any thoughts they have for the future, and becoming angry and insulted if you insinuate that there could be trouble ahead. Of course, underneath the anger may lie a fear they cannot face. Some will close any discussion about the future with the flat statement, "Oh, don't worry about me. I'll be gone soon enough." Or they may loudly deny that their health could ever fail them.

> Emma Dexter, at 77, was admired by her younger relatives and friends. Widowed and still living alone in her comfortable apartment, she dined out, went to the theater and concerts, traveled, and continued to work as a volunteer at her favorite hospital. It dawned on her suddenly that some of her younger colleagues avoided discussing any subject with her that was related to old age, even the tragic problems of some of the elderly patients—sensitive that they might be personally upsetting to her. As soon as she realized this, Emma quickly reassured them at a coffee break.
>
> "Don't worry about my feelings," she said. "Old age isn't a touchy subject with me. I never believed I'd enjoy it as much as I do. I love talking about it—even the problems I have. Ask me anything you want."
>
> "Are you sure, Emma?" asked a young volunteer tentatively.
>
> "Of course," she replied.
>
> "Well, then, I've often wondered—when one of these awful stroke cases comes in, does it worry you? Do you think about yourself and what could happen to you?" the younger woman said.
>
> "That," replied Emma, turning on her heel and walking out of the room, "is a subject I never think about."

Your parents may share Emma's feelings, and if they have any plans for their old age tucked away in the back of their minds, they may refuse to talk about them. Their feelings should be respected, and they should not be forced too suddenly into a discussion of the future. But the subject need not be dropped completely. You deserve to know what they are thinking, particularly if you are likely to play a part in their plans. In fact, *not* looking forward with parents can cause adult children extra anxiety—in addition to the worries their jobs, children, and marriages already impose.

Tom's parents had always firmly declared, "We never want to be a burden to you!" But after his father died suddenly of a heart attack at age 75 and Tom's work with a biotech company required him and his family of four to move to North Carolina, he began to worry that his mother back in Rhode Island might, in fact, become a burden. What was her financial situation, really? Would she need his support some day? Would she agree to sell her house? As it was, Tom and his wife, Jen, were struggling to save for their own children's college educations. For his own sake as well as hers, he needed to talk with Mom.

When the casual approach does not serve to open a real discussion of your parents' plans or anxieties about the future, a more direct approach may be necessary. Tom broached the subject with his mother by saying, "Mom, Jen and I have been doing a lot of thinking about you. You're doing fine now, and we hope things stay this way, but you never talk to us about what you'll do if you get sick. We'd like to know what you're thinking and what you'd like us to do." Another way to inch into the conversation is to share with your parents any steps you have taken to prepare for the future. By sharing your plans with them, you may make them feel less patronized and more willing to share their plans with you.

If nothing works and your parents steadily refuse to share their plans with you or even to plan at all, you can do some exploring on your own so that you will be ready with some reasonable alternatives if a sudden crisis arises.

If nothing works and your parents steadily refuse to share their plans with you or even to plan at all, you can do some exploring on your own so that you will be ready with some reasonable alternatives if a sudden crisis arises. Forethought on their behalf should focus on four major areas: their health and safety, their functional abilities, their social world (including the big question: "Should they live with you?"), and what may be the most crucial of all, their finances. As the old adage goes: "An ounce of prevention is worth a pound of cure"— applicable for the young as well as the old.

Prevention Measures to Facilitate Health and Safety

Regular medical checkups are important for all of us, but should occur with greater frequency in older adults (at least once a year, according to the American Academy of Geriatrics). A seemingly healthy 75-year-old may have an undetected condition that can lead to a catastrophic illness or further physical deterioration. Early detection and early treatment can prevent some conditions from progressing further. Incipient diabetes and high blood pressure, for instance, can be brought under control if they are detected early. They do not need to become fatal or incapacitating, and preventive interventions, such as weight control, increased exercise, and certain medications, can make this possible.

Basic health education is essential for everyone. In fact, many sociable older adults learn a great deal from each other as well as from the Internet and newspapers. Yet too many others, old and young alike, remain medically in the dark, unaware of the danger signals of a health crisis. Health awareness also includes the importance of good nutrition. Medical studies repeatedly show that poor nutrition is the cause of many problems formerly attributed to the aging process. Since older people living alone tend to eat only the foods they like and that are inexpensive and easy to prepare, gradual decline may come as much from inadequate diet as from the aging process. There are those who may hardly eat at all if they have no one to eat with, and some may just pick at some cheese and crackers. When they become seriously ill and are hospitalized, they often not only recover from their illness but also regain much of their former strength. Bland as it is, the balanced diet offered by hospital dietitians has been known to revitalize the very patients who complain the loudest: "The food here is terrible! I wouldn't give it to a dog!"

Close attention also needs to be paid to the hazards of the overuse of alcohol in older adults, whose tolerance level decreases with age, and to potential problems with prescription and over-the-counter drugs that they may be taking (discussed in Chapter 12).

Provisions for personal safety are equally essential. It is never too soon to ensure that the home is outfitted with simple installations, such as grab bars in the bathroom and railing on outside steps. The normal vision changes that occur in later life require good lighting in critical areas, such as stairways, as well as high contrast on telephone keypads and caution in operating a vehicle. Night driving, for example, becomes increasingly difficult for many older people, and they may have to alter their driving habits to ensure their safety and the safety of others.

Even if we cannot stop the aging process, we do have the power to stem the tide and be in control of our own bodies and behaviors to the extent possible. Bodily care and safety may not make older people live longer, but surely it will help them to live better and feel more youthful. As T. Franklin Williams, MD, former director of the National Institute on Aging, put it: "the trick is to die young as late as possible."

Developing New Interests for Older Adults

Progressive arthritis may be a painful blow to a woman who is known for her fine embroidery. Failing eyesight can disrupt the life of the avid reader, and loss of hearing may end hours of joy for the music lover. The active 65-year-old who still spends hours on the tennis court may at some point need to take up a less strenuous sport. "When Dad's painful old knee injury kicked up again, he finally hung up his tennis racket," says one son. "So for his birthday, we got him a kayak for the lake, and he loves it—especially at the calm, sunset hour, when the fish jump."

If your parents have to give up some of the pastimes they've enjoyed the most, you and they will usually see it coming. Fortunately, much more is known today about engaging activities that can be undertaken successfully, even by disabled older people, who are continually disproving the old adage "You can't teach an old dog new tricks." Today 60-, 70-, and even 80-year-olds are proving it is not too late to take up music, painting, yoga, meditation, pottery, indoor gardening, or creative writing. An instructor at a correspondence school for writers reports that many of her most imaginative students are 65 and older, and some are in their 80s.

Opportunities for paid or volunteer work may be found through government programs or groups such as the Retired & Senior Volunteer Program (RSVP; visit www.cssny.org/rsvp/). Senior citizen centers in the community often provide a variety of activities, from stretch classes to book groups to instruction in basic computer

Safety First—and Other Initial Steps

Although he lived many states away, Tom took the following thoughtful steps to help prepare his still-independent mother—and himself—for the future:

Helped Make Her Home "Age-Appropriate"

- Installed grab bars in the tubs and showers
- Eliminated slippery area rugs
- Carpeted the stairs
- Removed the steps that led to the kitchen and installed a ramp with banisters, in case she had to use a wheelchair or walker.

Improved Means of Immediate Communication

- Convinced her to carry her cell phone when driving and at other times in case of an emergency
- Programmed her cell phone with emergency numbers in the phone's "contacts" list

Did Critical Advance Paperwork

Tom copied the following information, with his mother's help, and filed it at his own home:

- Names and phone numbers of her close friends and neighbors
- Addresses and phone numbers of her physicians and lawyers
- Her will, her living will, and her health care and power of attorney proxies
- Information about her health insurance, pension, bank accounts, and investments, and an extra key to her safe deposit box ("Penny's Personal Papers Inventory" in Appendix C can serve as a guide)

If your parents are secretive, particularly about their financial affairs, ask them to fill out *Penny's Personal Papers Inventory* and file it in an accessible place.

skills. There is a lot of time to be filled in the later decades, even when energy is limited. Encouraging your parents to find gratifying activities can have a salutary effect on their total health and well-being.

Facing the Dreaded "What If?"

Somewhere, deep in our souls, we all believe "it won't happen to me—or mine." And it may not. Yet any discussion of future health care has to touch on the dreaded subject of debilitating conditions or catastrophic illness. Either situation, if mentally or physically incapacitating, may make it impossible for an older person to care for himself or herself. Naturally, this is the most painful topic to discuss, and some parents cannot face it at all. Your mother may be skirting the subject when she talks to you about how she will live "after Father is gone." But she may not be able to move farther ahead and discuss what could happen if she has a stroke "that paralyzes me." On the other hand, it is sometimes the younger generation who can't bear to think of illness and disability striking their parents. "When the time comes that I can't walk anymore," a severely crippled mother might begin—and then be quickly interrupted by her daughter with, "Oh, Mother, don't talk that way. It's not going to happen."

But what if Mother has already done a lot of thinking about the future? She probably has some strong feelings about her preferences—for a good long-term care facility, perhaps (Chapter 10 deals with this choice)—and really wants to voice them. These preferences should be explored whenever possible, because you can be a big help in focusing or facilitating them. Parents who dread the idea of nursing homes may hope to remain right where they are. An investigation of how much outside care is available in a given community could be reassuring and can establish whether this hope is realistic. (Chapter 9 reviews these community resources.) Or a parent may imply that she hopes to move in with you, another relative, or a special friend. If you already know that such moves will be impossible, make it clear as soon as you can and then move on quickly to alternative plans. And beware of making promises that can't be kept, such as "I promise never to put you in a nursing home." Especially beware of deathbed promises. You may rue the day when, in tears, you vowed to your dying mother, "Of course, I'll bring Dad to live with us." Deathbed promises can put a stranglehold on the living, producing the same chain of disastrous consequences as the question discussed earlier: "How can I say no?" When such promises have to be broken, an adult child may be accused of bad faith by the rest of the family and by an even more severe judge: himself or herself.

Nothing is lost by anticipating future problems and making a tentative plan of action. Like insurance that may never need to be used, the plans are comforting to have in reserve. They may never need to be activated if your parents are spared disabling illness. But if disaster does come, you will not have to go through the additional trauma of being caught unprepared, floundering helplessly, and having to resort to makeshift, unsatisfactory solutions.

Nothing is lost by anticipating future problems and making a tentative plan of action.

Living Arrangements—What Are Their Choices?

The future well-being of the elderly depends greatly on the social supports they will be able to rely on. Who will be around in the future for your parents to turn to for affection and companionship? What continuing contacts will be possible with friends, family, or other meaningful groups? Where will they get help with chores, transportation, and small emergencies? How accessible is their housing to their church or temple and community recreational activities? Discussions of advance planning with your parents should include all of these questions.

"Aging in place," a term coined by gerontologists, recognizes the strong desire of older adults to grow old in their own homes and familiar surroundings. According to the 2000 census, 90% of people age 60 and older preferred to stay in the same home or county. One result of this desire is a new concept among neighbors who organize a "support community," setting up a system combining volunteers and professional helpers for services—transportation, home maintenance, home health care, social activities, and even legal advice. Pioneered by the Beacon Hill Village in Boston, the idea has caught on in other neighborhoods as well. "I don't want to be packed off to some ghetto for old people," said one healthy member, age 67. "We're helping to form a support community now so we won't have to leave our homes later."

More often, physically disabled or financially strapped older people suffer isolation. They may not be able to visit friends easily or have friends visit them. Furthermore, if they live far from medical services, it may one day cost too much in physical and financial terms to get essential medical care.

In some cases, moving to a different location could provide greater safety and easier social contacts. Even if that necessity seems clear to you, you may still have a hard time convincing your parents. Point out to them that their friends are slowly vanishing, their neighborhood is going downhill, or the house is really too big for them to maintain—and still they insist on staying "at home." Because their home means so much to them, many older people willingly put up with loneliness and serious inconvenience so that they can stay right where they are.

But if your older parents are ready to give up the old homestead, where would they go? Any move, particularly a distant one, should also be weighed carefully.

Unable to face another winter shoveling snow, Ed Meyer moved to a condo on the Caribbean island of St. Kitts, where his oldest friends also had a home. The sunshine and the views were splendid, the medical services elementary. Two years later, when chest pains and tests revealed blocked heart arteries, Ed had to be flown to a Miami hospital for an emergency bypass operation. After his initial stage of recovery, he and his family faced the next question: now where?

A community several thousand miles away may make sense for the stage when your parents are "young-old." But it may not be the best solution when they become "old-old." What if they become incapacitated far away and need your help? What if they need a nursing home and there is none convenient in their new location? Before your parents make a move to a distant place, it is important to voice your reservations in advance. "It's your move," you might say pleasantly, "and I'm not going to stop you. But remember, if you're way out there, I can't promise I'll be able to visit as often as I do now—and you'll hardly ever be able to see Aunt May and Uncle George."

Should They Live with You?

This question can provoke stabs of guilt in even the most resilient children. Somewhere way back, many of us formed the belief that, yes, indeed, aging parents *should* live with us—and that there is something lacking in us if we don't make it possible. In Lou Meyer's short story "Live a Little," published in the *New Yorker* in 1980, the narrator describes meeting Abrams, an outspoken elderly resident in his mother's nursing home:

> There are tears in Abrams's eyes as he turns to me. "How is it, young man, that your poor mother, a veritable jewel among women, is spending her remaining years living here in the Home? Wasn't there a small place for her in your house? Under the sink? On the piano? In a dresser drawer?"

We can laugh at Abrams's words, but accompanying the laughter may be a prick of guilt. It can be painful when you have to admit that you cannot ask your mother or father to live with you. You may have perfectly legitimate reasons, such as insufficient living space, ill health, or no settled home. Or perhaps there are long-standing personality clashes: "She'd drive me crazy in a minute," or "My marriage couldn't take it." Then how much more painful it would be to take such a giant step, invite your mother to live with you, and then find out later that it just plain doesn't work. What seemed a loving act may result in lasting bitterness and strain between you.

If you are feeling, however reluctantly, that you *ought* to ask your mother to live with you, it might be comforting to know that other people share that reluctance. National surveys consistently show that the majority of adults in the United States, young and old alike, consider it a bad idea for elderly parents and their children to live together. Only a small percentage of elderly parents live with their sons or daughters. You probably assume that the strongest opposition to such an arrangement comes from the younger generation, but surveys show that the older the parents, the less likely they are to favor living with their children. They do not want to be

If you are feeling, however reluctantly, that you ought to ask your mother to live with you, it might be comforting to know that other people share that reluctance.

Should Mother Live With You? A Test for Both the Parent and the Family

- Most important: how does your spouse feel about it?
- What kind of financial arrangements are being considered?
- Is there enough living space for everyone to be comfortable and have some privacy?
- Will she depend completely on your household for companionship and entertainment?
- Can you *really*, *honestly* expect to live comfortably together? Do your personalities clash?
- When she visited you in the past, did you always count the days until she left?
- Can she take a back seat in the running of the household and the rearing of the children?
- Would she, because of temperament, education, or social experience, feel continually out of place in your home? With your friends?
- Will you be able to provide ongoing, accessible, competent medical care?
- Do you treasure your privacy?
- Would it be wise to uproot her from her familiar surroundings? Her friends? Her church? Her doctor?

If you and your mother manage to pass this test well, you have a good chance of creating a successful two- or three-generation family. If you fail the test, it is better to know it before you find yourself tied into a situation that is unworkable for everyone.

burdens. In fact, many declare flatly, long before the issue comes up, that they will "never, under any circumstances," live with any of their children. Some parents even mean it. Ironically enough, it is often the children of those very parents who press the invitation most strongly.

And yet, multigenerational families living in one household do occur, often for financial or cultural reasons. In some cases, a healthy older person can be a great help to have around, able to shop, cook, or provide child care. Rather than asking a parent to live with them permanently, some children think a part-time invitation is the best solution: "Mother lives with us in the summer, and then she goes to my brother Vic's until New Year's. She's at Beth's all spring. We've decided that's the best arrangement for all of us." It may well be a good arrangement for the children, but what about Mother? Older people usually function best with stable roots and less change. Mother, in that case, must have felt she was on the road all the time. A more permanently satisfactory situation might have been possible.

Should a parent plead to live with you, try to avoid emotion and base your choice on cold, careful analysis of your own situation, the wishes of the rest of your immediate family, and the history of your relationship. Is there adequate living space so that all generations can have some comfort and privacy? You must also consider whether the older person will be completely dependent on you for social contacts, or will be able to maintain important relationships with his or her church, community groups, and friends.

Most of all, do not move into the future on the basis of unspoken or unaired assumptions.

Kathleen Graham lived comfortably with her husband until his death. She was left financially well off and remained healthy enough to keep her own apartment, but it was generally assumed by her children and relatives that she would move in with her only daughter if she ever became incapacitated At least, that was assumed by her three sons. Margaret, the daughter, by remaining silent, seemed to share the family assumption. In reality, Margaret was far from eager for the move, and her husband and children were equally against it. Whenever she visited, Mrs. Graham usually managed to tangle with her son-in-law and upset her grandchildren. To complicate things, Mrs. Graham had a hidden competitive relationship with her daughter that made it difficult for Margaret to accept comfortably her role as mother and wife.

But Margaret kept quiet out of her sense of duty, her guilt, and her concern over what everyone else would say. No alternative plans were made, therefore, and when Mrs. Graham suffered a paralytic stroke, she was brought to live in Margaret's house after she had made a partial recovery. Her presence caused all the problems that Margaret had anticipated and feared previously, as well as new problems resulting from her mother's illness. Eventually, Mrs. Graham had to be resettled in a nearby nursing home. She felt betrayed as long as she lived, and Margaret never completely recovered from her feeling of failure.

Should They Live Near You?

Many adult children prefer that their parents live near them in anticipation of the time when one or both need help. Over and over again, the story is told of a son or daughter, whose parents have moved away from them to a warmer climate, having to commute long distances to help out when the parent becomes ill or disabled. Yet in this mobile society, it is often the children who must move, and who subsequently urge the parent to move near them.

In questioning whether parents should settle near you, many of the same issues about their ultimate welfare, such as community, medical, and social supports, apply.

In questioning whether parents should settle near you, many of the same issues about their ultimate welfare, such as community, medical, and social supports, apply. In particular, would it be wise to uproot them from their familiar surroundings? Undoubtedly, having them near you is preferable to traveling long distances to see them or arranging for care from afar. One solution is inviting them to move to a retirement community or long-term care facility near you.

Sarah moved from California many years ago and lived near her children and grandchildren in a New York suburb. Her own parents, now in their late 80s and growing more frail, were still living in their California home of 50 years. The anxiety of being so far from her parents and the wearing trips back and forth to California led Sarah to investigate a well-regarded retirement community near her home. However, she ran into a stone wall when she began broaching a possible move to her parents. Her mother was eager to move, but although Sarah pointed out all the advantages to her father, including pleasant apartments, meal service, and activities, he refused to discuss the matter any further. Finally, Sarah gave up and dropped the subject. But several months later, her father indicated that this "community living business" might not be a bad idea, and a plan was made to visit the residence.

After Sarah's suggestion was rejected, she stepped back in frustration. But this move gave her parents the time they needed to consider their options.

Another solution, if you and your parents want to live *near* each other, but not *with* each other, is an "in-law" apartment attached to a home or located over the garage. You have the advantage of both proximity and privacy. Modular homes that can be attached to your home or placed on your property are also a possibility. Known as ECHO Housing (Elder Cottage Housing Opportunities), these units cost about $25,000.

Should They Live with Others?

Those unfamiliar with the problems of old age automatically assume that when elderly parents can no longer live alone, there are only two choices for them—live with a child or enter a nursing home. That assumption is wrong. As Sarah's situation illustrates, there are other options. Special housing for the elderly is becoming increasingly available throughout the country. Sponsored by church organizations, community groups, and private investors, these facilities admit the relatively well and "independent" elderly and provide them with easy-to-care-for living units. Most also offer meals, housekeeping services, and recreational activities. Most important, perhaps, is the fact that they provide safety, companionship, and recreation. In some instances, assurances of care in the case of illness and disability are included. Advanced planning for special housing—when a parent is relatively healthy and active—is essential. A very disabled or ailing older person usually will not be admitted to these types of residences, which include:

- *Continuing Care Retirement Communities.* In these communities, older adults can live independently in their own quarters, but available to them are recreational programs, at least one meal a day, and health care and assistance if illness occurs. A skilled nursing facility home for around-the-clock care is part of the community or located close by. Those that include both skilled nursing and assisted living accommodations are usually referred to as "three stage" retirement communities. The guarantee of continuing care as an elder grows older and increasingly frail is a significant advantage of these communities. However, they are not inexpensive and thus are limited to those with financial resources. The older adult usually pays a significant upfront fee and monthly rent, or turns over his or her assets for long-term arrangements. Some of these facilities are located near residents' former homes, enabling them to age in place to some extent. Facilities under religious auspices may have significance for your parents if religion has played an important role in their lives.

- *Assisted Living Facilities.* These facilities are intended for the older person who can live in his or her own private quarters, but requires some supervision and help in managing. One or two meals a day in a congregate dining room are provided, as well as recreational programs. Monthly rental fees can range from $600 to over $4000. There is no guarantee of continuing care if an older person's condition deteriorates to the extent that he or she requires intensive or around-the-clock care. Some facilities maintain a home health care service, the costs of which are added to the monthly rent. Separate nursing home care may be required.

  Of benefit to older people and their families is the Continuing Care Accreditation Commission (CCAC), which sets standards for and accredits continuing care and other aging services. This accreditation helps ensure that a retirement community or other facility provides quality care. CCAC recently became a part of the long-standing Commission on Accreditation of Rehabilitation Facilities (CARF), which has available a list of accredited continuing care facilities (www .carf.org). The accreditation of assisted living facilities is expected to be implemented soon.

- *Subsidized Housing.* Subsidized housing (or "senior apartments") under charitable or government auspices is in short supply and only available to low-income elderly. Some services are available, but the waiting lists are long.

- *Shared Housing.* These arrangements are proliferating and include two or more unrelated older persons who decide to live together and share expenses, or more formal group living arrangements sponsored by community organizations. Akin to these arrangements are older couples or singles who live in proximity to others their age and share services as well as look after each other.

- *ECHO Housing* (Elder Cottage Housing opportunities) are temporary homes placed on the property of a single family house. Designed specifically for older adults, these homes allow for both privacy and close proximity to family members.

  Information about subsidized housing, shared housing, ECHO Housing, or other housing arrangements for older adults in your (or your parents' community) can be found at your local or area office on aging. You can locate this office at www.eldercare.gov or call 800–677–1116.

- *Naturally Occurring Retirement Communities* (NORCs). NORCs are housing developments, apartment buildings, or neighborhoods in which residents have lived for many years that now have a high concentration of older adults. Targeted health and social services are now provided to low-income elders in some of these communities as a result of public and private partnerships. You are fortunate if your parent lives in a NORC that is targeted for these services. You can read more about NORC supportive service programs at www.norcs.org.

Some older persons choose not to live in housing that includes only their own age group. They prefer to live near old and young alike. Yet a move may still be wise for them for reasons of safety, accessibility to services, social stimulation, and ease of housekeeping. When one member of an aging couple is debilitated and the other is not, the safety and supports mentioned earlier can relieve the active partner of constant concern, and give him or her more freedom to enjoy life, while still remaining at a spouse's side.

Certainly, the pros and cons should be weighed when considering any move. After you have found a perfect retirement community near your home, have you stopped to wonder whether the place will be equally perfect for your parents if it forces them to relocate from their familiar surroundings? The director of a retirement complex in a large midwestern university town reported that the majority of the residents made good adjustments, enjoying the range of activities and new friends. The poorest adjustments were made by those who had moved from a different state to be close to a son or a daughter. Having left homes, friends, and longstanding routines far behind, they had nothing familiar in their new situation except their children. Their children replaced the burden of long-distance worry with a different burden—boosting their parents' morale. This is why the ideal time for such a transition is when parents are active enough to make new friends and enjoy the offerings of the area—one reason why retirement communities have mushroomed near college towns.

What about Your Own Preparedness?

You may have been giving serious thought to your parents' old age and anticipating their future needs. But at the same time, have you given any thought to your own? You may be in fine shape now, at 40, 50, or 60, but your parents could live another 10, even 20 years or more. How much extra money or energy will you have to share with them then? You may be single or childless now and in a position to do a great deal for them, but what if you were to die young? The current extended life expectancy of older people creates the serious possibility that they will outlive their own children, a tragic but not uncommon occurrence.

If, when you contemplate your own situation 10 or 20 years from now, it seems unlikely you will be able to do much for your parents, it would be better to discuss this openly. If you remain silent, they may assume they can count on you and make no alternative plans for themselves. Adult children too frequently play games with their parents, sending out the message that they feel their parents want to hear rather than one that is accurate. An inability to send the correct message may stem from a daughter's need to be a "good parent" to her own parents, or from a son's need to prove that he is a better parent to them than they ever were to him.

> The Dodsons were a well-to-do couple with an apartment in Boston and vacation homes in Newport and Palm Springs. They suffered financial reverses in their later years, so at the time of Mr. Dodson's death, his widow was left literally penniless and quite resentful of her dead husband. Her son,

however, was able to recoup a small part of the family fortune through his own ingenuity, and for 10 years he was able to support his mother in an elegant apartment hotel with a live-in companion-housekeeper. After a time, the son suffered his own financial reverses and his health deteriorated. He continued to support his mother, although he could barely support himself and his family. Because of his own strong need not to seem a failure to his mother, as his father had been, he never admitted the financial drain she made on him. But eventually, he was forced to tell her that he was incapable of supporting her any longer. His mother was bitter and resentful, feeling, with justification, that if she had been told of the problems earlier, she could have made better plans for herself.

Preparing Does Not Mean Interfering

This chapter began with a strong warning against interfering with the successful lifestyles your parents may have developed. It may seem that a contradictory position has been taken in suggesting that you help them consider their future. Actually, there is no contradiction here. The goal is to encourage adult children and their aging parents to become partners in planning for the best choices possible. Family members can express their caring concern by helping to gather information and guidelines, suggest alternatives, and raise cautions. Parents, of course, will make the final decisions.

If they view your efforts with distrust and resentment, it may mean that they are simply not ready to start thinking ahead at the same time you are. On the other hand, they may respect, and even welcome, your opinion. If not, if all attempts fail and you make no progress at all, you'll at least have the comfort of knowing that, having explored some plans on your own, you'll be better prepared if the day comes when they cannot manage on their own.

The goal is to encourage adult children and their aging parents to become partners in planning for the best choices possible.

Bob Morris on Planning Ahead

There was no preparation. Even though I was lucky to have a brother who was very efficient—and very well off, and very responsible—we were blindsided by the conditions of the home that they had lived in their whole lives and didn't want to leave; we were blindsided by their inability to commit to having real help; we were shocked that they spoke of possibly moving to, you know, an assisted living community—and then changed their minds. And we absolutely did not know how to get into their home and make things better.

There were discussions for years about what to do. Maybe they could move to a residential community nearer to us. Or, maybe somewhere else? Well, in my house, the constant note that my mother had sounded was that a parent in a nursing home was a sinful thing. There was always that sword of Damocles hanging over our heads. They were discussing options, but never taking any action. You know, I think the only thing that we knew to do was to make sure that there was a living will in place. And other than that . . . nothing. Nothing.

We were just a classic textbook case of terrible, poor preparation. No safety bars in bathtubs until a couple of accidents happened; no help in the house; no thought, until things had just gotten so desperate. I'll tell you what happened in our case. My brother just swept in. He contacted and contracted with the assisted-living place that was near him, and he said to my parents, "That's it. Game over—you're in. You're out of this house—you're moving here to the city." My kids will come and see you all the time—we'll be around to visit you all the time. It's a lovely building on a beautiful block, and this is how it's gonna work."

Yeah, we were blindsided.

8

Stepping Up to the Dollars and Sense

Eighty-year-old Fran and her 85-year-old husband, Steve, lived quietly and comfortably in their own apartment not too far from their two sons. The brothers, much to their frustration, knew little about their parents' finances and were concerned how they might manage if either needed nursing home care. When their sons broached the subject of finances, Fran and Steve responded firmly, but nicely that such matters were not their business. Realizing that their parents would brook no interference in their lives, the sons decided to make a present to them—the services of a financial advisor. A frugal couple, Fran and Steve were very pleased with this gift, which helped them keep control of both their finances and their privacy.

MONEY CAN BE A TOUCHY SUBJECT, EVEN IN THE closest of families. Some men are unwilling to discuss their finances even with their wives. Widows may be equally secretive with their children. Adult children can avoid the subject for fear of stirring up bad feelings. There are still people who claim, proudly or smugly, "We don't discuss money in our family." That may have been a sign of good breeding in Victorian times, but these days, it can be a prelude to disaster.

Older adults can be secretive if they feel—sometimes correctly—that their children are prying to discover what inheritance can be expected. In the case of some affluent elders this can be substantial. While the family is relieved of concerns regarding medical expenses and the costs of long-term care, other worries may arise as adult children witness a dwindling inheritance or sibling conflict erupts over whom an aging parent is going to favor in his or her will.

Older adults can also be secretive if they are ashamed of having so little money. However, if approached tactfully, they may be willing to explore their financial future with you, or at the very least, like Fran and Steve, consult a financial advisor.

There is no need to imply that you question their ability to manage intelligently, but you may be able to point out pitfalls ahead that they have not considered, or benefits that are due them that they had not heard about. Some older people are fully aware of the economic realities that can face them as they age, but others may not realize that an ever-increasing proportion of their limited income will have to be devoted to health needs as time goes on. They may not have taken into consideration how inflation affects a fixed income by steadily eroding its buying power. It is also important to consider how they will be able to cope with the expenses of a serious illness, and to find out exactly how much of the cost will be covered by insurance.

Financial Preparedness

Whether or not your parents are willing to discuss the details of their own personal income and assets, you may find it helpful to inform yourself about the variety of financial supports available for older adults. Once you know what these supports are—the range of their coverage, who is eligible for them, and how they are administered—you will certainly have a more realistic understanding of your parents' current and future financial possibilities. But always remember that what you learn today may be changed tomorrow. The entire financial picture for older Americans is in a state of flux. Costs and benefits change from one year to the next. It is hoped that benefits will continue to change for the better, but there is always the danger of cut-backs in an uncertain economy.

Social Security

Social Security (also known as Old-Age and Survivors Insurance) has been a major source of income for older Americans for over 70 years. In 2002, it accounted for an average 39% of aggregate income for those 65 and older. (Pensions accounted for 19% of their income; personal assets, 14%; and earnings, 25%.) Eligibility for Social Security benefits is based upon the older person's work history, but benefits are also paid to family members and surviving members of retired workers and to disabled workers under the age of 65. In 2004, benefits were paid out to 48 million people.

You may feel somewhat reassured if your parents tell you that they are receiving money both from Social Security and from pension funds. But even though the intent of the Social Security Administration, when it was established in 1935, was to provide some ongoing financial security for Americans after retirement, inflation has turned that hope into a pipe dream for many, despite mandated annual cost-of-living adjustments. Pension checks and Social Security checks, even in combination, often cannot keep up with rising prices.

Pension checks and Social Security checks, even in combination, often cannot keep up with rising prices.

If your father retired before he was 65 (this is permitted after age 62), his checks are reduced accordingly. If he delayed retirement until after 65, his benefits are slightly higher. However, the age of eligibility for full retirement benefits is changing, except for those born in 1937 or earlier. For those born in later years, the age of eligibility increases incrementally, to the point that, currently, anyone born in 1960 or after will not be eligible until age 67.

If your mother is still alive and has been working, she is entitled to her own Social Security. If she did not work and make independent contributions, she then qualifies as your father's dependent and collects an amount equal to half his check. In other words, two people are thus entitled to one-and-a-half payments. If a wife who has worked finds that the Social Security benefits she would receive as her husband's dependent are higher than her own benefits would be, she may choose to be considered his dependent. This means, however, that she forfeits all contributions that she and her employer have made to the Social Security fund. (The same is true for a husband who chooses to be considered his working wife's dependent.)

What if both of your retired parents worked and both are receiving Social Security benefits—and then one of them dies? The survivor, either widow or widower, may then receive a survivor's benefit equaling the larger of the two. If the greater earner is the survivor, this benefit adds nothing. But in many cases, longer-living women—who were generally lower wage earners and may have had some gaps in employment for child-rearing—benefit. Of course, the death of a spouse also means that a household once counting on two Social Security checks now has only one.

If your mother has been collecting her own benefits and decides to remarry, her checks will not be affected. But if she has been collecting as your father's widow, she again has two choices: she can collect as your dead father's dependent, receiving half his benefits, but *losing her widow's status, which may have provided a larger amount*—or she can collect as the dependent wife of her second husband. She will obviously choose the system that pays better. But she may decide to choose neither and turn down a second marriage because it costs too much and she cannot afford the luxury.

> Five years after her husband's death, Carol Benson met Ron, a delightful retired accountant, at her bridge club. They dated for a year, and Carol, happily in love for the second time in her life, felt younger than she had in years. He was not wealthy, but loving and kind, with a great sense of humor. When they discussed marriage, however, it became clear that tying the knot would deprive her of her survivor's Social Security check—larger than her own had been—which she counted on to get along. Her other choice would be to become Ron's dependent, which also meant a loss of income. Although their children approved of Ron's and her remarriage, the two planned their future together with financial realities in mind—they lived together, but not as official husband and wife. At first, their church-going children were appalled. But they eventually got over it, saying, "Hey, it's Mom's choice and life."

By pooling their resources, Carol and Ron gained a somewhat greater state of financial security. Such a decision is particularly hard on older people with traditional values. But according to current Social Security regulations, no matter which way the pie is sliced, people— usually women—who did not work come out receiving the smaller share.

What does all that mean in cold cash? In June 2007 the average monthly Social Security payment for retired workers was $1,050. The maximum monthly payment, currently capped at $2,116, is an insufficient income on its own for many older Americans. Yet for many others, Social Security payments are the lifeline that keeps them from poverty. It has been estimated that, without Social Security benefits, the poverty rate among older women and persons of color would be more than 50%. It is little wonder that increasing numbers of older adults are continuing their careers or finding new jobs to supplement their retirement income.

It is important to note that if your father opted for early retirement benefits between ages 62 and 64 and keeps on working, he is subject to the Social Security earnings test that allows him in 2007 up to $12,960 in annual earnings without his Social Security benefits being affected. In 2000, the Senior Citizens Freedom to Work Act eliminated the earnings test for beneficiaries 65 and older. Although early retirement has become increasingly popular, a countertrend is currently under way. Eighty percent of younger workers now expect to work after the age of 65.

Any confusion that you or your parents feel about their benefits, entitlements, or eligibility can usually be cleared up by a visit to your local Social Security office, listed in the telephone directory under U.S. Government, Department of Health and Human Services, Social Security Administration. A staff member should be able to answer

---

Information on Social Security Benefits

- Visit your local office.
- Call 1-800-772-1213.
- Visit www.ssa.gov.

your questions and also to supply you with a variety of free pamphlets explaining the workings of Social Security.

Social Security in the Future

There is much apprehension about the future solvency of the Social Security system. Admittedly, it faces challenges, especially from the anticipated explosion of the over-65 population as the baby boomers enter the ranks of the elderly. The architects of the system established in 1935 expected that monies coming into the Trust Fund—contributed by the workers of America, the employers, and the self-employed—would always be greater than payments going out to support the retired, over-65 segment of the population as well as younger people who were disabled. But in those days, the ratio of old to young was much lower. This ratio has been steadily shifting over the years. In 1950, for every retired person collecting benefits, there were 7.5 workers. In 1986, there were 5; and in 2000, 4.5. By the year 2020, there may be only 3.3 workers for every beneficiary. Legislators are debating a variety of different solutions to shore up the threatened system, including further raising the age at which benefits may begin. While significant revisions may be made in the future, the chances are minimal that these will affect any retired person already receiving Social Security benefits.

While significant revisions may be made in the future, the chances are minimal that these will affect any retired person already receiving Social Security benefits.

Pensions

Unless your parents have other assets, the only way they can get along reasonably well is if they have Social Security and adequate pension benefits—and many pensions are far from adequate. A variety of retirement systems do provide reasonable incomes for retired personnel: the federal retirement system, the Teachers Insurance and Annuity Association, veterans' pensions, and many union and company plans. There are also a number of private pension plans for self-employed men and women.

But many workers arrive at retirement age with no pensions at all, or find when they near age 65 that the pensions they had been counting on vanish before they can reap the benefits. The faithful worker is not always rewarded when he retires. An assistant secretary of the Department of Labor testified at a congressional hearing in 1969, "*If* you remain in good health and stay with the same company until you are sixty-five, and *if* the company is still in business, and *if* your department has not been abolished and *if* you have not been laid off for too long a period, and *if* there is enough money in the fund, and *if* that money has been prudently managed, you will get a pension" (Thomas R. Donahue, quoted in the *Washington Post*, November 24, 1970). The statement is still true today, nearly 40 years later. Factories and plants may close down, leaving employees near retirement and unprotected. Pension rights may be lost if an elderly worker is laid off, retires too soon, or transfers to another job. The money that such workers have paid into a pension fund may be forfeited. Pension reform legislation was introduced with the Employee Retirement Income Security Act of 1974, popularly known as the Pension Reform Act, which established an Office of Employee Benefits Security under the Department of Labor to investigate questions and complaints from individuals about their pension rights.

Social Security was never intended to serve as the total financial support of older Americans. It was expected that it would be supplemented by other sources of retirement income—especially private savings and pension plans. These three sources of income are referred to as the "three pillars" of retirement income. But too many older adults in the United States are supported by one pillar only: Social Security. This explains why too many live at, below, or near the

Information from the Department of Labor on Pension Rights

- Call toll-free 1-866-4-USA-DOL.
- Go to www.DOL.gov, and click on "Health Plans and Benefits."

poverty line. At times of expanding economic activity, when workers were needed, benefits such as pensions were added to attract them. That is less the case today. Some companies provide a 401K, a tax-sheltered savings plan to which both the employee and the employer contribute, but many do not, leaving workers to provide for their retirement however they can. How to increase participation in retirement programs is a major challenge facing policymakers who are working to improve the financial security of future retirees.

Supplemental Security Income

What can be done if your parents' monthly income, including Social Security, is inadequate? They may be eligible for additional income under the federal Supplementary Security Income program (SSI) that is administered through the states. Effective January 2007, the SSI payment for an eligible individual is $623 per month and for an eligible couple $934 per month. A number of states provide a supplement to the basic SSI payment. Your father, at age 65 or over, is eligible for minimum SSI benefits if his monthly income falls below a certain level. He does not have to be destitute to apply; but there is a resource limit for individuals and couples. For information on SSI and the program in your state visit www.ssa.gov/notices/supplemental-security-income/.

Since SSI became the nation's first federal public assistance program in 1974, the number of older recipients has grown to 1.8 million. Participation rates, however, are low for low-income older persons. It has been estimated that only 40%–60% of older persons eligible for SSI actually participate in the program. Some are unaware that such a benefit exists; others have modest savings tucked away, just enough to make them ineligible. But many are too proud and independent-minded to accept assistance. While SSI was intended to be a supplement to Social Security rather than a welfare program, it does not seem to have been able to shake off the stigma of welfare.

Social Security and Supplemental Security Income

How Are They Similar?

- Both programs are run by the Social Security Administration of the Department of Health and Human Services of the U.S. government.
- People can get both if they are eligible for both.
- Anyone who is dissatisfied with a ruling under either program has a right of appeal through the Office of Hearings and Appeals of the Social Security Administration (Ask for details at your local office.)

How Are They Different?

- Social Security is a program of insurance wherein benefits depend on average earnings over a period of years. Supplemental Security Income (SSI) is a program of *assistance* wherein benefits depend on need.
- Social Security benefits are paid from contributions made by the working population under 65. The money for SSI assistance comes from general funds of the U.S. Treasury: personal income taxes, corporation taxes, and other sources.
- Social Security is uniform throughout the United States. SSI varies from state to state.

Non-Cash Supplements

Some financial aid is provided for the older adults through programs that offer, instead of money, opportunities to cut down on expenses.

- *The Elderly Nutrition Program*, authorized under Title III of the Older Americans Act, provides grants to state agencies on aging to support congregate and home delivered meals to persons 60 years and older. Designed to address nutritional deficiencies and social isolation among older adults, the program has expanded significantly in recent years particularly in home-delivered meals. Congregate meals for older adults able to travel are provided in senior centers and other community facilities such as churches and temples. While the program is targeted to persons with the greatest social and economic need, everyone over the age of 60 is eligible. Older persons are encouraged to contribute toward the cost of the meals, but cannot be denied services for failure to contribute.

- *The Food Stamp Program*, operated under the U.S. Department of Agriculture, assists low income individuals and families in purchasing the food they need for good health. Eligibility for the program, like SSI, is based upon income and resources. Benefits are provided on an electronic card that is used like an ATM card and accepted at most grocery stores.
- *Tax Relief.* Taxpayers over the age of 65 are allowed some benefits under the taxing regulations. There are provisions in the federal tax code that benefit older people including exclusion of certain pension benefits, the one time exclusion of up to $125,000 in capital gains from the sale of a primary residence after age 55 and a tax credit for low-income elders with few or no Social Security benefits. A number of states also offer property tax relief.

Depending on where they live, older adults may find a variety of ways to save money. Some communities give out half-fare or free transportation cards; some supermarkets issue their own food stamps providing a 10% reduction on total costs; some movie houses offer half-price tickets at certain hours. Many of these commercial businesses do not make public announcements of reduced prices for elderly shoppers. The only way to find out is to ask. There is no overall nationwide policy on these non-cash benefits, which vary greatly from location to location.

Information on Non-Cash Supplements

Contact your local Area Agency on Aging office.

- Call toll-free 1-800-677-1116.
- Go to www.eldercare.gov.

Reverse Mortgages

When Phil and Donna Rose bought their $20,000 home in 1950, they took out a 30-year mortgage. Thirty years later, they made their last monthly payment and had a mortgage-burning party to celebrate. In 1980, they not only owned their house free and clear, but also after years of skyrocketing housing prices, their $20,000 property was now worth over $100,000. By the time they retired in 1995, they felt as if they were sitting on a gold mine. But were they?

Their combined retirement income of $60,000 seemed adequate at the time to cover their own needs, but they had not taken into account their house's needs. Over the next few years, they had to dip into their modest savings to pay for a new roof, a new septic system, and repairs to their sagging porch. In addition, their property taxes rose sharply after a recent community-wide assessment. When their old heating system broke down and needed to be replaced before winter, they were stymied. Because of the high value of their house, they could easily qualify for a home equity loan, but they would not be able to cover the loan's monthly installments. The only options they saw were to sell their treasured family home and move or to continue to let their house eat up the dwindling savings they had hoped would protect them when they were really old. Terrified of losing their financial security blanket, they decided to sell their house and move. Zoning in their town, however, did not permit apartments, so they had to move to a nearby town to find one. It was only 3 miles away, but Phil and Donna felt cut off from friends, relatives, and patterns of living built up over half a lifetime.

Many older people—single individuals and couples—face Phil and Donna Rose's dilemma: they are house-rich, but cash-poor. A surprising number of older homeowners (78%) own their homes free and clear, having paid off their mortgages years ago. But not everyone chooses to hang on to the old homestead. For many, it's "Who needs to rattle around in this empty place with the children gone?" or "John can't handle the stairs anymore!" or "It's our last winter with snow and ice. We're off to Florida!" or "This place is worth $250,000;

let's take the money and run!" But probably just as many love their homes, seem able to manage normal maintenance, and are determined to live right where they are forever! Sudden, catastrophic household repairs can put an end to these dreams and force the elderly owners to move.

There is now a third option to add to the two that were available to the Roses: reverse mortgages (or RMs; also called *reverse annuity mortgages*, or RAMs). RMs vary in design, but all have a similar purpose. They make it possible for people age 62 and older to tap the equity in their homes rather than in their savings accounts. With an RM, a homeowner receives income from a bank or another lending institution as a lump sum, a line of credit that can be drawn on when needed, or a monthly amount for a certain period or for life. Unlike a regular mortgage, a home equity loan, or a home improvement loan, which has to be paid back with interest in monthly installments, an RM imposes no repayment obligations. At the end of a certain period, or when the owner moves or dies, the home is sold; the total amount borrowed, plus interest, is deducted from the selling price and is returned to the lender. With some RMs, the owner must share with the lender some portion of the amount the house may have appreciated over the years since the loan was signed. An RM, of course, means that heirs will receive diminished legacies.

According to the Reverse Mortgage Lenders Association, increasing numbers of older adults are taking advantage of RMs. By 2007, lenders were issuing 2000 more RMs a month than they had a year ago. An RM seems like the answer to elderly homeowners' prayers, but like all other sure-fire schemes, RMs have their own loopholes, limitations, exceptions, and abuses. One potential downside, for example, is that closing costs can be comparatively high. Caution is required, and consultation with a knowledgeable financial advisor is an important first step.

Who Pays the Medical Bills?

Your parents may be hale, hearty, independent, and contented at the moment. You may be amazed at how well they seem to get along, even though you are pretty sure they do not have much money. But that reassuring situation is not likely to continue if either one or both develop a chronic condition, a general state of poor health, or a se-

Obtaining a Reverse Mortgage

Reverse mortgages are widely available from different agencies. Most popular are Home Equity Conversion Mortgages, which are federally insured loans requiring mandatory financial counseling sessions for the borrower. There are also privately backed reverse mortgages and other options discussed on the web sites of the American Association of Retired Persons (AARP) and the National Center for Home Equity Conversion:

- www.aarp.org/revmort
- www.reverse.org

rious illness. In that case, they will see doctors more frequently and will need to spend more on drugs (the largest single medical expenditure) as well as other health-related items. No other expense is more draining for older adults and more potentially disastrous than the cost of health care. Government and private insurance programs, while helping to meet some health care costs, are by no means able to cover all of them. There are often loopholes and gaps in the coverage for the medical and skilled nursing care of people with acute illnesses, and—short of Medicaid assistance—there is little in the way of coverage for the costs of long-term care of older adults with chronic illnesses.

No other expense is more draining for older adults and more potentially disastrous than the cost of health care.

Your parents, like the majority of older Americans, probably rely heavily on one of two government programs that help to defray medical costs: Medicare and Medicaid, both established under the Social Security Administration. They may also carry some additional private medical insurance to fill gaps left uncovered by Medicare.

Medicare

Medicare, enacted in 1965, is a federal health insurance program tied to Social Security eligibility or Railroad Retirement Benefits. It is an entitlement program that covers persons regardless of income or prior health condition. From its inception, Medicare has provided hospital insurance coverage and outpatient medical insurance. The program, however, has undergone several major changes. These include the 1983 authorization of the Prospective Payment System, which replaced the fee-for-service-system for determining hospital charges; the expansion of the role of private plans under the Balanced Budget Act of 1997; and, most recently, coverage for prescription drugs under the Medicare Prescription Drug, Improvement and Moderation Act of 2003, known as Medicare Part D.

Currently covering 35 million men and women over 65 and 6 million younger people who are physically disabled, the Medicare program is divided into four sections:

- Part A, a mandatory *hospital insurance program* that helps pay for medically necessary inpatient hospital care, including prescription drugs. It also contributes to limited post-hospital care in a skilled nursing facility.
- Part B, *supplemental medical insurance* that helps pay for the outpatient services of physicians and some other practitioners. It is available on a voluntary basis to those covered by Part A, over 90% of whom are also enrolled in Part B.
- Part C, *Medicare Advantage*, offered by managed care companies, including health maintenance organizations (HMOs). Participants must be enrolled in Medicare Parts A and B.
- Part D, *the outpatient prescription drug program*, providing coverage for outpatient prescription drugs through private plans.

Parts A and B Coverage—The Original Medicare Plan

This is a fee-for-service plan that covers many health care services. Contrary to popular assumptions, a Medicare card does not arrive on your parents' doorstep along with the birthday cards the day one of them turns 65. They must apply for membership. Medicare is *not* automatic, and it is *not* free. The average yearly medical bill for someone over 65 is over $4000. Of that sum, Medicare pays only a part. The individual is still responsible for coinsurance, deductibles, and copayments, which can add up. Called "gaps" in Medicare cov-

Additional Information on All Four Medicare Benefits

- Call toll-free 1-800-Medicare (1-800-633-4227).
- Go to www.medicare.gov
  www.aarp.org/medicare
  www.medicareadvocacy.org
- For information specific to Medicare Advantage Plans (Part C), go to:
  www.medicare.gov/choices/overview.asp
  www.medicare advocacy.org
- Also consult the Medicare handbook, *Medicare and You,* 2007
  (PDF version available on www.medicare.gov)

erage, these costs can be covered by private insurance policies (discussed later in this chapter.)

But even after these "gaps" are covered, Medicare does not necessarily pick up all of your parents' medical expenses. Medicare regulations contain a series of "nots": Medicare does *not* cover care that is considered "unreasonable and unnecessary." This would apply to procedures such as face-lifts, tummy tucks, and other forms of elective plastic surgery. Medicare does *not* cover hearing aids or tests, dental care, routine foot care, and eyeglasses. This is a long list of "nots," and it excludes relief for some of the very conditions older people are most likely to suffer from. (The one exception in this list of "nots" is that Medicare allows one new pair of glasses per year to patients who have had cataract surgery.) It is a good idea to check with your local Medicare office on coverage issues. Medicare is administered through regional carriers and can vary in its interpretation of coverage regulations.

What is certain is that Medicare does *not* cover long-term care in a nursing home, or the older person's home, which can spell financial disaster or reliance on Medicaid assistance. While Medicare covers some skilled nursing care and rehabilitation for a limited time following hospitalization, it does *not* cover extended care in or out of a nursing home or support services in the home, such as homemakers, chore services, personal caregivers, and home-delivered meals. The costs for long-term care, either at home or in a nursing home, must be borne by older adults, either through their own funds or through private insurance. As discussed in the next section, the Medicaid program covers long-term care for indigent older adults. There are also community programs discussed in the next chapter that help allay some of these costs.

Keep in mind that medical bills will be disallowed if your mother or father receives care from persons or organizations whose services are not certified by Medicare. You or your parents can check the Medicare status of any service or physician you consult by asking directly or calling your local Social Security office. Not all doctors and medical services are willing to accept the fees established by Medicare, so it is wise for you or your parents to make it a practice to ask in advance whether the professional consulted accepts Medicare assignments. If not, your parents will be expected to cover the bill themselves, then apply for Medicare reimbursement, and finally, coinsurance payment, *if they carry another policy.* The process may be slow, and even when the reimbursements arrive, they *will not* cover the total amount paid. If your parents cannot afford to pay the extra amount above what Medicare allows, they may have to find another doctor. In most states, agreeing to accept Medicare fees is purely voluntary on the part of doctors and other health professionals.

There is much confusion about how Medicare works, what services are covered, and even how to fill out a Medicare form correctly. If you and your parents share this general confusion, you are likely to find some clarification in *Medicare and You 2007* and other publications available free at any Social Security office or on the web site www.medicare.gov. You will find spelled out which services are covered, the range of payments allowed, how to submit insurance claims, and the addresses of organizations across the country selected by the Social Security Administration to handle claims.

Your parents may be surprised to discover that they have rights. They do not have to accept without protest decisions they feel are unfair in their own individual circumstances. They have the right to appeal any decision about their Medicare coverage, whether in the original plan, a Medicare Advantage plan, or a Medicare prescription drug plan. The process may be time-consuming, and it may be months before the outcome is known. Information about Medicare appeals is listed on www. medicare.gov or can be obtained by calling toll-free 1-800-Medicare (1-800-633-4227).

The *Prospective Payment System* was developed by the federal government to help stem hospital costs, which have been escalating steadily and are responsible for the lion's share of the total Medicare expenditure. Under the old system, the government paid hospitals for the care given Medicare patients. With the Prospective Payment System, hospital reimbursements are based on average costs for specific diagnoses, which are referred to as Diagnosis Related Groups (DRGs). This is how the system works:

> Seventy-year-old John Grant is admitted to the hospital for a gallbladder operation. The surgery goes well; he recuperates quickly and is discharged on the fifth day. Pete Fletcher, also 70, also undergoes gallbladder surgery. He recuperates slowly, but nevertheless is discharged on the seventh day. His family is furious that the hospital has "kicked out" a frail old man and "dumped" him on his relatives, who are ill equipped to give him the kind of nursing care he needs.

How did this happen? The Medicare reimbursement had been determined under DRGs to be a certain dollar amount for a gallbladder operation and for a hospital stay not to exceed a certain number of days. If the hospital had kept Pete longer, the reimbursement by Medicare would still have been a preset dollar amount and the hospital would have had to carry the costs for the extra hospital days. In contrast, John was discharged sooner than the DRG's allotted time, thereby lowering the costs, but the hospital still received the preset dollar amount and therefore made money. When there are serious complications, a patient may be kept in the hospital longer than the time the DRG has set, and Medicare may pick up some of the extra costs, but this does not happen routinely.

If you think the hospital is sending your parent home too soon, call 1–800-Medicare and ask for the Quality Improvement Organization (QIO) to review your case. Your parent may be able to remain in the hospital at no charge during the review. As stated on the Medicare web site, "The hospital cannot force you to leave before the QIO makes a decision."

Part C—Medicare Advantage Plans

Private Medicare plans subsidized by the government have expanded in recent years, and in addition to HMOs, include regional, Private Fee-for-Service Plans; Medicare Special Needs Plans; and Medicare Medical Savings Account Plans. These plans are attractive because their relatively low out-of-pocket costs provide all of the benefits provided by traditional Medicare plans, or more, such as eyeglasses. On the downside for some enrollees is that the copayments for some services may be higher, and in some cases, coverage is restricted to physicians, hospitals, and specialists participating in a plan. Under traditional Medicare coverage, consumers have a far wider range of choices. Another downside is the questionable stability of these subsidized private plans. While traditional Medicare programs continue to be the choice of many beneficiaries, there has been a recent surge in enrollment due to aggressive marketing, described in a *New York Times* article (May 7, 2007) as "improper hard sell tactics" on the part of insurance companies.

Part D—Prescription Drug Coverage

The Medicare Prescription Drug, Improvement and Modernization Act, enacted in 2003, created a new drug benefit as Part D of Medicare. It was inaugurated in January 2006. Under Medicare Part D beneficiaries have a choice. They can remain on the tradition fee-for-service Medicare plan and enroll in one of a number of private prescription drug plans. Or they can enroll in a Medicare Advantage plan for all Medicare-covered benefits including prescription drug coverage.

Traditional Medicare drug coverage has three phases. Plans can vary, but, for example, in phase 1, the initial coverage period, an older person can pay a deductible and 25% of drug costs, up to $2250. Then comes phase 2, known as the "donut hole." Once your parent's drug costs exceed $2250, but are less than $3600, he or she may have to pay the total cost of the drugs. In phase 3, once those costs reach $3600, known as the "catastrophic phase," your parent will pay only 5% of the drug costs. The "donut hole" of phase 2 is the most criticized part of Medicare Part D, and some states have made independent efforts to provide support during the gap.

For low-income elders, Medicare will provide additional assistance, but beneficiaries have to meet income and asset tests to receive this assistance. You can apply online by visiting the "Help With Medicare Prescription Drug Plan Costs" section of the Social Security Administration's web site (www.ssa.gov).

There are a wide variety of Medicare D plans to chose from, each with its own provisions. One or two even cover the "donut hole." Social workers on the front lines of advising older adults about their entitlements note that Medicare Part D is confusing and complicated, and changes take place every year. Even the formularies—meaning the lists of permitted drugs—differ from plan to plan. Moreover, the formularies are allowed to change, and do change, year to year, protecting the suppliers, but not the consumers. Because of the difficulties faced by consumers, further changes to Medicare Part D will undoubtedly occur. The *AARP Bulletin* and other sources listed in this chapter and Appendix A can keep you updated.

> Social workers on the front lines of advising older adults about their entitlements note that Medicare Part D is confusing and complicated, and changes take place every year.

Private Health Insurance

Medigap Policies

Because it was originally assumed—incorrectly—that Medicare coverage would carry the major burden of medical expenses for older adults, many workplace health insurance policies for retirees cease coverage when insured individuals reach 65 or become eligible for Medicare. And, as some retirees have experienced, even continuing health coverage provided to them at retirement is dependent on the health of the company they worked for.

> When Sam Loomis retired at age 62, the large automotive supply company he'd worked for was one of the most admired in the country, often written up as a model of success. Ten years later, Sam's excellent retiree medical plan, in combination with Medicare, paid for a mitral valve replacement for his

heart. At age 76, Sam was diagnosed with prostate cancer, requiring expensive radiation treatments. By then, his former company, suffering from the general decline in American auto manufacturing, went on the skids and filed for bankruptcy. All retiree medical plans were canceled, leaving Sam to pick up the percentage of costs not covered by Medicare.

The gaps in Medicare coverage have proven to be so costly that many older people carry, if they can afford it, some type of supplementary medical insurance to help defray extra costs, including medical deductible and coinsurance costs, additional inpatient hospital days, outpatient services, and extra post-hospital days in a skilled nursing facility. Supplementary health insurance policies are available to older adults from a number of insurers. They have a variety of names, such as "65-Plus," "Medicare Tie-In," "Supplemental Coverage," "Medicare Plus," or "Medigap." The policies are usually handled by the same carriers that handle Medicare claims. More information can be found in the handbook *Medicare and You* available on www.medicare.gov or call 1–800-Medicare.

While "Medigap" policies may cover Part A or Part B of Medicare deductibles, they usually only cover services also covered by Medicare. Julia Lienart, a 77-year-old widow suffering from serious macular degeneration, had a bill of $800 for optical devices. Knowing that Medicare did not reimburse for these devices, she blithely sent her entire bill to her supplementary medical insurance company. The bill was returned very quickly with a note stating anything *not* reimbursable by Medicare was *not* reimbursable by that company either. The supplemental policies also have a long list of "uncovered" services and equipment, most of which are the very ones likely to be needed by an older person: dental and foot care, eyeglasses, hearing aids, routine physical examinations, and—the most catastrophic health expense of all—long-term care, either at home or in a nursing home.

Many people realize only at retirement or shortly before that their company health insurance will end the moment the gold watch is presented. At age 65, they may have to start shopping for supplemental coverage, which may be hard to find and hard to pay for on their retirement income. They may discover that cost is not the only problem. Some insurance companies may refuse to cover anyone with "a preexisting condition" or allow coverage to go into effect only after 60 or 90 or more days.

Long-Term Care Insurance

Long-term care refers to a variety of medical and nonmedical services to people who have a chronic illness or disability. It includes medical and skilled nursing care and essential support services that provide help with various activities of daily living, such as bathing, toileting, and dressing. Long-term care can be provided in the home, in assisted living, or in a nursing home. As has been emphasized, Medicare pays only for medically necessary services provided at home or in a nursing home, and only for a short time, or intermittently—but not for long-term care services. Medicaid, however, does cover these services for low-income older adults, both in the home and in the nursing home. But older adults with financial resources must bear the hefty costs of long-term care on their own—costs that can total tens of thousands of dollars per year. For these elders long-term care insurance is becoming increasingly available. While your parent may not be eligible for coverage at his or her advanced age (although some healthy elders are), you should be considering coverage for yourself.

Long-term care insurance is becoming increasingly available. While your parent may not be eligible for coverage at his or her advanced age (although some healthy elders are), you should be considering coverage for yourself.

About 7 million Americans now have long-term insurance policies that cover a range of services, including extended care at home or in an adult day-care center, assisted living residence, or nursing home. Insurance coverage is usually triggered when a person cannot perform at least two key activities of daily living such as feeding and bathing or has a diagnosis of dementia. A number of insurance companies are now providing these policies. Consultation on the provisions of these policies is strongly recommended. While they vary in what they cover, they are not inexpensive. For information on Medigap and long-term care insurance programs, call your state health insurance program. The number is available through your Area Agency on Aging office or at www.medicare.gov/contacts/static/allstate.

Medicaid

This state-administered program for financially needy patients draws on state and federal funds. Each state designs its own individual program within the broad framework of federal regulations, so there is great state-to-state variation. In most states, those individuals who receive Supplemental Security Income are also eligible for Medicaid, but eligibility does not mean automatic coverage. SSI recipients must apply for Medicaid at their local office. Those with unbearably heavy medical bills must "spend down" to whatever dollar amount determines Medicaid eligibility.

In most states, spending down occurs in two ways. The first type applies to people who live at home, but have continuing high medically related expenses. If paying these costs depletes their resources enough, older individuals or couples can apply for Medicaid assistance under the "medically needy" program of their state. There is state-to-state variation in the figures used to define "medically needy." If an individual or couple meets the requirements of their state's program, Medicaid will help to pay medical expenses on an as-needed basis—or as long as the illness or chronic condition continues.

The second type of spending down accepted by all states occurs when nursing home residents have used up all their resources to cover the cost of their care and cannot continue to pay these charges. At this point, elderly residents can apply for Medicaid. If their applications are approved, the residents must contribute all their monthly income (including Social Security checks) toward their nursing home care, except for a small "personal needs allowance."

Obtaining Medicaid

To determine if your parent is eligible for Medicaid:

- Go to www.cms.hhs.gov and click on "Medicaid" and then "Medicaid Information for Consumers"
  or
- Regional offices can be located at http://cms.hhs.gov/ RegionalOffices/

Medicaid will then pick up the balance, which is determined by a set daily rate that the nursing home has agreed to accept from the state for all Medicaid residents.

When the need for expensive long-term care is looming, there are older persons who seek to protect their assets to be eligible for Medicaid assistance. They may make a gift of property or funds to their children or place their funds in irrevocable trusts. In the past, when a person applied for Medicaid, officials examined an applicant's finances for the past 3 years. This time limit has now been extended to 5 years, known as the "look-back period." If funds have been given away within the last 5 years, then the older person will not be eligible for Medicaid until the amount transferred has been spent on the parent's long-term care.

Spending down can be tragically humiliating and disruptive to couples when one partner remains at home and the other is in a nursing home or about to enter one. Years ago, the state considered almost all of a couple's total income and assets when determining Medicaid eligibility. In some tragic instances, couples would go through divorce proceedings to preserve some assets.

In 1988, Congress enacted provisions to prevent what had come to be called "spousal impoverishment." With variations in policies among the states, the spouse who remains in the community is allowed to keep whatever income he or she needs to live on. Every state Medicaid program receiving federal funds must supply certain basic services: inpatient hospital care, outpatient hospital services, laboratory and X-ray services, physician services, skilled nursing facilities, rural health clinic services, and some home health care. A wide variety of optional services may be available in the state where your parents are living. These optional additions can include clinic services, prescribed drugs, dental services, prosthetic devices, eyeglasses, private-duty nursing, physical and speech therapy, emergency hospital services, ambulance services, and services by an ophthalmologist, podiatrist, or chiropractor. Case management and other home- and community-based services may also be included. In fact, Medicaid is the primary government payer for care provided in a nursing home. Despite the wide scope of health-related services offered to Medicaid recipients, it should be remembered that all these services, basic or optional, may be limited in scope or availability and may vary from state to state.

Medicare and Medicaid

How Are Medicare and Medicaid Similar?

- Both programs are designed to help defray hospital and medical bills.
- Both programs are part of the Social Security Act.
- An individual may be eligible for both programs.

How Are They Different?

- Medicare is a federal program. Medicaid is a federal-state program. Medicare is uniformly administered by the Social Security Administration throughout the United States (although rules may vary according to regional carriers.) Medicaid programs vary from state to state within federal guidelines and are administered by local social service departments.
- Medicare is an insurance program available to persons over the age of 65 and younger persons with disabilities. Medicaid is an assistance program available to financially needy people of all ages according to standards of eligibility set by each state.

What Can You Do?

In the past, children who had some financial means were held legally responsible for their elderly parents' support by laws of filial responsibility. Heartbreaking stories were reported of entire families wiped out by the illness of one elderly relative. Money set aside for Johnny's education sometimes had to be used to keep Grandma in the nursing home. Federal regulations prohibit relative responsibility as an eligibility condition for Medicaid, with *some* exceptions for spouses or the parents of children under age 21. In administering SSI, however, states *may* hold adult children responsible for their parents. These regulations have been difficult to enforce, and there is a right of appeal to the Office of Hearings and Appeals of the Social Security Administration (www.ssa.gov).

Whether "filial responsibility" has a legal hold on you or not, you may feel it anyhow and wonder what you can do to help when your parents are living under financial privation. If you have plenty of assets, you may be able to take over and support them. But even if you have financial problems of your own, there are a number of ways to help.

- *Keep Them Informed.* If you inform yourself about available programs, you may be able to show your parents how they are eligible for greater benefits, including non-cash supplements. (Don't be surprised if they are better informed than you are.)
- *Override Their Pride.* The older generation is often too proud to apply for assistance that is due them, fearing the hated stigma of welfare. You may be able to convince them that supplements are not "handouts," but returns from their own contributions as taxpayers.
- *Encourage Them to Work.* Your father and mother may be retired from their lifelong careers, but if they are healthy, there is nothing to stop them from taking a second job or starting a second career. If they want to try this, instead of dissuading them, explore with them the possibility of part-time employment, which might provide a necessary financial boost without overtaxing their energies. Opportunities are limited, but a few communities have employment agencies dealing exclusively with retired applicants. Title V of the Older Americans Act established the Community Service Employment Program, which makes funds available to projects employing the elderly. Contact your Area Agency on Aging office for more information (www.eldercare.gov).
- *Make Small, Regular Contributions of Your Own.* They may refuse it out of pride, but you may be able to persuade your parents to accept small amounts from you and others in the family. Life at the poverty level is grim for anyone at any age. A few extra dollars a month contributed by family members could make day-to-day living a little less dismal. But keep in mind that those extra dollars may be considered as income when Medicaid or SSI eligibility is being determined.

Seek Legal Counseling—"Elder Law"

Your family lawyer, well trained in wills and estates, may know little about the intricacies of Medicare and Medicaid regulations and even less about the financial problems of aging. Because of the complications involved in arranging the affairs of older people, a new legal specialty—"elder law"—began in the 1970s and has been steadily growing ever since. A lawyer specializing in the legal problems of older adults can help clients understand various options open to them under government programs, as well as counsel them on legal steps they can take to protect their assets in the event of serious or chronic illness. They can also advise you on the steps to take if a parent can no longer act on his or her own behalf, and help prepare end-of-life directives, such as power of attorney, power of medical attorney, and living wills (as discussed in Chapter 6). You can locate an elder law attorney in your area by checking the web site www.elderlaw answers.com or the web site of the National Academy of Elder Law Attorneys at www.naela.com.

Because of the complications involved in arranging the affairs of older people, a new legal specialty—"elder law"—began in the 1970s and has been steadily growing ever since.

Some older people cannot afford a lawyer to advise them on their rights and to safeguard their assets. When problems needing legal intervention arise, however, help can sometimes be found through your Legal Aid Society, which provides low-cost advice for all age groups. Area Agency on Aging offices are good sources of information on where to find legal help. AARP also offers low-cost legal consultation.

Your parents may seek legal advice themselves to put their affairs in order. Some older people, however, reluctant to think about the future and what may lie ahead, refuse to consider advance planning. If a crisis comes, and your father is obviously unable to handle his funds or pay his bills, you may be forced to get legally involved. He may go off on crazy spending sprees or be threatened with eviction for nonpayment of his rent. He needs some kind of protection. After consulting his lawyer or another legal professional, you may be advised to select one of three commonly used procedures that can be put into action quickly: power of attorney, joint tenancy, or inter vivos trust. All three require that your father be sufficiently alert—and willing—to enter into a contractual agreement.

1. Power of attorney is used most frequently. If your father gives you power of attorney, he thereby allows you to manage his funds. Power of attorney will be terminated if your father becomes incompetent, unless he has stated in writing, while competent, that the document should remain valid in the event of his incompetence.

2. Joint tenancy is also frequently used and does not have the same limitations as power of attorney, because each party has total control over the funds, regardless of the competency of the parties involved. If your father is able to enter into a joint tenancy contract with you or another responsible person, and deteriorates thereafter, the joint tenancy continues.

3. An inter vivos trust is the most sophisticated of the three and provides the greatest flexibility. Using that procedure, your father may create a trust for himself, naming himself as trustee, but at the same time providing for a successor trustee (you or another person) to take control if he becomes incapacitated.

Each of these legal procedures has its own drawbacks and limitations, all of which should be reviewed with a lawyer. They may also be costly, but the most important problem to be faced is that most older people are reluctant to turn over all, or even a portion, of personal control of their own financial affairs. You may be caught in an uncomfortable dilemma if your father is reluctant to accept any advice from you. Either you insist on helping him, thereby antagonizing him and making him feel more powerless than ever, or you sit back and do nothing, watching him squander his money or face exploitation by others. A third alternative is to seek counseling (see the resources in Appendix A). Not infrequently, you can arrive at an approach that will protect both your father's resources and his self-esteem.

Pulling Your Plans Together

In the past two chapters, we have discussed the variety of steps you can take to prepare for the physical, mental, and financial challenges that may lie ahead for your parents. Difficult conversations may have to be initiated. Although your plans may never need to be executed, it's far better to look ahead than to be "blindsided," as were Bob Morris and his brother.

A helpful guide in planning is Penny's Personal Papers Inventory (Appendix C), designed by social worker Dr. Penny Schwartz of the Mount Sinai Medical Center in New York. Taking this inventory can be a joint activity for you and your parents. Or you can ask them to fill it out themselves and update it every year. Some parents who wish to preserve their privacy could simply keep the inventory in a safe place, to be released to you if the need arises.

Whatever your parents' current level of finances and information, keeping up to date with potential benefits, with their often glaring gaps, and with changes that are likely to occur—in both their own lives and in public programs of support—will help both generations to be more ready to cope with the future. One sure thing about the future is that it keeps on arriving.

Bob Morris on Not Wanting to Know About $$$

I think that there are situations in which the parents don't want their kids to know about their assets—and then there are other times when kids don't want to know about their parents' assets. In my father's case, between what my mother had left behind and what he had saved, there was close to a million dollars in assets. And for years, he wanted me to sit with him and kind of go over the details.

I didn't want to deal with the 800 bank account deposit slips lying around his apartment that looked like the yellow brick road. I didn't think it was any of my business. I was self-sufficient enough—a struggling writer making enough to get by—and had a comfortable enough life that I didn't want to know that there was all this money that he was planning on leaving to me. I thought it was unseemly to know about that, because I was afraid that I was going to start thinking about it too much.

You know, you struggle to be autonomous in life, and I worked very hard not to be dependent on my parents. It's enough that they put me through college. But I didn't go to them for handouts and freebies. It made me feel good to be independent—and it probably made them feel good, too. They were generous people, but they didn't need to be.

I think a lot of kids don't want to know about their parents' finances. But I'll tell you one thing. When I knew what he had, and then when that last miserable year kicked in, and it was costing him $100,000 a year at least, between assisted living and aides, it was a great comfort to know that he could afford it.

9

Stepping In—When They Cannot Manage and You Can Help

"Timmy, it's bath time. Did you pick up all your toys?"

"Yup."

"Timmy! You did not! What's all over the floor?"

"Nothing! Just a couple of marbles. I picked up my cars."

"Get those marbles, too. Right now! You know Grandma's coming at 6 o'clock to sit with you. Come on! Hurry!"

"All right, all right! I'm doing it as fast as I can. What's the big deal about a couple of little marbles?"

ONE OF TIMMY'S MARBLES DID MAKE A BIG DEAL. Grandma stepped on it as she walked in, turned her ankle, lost her balance, and fell. That night, instead of Grandma sitting with Timmy, Timmy's family sat in the hospital while Grandma's broken hip was set. Before she stepped on the marble, she had been a self-sufficient 79-year-old, ready to help out whenever one of her children needed her. Afterward, the tables were turned, and it was clear to them that she needed their help for the first time. But that was the only thing that was clear. It was unclear how much help she would need, what kind of help, and for how long.

The story of Timmy's grandmother is not unusual. A widow or a widower, or an older couple, may move along through the years functioning reasonably well and presenting few, if any, problems to their children, who accept the status quo and give little thought to its impermanence. But one day, a crisis can occur with little warning. A stroke can render an older person partially or totally incapacitated in a matter of hours. Even minor falls can result in serious fractures.

More often than not, however, an approaching crisis gives off warning signals. Telltale signs appear months, possibly years, in advance, and are all too often ignored or denied by everyone. (As noted in the previous chapter, when the signals are picked up early, some crises can be averted.) Your father may be suffering from a number of conditions that limit rather than incapacitate him, although it is obvious to everyone that his normal resiliency is declining, his social world closing in, and his friends dying off. He may also have hidden clinical conditions that surface only after a serious accident or a physical or emotional trauma.

Events that commonly precipitate a crisis are the death of a spouse, an acute illness such as pneumonia or a severe bout of the flu, a serious fracture, or a frightening car accident, even though no injury is sustained. The extent of permanent disability left after such a crisis is unpredictable—especially at first. Since the recuperative powers of two convalescents can be very different, one may return to a life of self-sufficiency within a matter of months, while the other may need to rely permanently on the help of others.

Diseases are not necessarily crises in themselves. The crisis develops when a disease interferes with an older person's ability to manage. The day that your mother learns she has cancer may be agonizingly painful for everyone, but the more serious problems arise when her illness begins to interfere with her normal routine and her ability to manage. An older man can live with his diabetes for years, but one day, the disease may progress to the point where amputation of a limb is necessary or his vision is seriously impaired. Arthritis may eventually make walking very difficult; glaucoma may advance to partial sight. Mental disorders as well—temporary, pro-

Diseases are not necessarily crises in themselves. The crisis develops when a disease interferes with an older person's ability to manage.

gressive, or permanent—must be evaluated in terms of the disability they produce. Your mother's occasional loss of memory may disturb her and upset you without seriously hindering her ability to take care of herself. But if she becomes increasingly forgetful or disoriented, it may one day become unsafe for her to continue to live at home alone. The amount of help older adults will need is largely determined by the impact on their physical and mental functioning. Their future depends a great deal on their resiliency as well as the supports available to them within their families and their communities.

This chapter addresses the steps that adult children and their older parents can take when, suddenly or gradually, it becomes apparent that help is needed if they are to make a go of it in their own home. There are many levels of such help, from "off-and-on" assistance from family members and others to regular daily care to around-the-clock care. And, these days, there are many more community sources to turn to for valuable help and advice than formerly. A crucial preliminary step in determining the level of care your parent needs, and making an appropriate plan, is a full and careful assessment of the situation.

When You Are Not the Responsible Relative

It is important to note that your role in helping your parents may not necessarily be a primary one. Of course, a single parent in trouble clearly needs your help. But in many older couples, the spouse or partner of an ailing parent is able to take on the main responsibility for his or her care. In fact, the majority of caregiving to older adults is provided by a spouse, often a wife. If your mother is increasingly frail and ill herself, she may welcome your help or may even be ready to turn over the responsibility for looking after your father and herself to others. But not always. As the longtime decision maker and loving support for her husband, and the one who knows him best, she may be very reluctant to give up this role—or even to share the burden with her children. Whether she seems able to carry out the daily tasks of caregiving or is nobly or stubbornly overrating her strength is something best determined by her closest family members. Steps to take when parents need your help and refuse it are discussed toward the end of this chapter.

Putting All the Pieces Together: The Assessment and Plan

In times of crisis, neither older adults nor their children can look into a crystal ball and see what lies ahead. The safest way to judge the future is to find out as much as possible about what is going on in the present. What does Mother have going for her? What does she have against her? This is the time to take a deep breath and slow down, even if Mother is in the hospital and her discharge is imminent. Don't rush things. Make sure that you and your parent—or both parents—are working as a team.

It's particularly tricky to attempt an intelligent assessment of long-term needs when older people are in the hospital. Since recovery is usually slower for them than for younger adults, playing for time is important. What looks hopeless today may seem hopeful next week. If the hospital discharges your mother before she is ready to go home, the family should make temporary, short-term plans until they can get a clear picture of the situation. A transfer to a rehabilitation facility may be the next step. Many nursing homes, and even some hospitals, have "step-down" accommodations where your parent can receive rehabilitation and continuing nursing care, giving everyone time to get a better view of her overall condition and to make future plans. Medicare may cover the cost of this post-hospital care for up to 100 days. You may even be able to bring your parent home with Medicare-covered home health care for a limited time.

The "geriatric assessment," a term used by professionals in the field of aging services, is considered to be a critically important intervention when appropriate plans need to be made. If a professional, such as a geriatric care manager, takes the lead in making an assessment, the family members and the older parents should be involved in this process as well. However, if professional help is not available for pulling together the various aspects of your mother's situation, or if your funds are limited, the responsibility may fall on your shoulders. In that case, you are still not alone: social workers and therapists, as well as the nursing and medical staff in either the hospital or rehabilitation facility, can be asked to help you evaluate your mother's needs.

The assessment process can be compared to putting together a jigsaw puzzle. Your mother's future is made up of a number of separate but interrelated pieces that reveal a clear picture only when all of them are fitted together. Is that broken hip healing well or poorly? Is she otherwise in pretty good health? What about her emotional strengths and weaknesses, her personality, her motivation, her finances? Perhaps most important of all is the question of how she will be able to manage at home—deal with stairs, shopping, and cooking. Even if there is every reason to believe that she could make a good recovery from a crisis, she will undoubtedly need some amount of help during the recuperative period. It's also sadly possible that, henceforth, she will never be able to manage completely alone in her home. Her future depends, to a great extent, therefore, on the care her family can provide or the help available in her community.

Alert families do not wait for a crisis to happen. The same kind of comprehensive assessment is helpful for older people who are not in the hospital but are already having serious difficulty at home. Although many medical procedures cannot be done in the home, an important part of the assessment can be made right there. When an elderly man is seen in his own home setting, it will be easier to understand how much help he will need if he is to remain there.

Although many medical procedures cannot be done in the home, an important part of the assessment can be made right there. When an elderly man is seen in his own home setting, it will be easier to understand how much help he will need if he is to remain there.

George Light, long divorced, was known as a superb cook, who delighted in entertaining friends and family at his table. Despite occasional bouts of rheumatoid arthritis and the need for medication to control a heart arrhythmia, George got about well, relying on his car. But both his living room and bedroom were on the second floor of his duplex, up a turning flight of stairs. As his arthritis became more severe, it became harder and harder for him to climb those stairs. Some nights he just couldn't make it, and he fell asleep in a lounge chair in the small TV room off the kitchen. His children worried: how could he continue to live there? In this case, it wasn't George who flunked an assessment, but his home. A move to a single-level condominium nearby enabled him to use a walker to move from room to room, and soon he was back cooking up a storm and sleeping well.

Although George loathed the idea of moving, and initially resisted it, his children and his best friend helped convince him to go along with it, and then his strong grandsons took over the strenuous parts of the move. Whether or not other family members will ultimately be the ones to give hands-on support to an aging parent, it is important to involve them when attempting to determine the future needs of an aging person. Your siblings, your spouse, your children, and even close friends may have good information to offer. As noted in Chapter 11, to promote family harmony at this critical time, the "buy-in" of significant family members should start as early as possible—and the best time is during the assessment.

Whether your mother's needs emerge gradually or occur as the result of a crisis, the best way to understand all the pieces in her situation, and how they fit together in the total picture, is to consider the different aspects of her life: physical, psychological, functional, social, and financial. That may seem like a lot to handle, but if you look at the big picture, you will have a clearer idea of the care she is likely to need, and you will be better able to plan accordingly. If you and she have done any contingency planning, as discussed in the last chapter, you may now be ready to put some of those plans into action.

Signs of Trouble

These are common signs that your parent may be having health problems:

- Loss of weight
- Difficulty in getting around
- Decline in self-care
- Confusion
- Unremitting anxiety and sadness

Still, "the best-laid plans oft go awry," and some contingency planning may have to be revised and adapted for her current situation.

The Physical Piece

After an illness, an accident, or a general physical decline, an older man may wonder, "What's happening to me?" and his wife and children may ask themselves, "How much damage has been done?" "Is he getting worse?" "How long can he go on like this?" "What can we do to help him?"

A thorough physical examination, including mental, hearing, and vision testing, is the first and most crucial step to be taken before any answers can be given. But you may hit a snag right there. Since the medical profession, in general, has given low priority to the problems of older adults, it is unsafe to assume that every physician is familiar enough with geriatric medicine to make an accurate or thorough diagnosis. And specialists will have to be consulted, as in the case of suspected vision or hearing loss. Illness does not always show the same familiar signs and symptoms in the old as in the young. The diseases of the elderly, as pointed out earlier, are often so closely intertwined that they present a confusing picture, difficult to interpret unless a physician has special knowledge and experience.

Unfortunately, there are doctors who, because of lack of geriatric training in medical school, lack of experience with older adults, lack of time, or lack of interest, tend to attribute an endless variety of symptoms to one cause—aging. "Your mother isn't getting any younger, you know," they may say with a shrug, as if that were the answer to everything she's suffering. It is particularly dangerous to pin the hopeless term "Alzheimer's" on confused, disoriented, and even hallucinating older patients. These days, more sophisticated tests are available to distinguish her symptoms from what may be a treatable, reversible brain condition resulting from any number of causes, including certain medications and malnutrition.

VISITING THE DOCTOR

If possible, it is important that you or another family member be present with your parent when diagnoses are rendered by a qualified physician. As many older people do, your mother may try to hide some of her worrisome symptoms and give the doctor falsely upbeat

If possible, it is important that you or another family member be present with your parent when diagnoses are rendered by a qualified physician.

responses. She may be confused and upset and miss much of what the physician has said. Or it may be hard for her, if alone, to stand her ground with a brisk doctor and insist that her questions be answered, her condition explained, and its treatment mapped out clearly. In case you also forget to raise some important questions when you have the doctor's attention, it's best to come with a list of questions written in advance. One critical issue to raise is the possible side effects and interactions of the multiple medications—including over-the-counter drugs—she is taking, including those prescribed by other doctors. (This concern is discussed in Chapter 12.)

It's not always easy to speak for a parent who doesn't speak for herself. Too many of us feel "cowed" before authority in the doctor's office. But, fortunately, the young and middle-aged generations of today are more firmly behind the movement supporting a patient's right to know. If you are dissatisfied with the answers you get—if they seem casual, unconcerned, or fatalistic—you may be able to get more helpful answers by consulting with another doctor. If your mother's eye doctor dismisses her deteriorating vision with the comment, "Nothing can be done about it!" perhaps he or she is right. But a vision rehabilitation therapist might be able to teach her how to make the most of her remaining eyesight. Or, if your mother's doctor dismisses her lower back pain resulting from osteoarthritis and insists that nothing can be done to help her medically or surgically, perhaps the doctor is right, but it's possible that a physical therapist could help her increase her strength and decrease her pain.

If your father is fortunate enough to have a competent, interested family doctor who has known him for quite some time, so much the better. A long-standing close relationship with an older patient can be particularly helpful in assessing changes in his overall physical condition. Your own knowledge of your father's medical history can be useful, too, especially with new doctors. If he had a mild, transient stroke 4 years ago from which he fully recovered, he may succeed in overlooking it—but you should bring it up.

But if he does not have a doctor you both trust, and you don't know whom to see, there are better ways to go about the search than flipping through the Yellow Pages or asking a friend, neighbor, or

Tips on Medical Care

- Select a physician with geriatric expertise or experience in treating older patients.
- If possible, accompany your parent to doctor's visits armed with knowledge of his or her medical condition and history and a list of the medications he or she takes.
- Make a list of your questions in advance.
- Seek a second opinion if the answers you and your parent receive from the physician are inconclusive, dismissive, or unclear.
- Seek a referral for psychiatric consultation if psychotropic drugs are prescribed.

Aunt Emma. There may be a nearby medical school, a hospital with a medical school affiliation, or even a reputable local hospital where you can find the names of doctors with geriatric experience. The county medical association or a local social agency or Office of the Aging may also have names of physicians with explicit experience in treating older patients. Some communities have compiled directories listing cooperating physicians and including information about their training, credentials, fees, office hours, and Medicare and Medicaid participation.

The Psychological Piece

The impact of illness and disability on an older person's mental and emotional state is too often ignored. Yet, this can sometimes cause as much damage to the patient as the physical condition itself. Some, but not all, physicians are careful to take that vital element into account as part of a general examination. There's no doubt that the incidence of depression increases with age and often goes hand-in-glove with their physical problems.

If your mother's emotional or behavioral problem seems serious, such as those discussed in Chapter 4, then obviously a psychiatric examination is necessary. The older adult with symptoms of memory loss, confusion, and disorientation may be experiencing the onset of

Alzheimer's disease; on the other hand, the condition could be temporary, caused by poor diet, medication misuse, or severe anxiety or depression, all of which are treatable. No diagnosis of an irreversible mental condition should be made summarily. In evaluating the emotional factors in your mother's condition, not only psychiatrists and psychiatrically oriented physicians, but also clinical psychologists, social workers, and nurses can be helpful. Here again, your county medical society or local hospital and social service agencies can point you in the right direction. Also see the web sites and phone numbers listed in the "Quick Reference Directory to Services in the Community" listed in this chapter and in Appendix A.

The Functional Piece

Physical and psychological factors account for only part of the total picture of an older man or woman in a crisis situation, because physicians are interested mainly in diagnosis and treatment. They can tell you what's wrong with your father, what caused his problem, what other conditions contribute to it, and what procedures will modify it. But they may fail to consider how the problem is likely to affect your father's personal life and his day-to-day functioning. "Be sure he keeps to his diet and takes his medication. Call me if you have any problems, and I'd like to see him again in 3 weeks," a doctor may say pleasantly as he dismisses you and your father.

But as you leave the office, your mind may already be swirling with the next questions. If he lives alone, will he be able to resume his daily routines—shopping, cooking, dressing, bathing, toileting? Will he be alert or coordinated enough to protect himself from all the potential hazards in his environment— the stove, the tub, driving? Can he manage the stairs, pay his bills, take his medicine regularly, keep to his diet? Will he call you or someone else if he is in trouble? Even more important is his motivation to regain independence. If he has lost motor skills, will he be willing to relearn them through exercise or physiotherapy? Is he receptive to using compensatory devices, such as wheelchairs or walkers?

Often local community agencies, such as your Area Agency on Aging or local senior center, family service agency, or hospital, can arrange for a trained staff member to make a home visit to assess how well your father is managing his daily routines in and out of the house. Without this assessment, you may too hastily assume during a crisis that your father is permanently disabled, and make plans that result in his becoming more helpless than he needs to be. Or, you may underestimate the extent of his disability, provide inadequate support, and invite a serious accident. The home assessment may be done by a nurse or social worker who may also act as a geriatric care manager, someone who can help you assess your father's needs. (See the "Quick Reference Directory to Services in the Community" box, on page 245, for contact information.)

The Social Piece

Another missing piece in the total picture involves the social supports available to an older person who hopes to live at home. Will a spouse or domestic partner be able to provide the care needed, or will they both need assistance? Sometimes one particularly devoted relative, such as an adult child, can take on the job. Some families set up schedules, take turns, and share the responsibility of caring for a disabled mother or father. Even friendly neighbors may be willing to pitch in and provide the extra support necessary. But don't assume or presume on others unless you are sure they are truly willing and able to make the commitment. From these sources, you may be able to put together a network of support for your parents. If not, it may become painfully clear that there is no way you and your family can provide all the care needed, and you will have to seek the help of outsiders.

The Financial Piece

Finances are a big piece of the puzzle. Money—or the lack of it—is most often a crucial factor in the planning process, speeding it up or blocking it completely. To remain in their own homes, older adults may be saddled with extra expenses to cover special equipment, special diets, and safety installations. Beyond that, they may also need to pay for a housekeeper, or home health aide. As described in Chapter 8, Medicare coverage for help at home is limited. Medicaid for low-income or indigent adults may cover some of these costs and provide some community supports. But if you, your parent, or your family—or some willing combination—has the financial resources to provide the needed extras, the chances that your parents with chronic disabilities will be able to abide safely at home are considerably greater.

Who Puts All the Pieces Together?

Even though an overall professional assessment makes sense in principle, it is sometimes close to impossible to obtain in reality. You may have trouble finding any competent help at all. Many professionals are ill equipped to offer the thorough physical, psychological, and social work-ups needed by millions of older citizens in trouble, even though the numbers of professionals and agencies offering this service, including geriatric care managers, have grown significantly in recent years. You and your family may have to be your own father's or mother's evaluator, putting the whole puzzle together yourselves from assorted bits of information, insights, and advice.

You and your family may have to be your own father's or mother's evaluator, putting the whole puzzle together yourselves from assorted bits of information, insights, and advice.

If so, the best way to proceed is slowly, deliberately, and watchfully. If you do not panic, you yourself may be quite adept at figuring out what is happening, since you've known your parents longer and better than anyone else. Obviously, arrangements must be made to care for a disabled person adequately during an emergency, but they should not be solidified too quickly into permanency. They should be subject to revision until the situation stabilizes and its long-term implications become clearer.

Nancy Adams laughs a little sheepishly today when she remembers all the terrible thoughts that galloped through her mind whenever she looked at her disabled father in the early weeks following her mother's sudden death. "I couldn't bear to look at him. He seemed 10 years older. All the progress he'd made in getting around after his car accident vanished overnight. Someone had to lift him from the wheelchair to the bed. He hardly spoke, barely listened to anyone. I kept asking, "How can he go on? He can't live alone here! He'll have to move in with us! I'll have to quit my job to take care of him! But I can't

do that! A nursing home, maybe? Never! Not that! But what?"
I found myself wishing he'd died, too. What was left for him?"

Luckily for Nancy, she didn't know which way to turn and therefore did nothing. She took time off from work to help her father through the first devastating effects of her mother's death. Then, slowly, everyone noticed that he seemed to be getting stronger, moving around a little better every day, eating more, taking notice, responding. A few months later, it became clear that with some additional help—granted, that was a problem to arrange—he would be able to live a somewhat independent existence. When he remarried a few years later, Nancy was a little ashamed that she had predicted such a dire future for him just a short time earlier.

Pessimism may, on the other hand, be warranted. Nancy's father was lucky, but many are not. Emergencies that pass leave some older people totally incapacitated. Radical changes must be made then, and families who have learned everything they can about the realities will be consoled to know that they had no other alternatives. They will be less likely to torment themselves months later with guilty self-accusations, all beginning with phrases such as "If only we'd realized..." or "We never should have..." or "Why did we...."

As the population of older adults grows, and promises to balloon as baby boomers enter the ranks of the elderly, professional and community concern is growing as well. More community agencies are serving older people, providing assessment and care management services, home care services, adult day care, and housing. The goal of these home- and community-based services is to enable older people to keep living in their own homes as long as possible. A great deal of attention has been given recently to providing older persons with a single entryway to the community where a thorough assessment can be made of their situation, and where the help they need, pooled from perhaps a variety of sources, can be coordinated and managed for them. The assessment is seen as a vital preliminary to good planning by these service providers, just as it should be seen by the family and the older person.

"Geriatric assessment units" are another important development. Usually sponsored by hospital centers, these units are few in number. Most notable are the services provided by Mount Sinai Hospital in

New York and Duke University Hospital in Durham, North Carolina. Their services, now being replicated in different parts of the county, include full psychiatric, medical, psychological, functional, and social workups that closely involve the family. For more information, see the "Quick Reference Directory to Services in the Community" box, on page 245 in this chapter, as well as Appendix A.

The Levels of Care?

Since crises vary in severity, duration, and extent, there are several different ways to cope with them. During the acute phase, older people, like younger ones who are seriously ill, need skilled, constant care. But once that phase has passed, other types of care are often more appropriate. It is important to find the right balance in your own situation. Too little care can make your mother overanxious; too much care can make her unnecessarily dependent. Complicating the matter is the fact that her condition will change in time, although not always for the worse. In that case, reassessment is necessary to determine the right care at the right time.

Off-and-On Care

This level of care is neither continuous nor intense. Your parents may need help only during special periods, such as while recovering

Your parents may need help only during special periods, such as while recovering from minor illnesses or accidents or after the death of a beloved relative or friend.

from minor illnesses or accidents or after the death of a beloved relative or friend. When an emotional flare-up is triggered by a crisis, they may benefit from counseling or individual or group therapy. Temporary care should be available for just the amount of time it is really needed—no longer, no shorter.

Undoubtedly, the best place to find occasional care today, as in years past, is still within the immediate family. That does not mean that you have to be around your parents all the time or that you have to take them into your own home. Simply knowing you're available when they need you can provide all the reassurance they need to get along on their own the rest of the time. Sons, daughters, and in-laws, as well as sisters, brothers, nieces, and nephews, are usually quick to respond to a close relative's crisis if they are nearby and in a position to help. Close relatives provide an all-important ingredient often missing in off-and-on care from outsiders: the loving comfort that gives the extra boost to an older person's recovery.

> Eighty-year-old Maude Evans had a cardiac condition and high blood pressure, but had been able to live by herself for the last 10 years. When she was feeling well, she could manage her small apartment, cook for herself, and visit her friends and relatives. Periodically, she suffered cardiovascular flare-ups, which required close medical supervision and a good deal of rest. At times, the flare-ups made her anxious and depressed; at other times, they were precipitated by an emotional upset. During those episodes, her daughter would visit her daily to take care of the house, prepare meals, and do necessary chores. Occasionally, during an acute phase, an aide was hired to stay with her. But as soon as her condition improved, Mrs. Evans was eager to have her house to herself again and to return to her former pattern of living. Just knowing that she had someone to turn to for help if things went wrong allowed her to manage alone when life was going smoothly.

Particularly crucial to off-and-on care are rehabilitation services following an illness or accident. Some older people can be restored to a degree of independent living if they are provided with physical or occupational therapy to restore functioning before it is lost. These services can be arranged privately or through social or health agencies, which will be described later in this chapter.

When off-and-on care is not available, the anxiety of having no one to turn to in case of emergency may be too much for an older person and his or her family to bear. Sometimes, too, conditions that could have been nipped in the bud degenerate into chronic conditions, ultimately requiring radical changes, such as nursing home placement, that are traumatic to everyone.

Supportive Ongoing Care

This middle-range level of care is needed by older people who have chronic disabilities that permit them to function in some areas, but not in others. Although their conditions are not likely to improve, older people with chronic disabilities are often able to get along at

Although their conditions are not likely to improve, older people with chronic disabilities are often able to get along at home if on-going care is provided in specific areas.

home if ongoing care is provided in specific areas. Your father's heart condition may prevent him from managing his apartment alone, but if someone comes in to prepare at least one meal a day for him, and do the marketing and heavy cleaning, he can probably remain where he is—and where he may vehemently insist he wants to remain.

Older adults with chronic disabling arthritis may also need ongoing supportive care, as well as those who have no one specific infirmity, but are just generally weakened by advanced age. Although physical chores are beyond them, they may be perfectly capable of thinking clearly, making their own decisions, knowing exactly what they want, and saying so, loud and clear. Supportive care may also be required for those who are physically sound, but because of minimal mental impairment, need someone to help them manage their routines or their money, or make complicated decisions. Their ability to make decisions for themselves in some areas, however, should never be underestimated or taken away, unless they are courting danger to themselves or others.

As in the case of temporary care, supportive care is often provided by children and close relatives. But supportive care is long-term, ongoing, and sometimes very demanding. As we discuss in the next chapter, some families may find it too heavy a burden, and the help of outside agencies and professionals must be sought.

24-Hour Care

Eventually, for some older people, the time does come when halfway measures are no longer enough. One day, after a stroke, a heart attack, or severe mental deterioration, your mother may no longer recognize you or anyone else, or she may be permanently disabled. Your father may not know where he is, or he may have lost control of his bodily functions. People in those tragic conditions require 24-hour care. Some, whose overall condition may not be so hopeless, are still disabled enough to require constant medical attention

Intensive care is also taken on by some families, either in the older person's home or in an adult child's home.

and skilled nursing. That is the point at which some families cannot manage and feel forced to consider institutionalization. But intensive care is also taken on by some families, either in the older person's home or in an adult child's home.

> Prior to her stroke, 78-year-old Alice Tarrant had lived with her daughter and her daughter's family. She had been a good-humored, cooperative person who blended well into the family, helping when needed and rarely interfering. She was an excellent babysitter, and she shopped and took care of the house while her daughter and son-in-law went to work every day.
>
> Her stroke left her paralyzed on one side of her body and unable to handle any of the activities of daily living, including bathing, dressing, feeding, and toileting. At times she was incontinent. But following her hospitalization, the family decided to bring her home. They bought a hospital bed and other equipment to make nursing care easier and hired a home health aide to come in every day from 9 o'clock to 5 o'clock. A visiting nurse stopped by regularly to check on Mrs. Tarrant's condition, and a local doctor made occasional house calls. Her daughter and son-in-law took over in the evening and on weekends, but other relatives came in regularly to relieve them when they needed a break. Fortunately, there happened to be a number of other relatives willing to share the responsibility, and no one individual was seriously overburdened. Mrs. Tarrant, although partially paralyzed, remained in her familiar setting, aware of her family and the love and concern that surrounded her.

Alice Tarrant was fortunate that outside help was available in her community and that so much "inside" help was offered by her extended family. One family member—a daughter, a son, a daughter-in-law, a nephew, or a sister—may be willing enough, strong enough, and dedicated enough to assume the major responsibility. But no one should impulsively volunteer to be a primary caregiver without a full understanding of the rigorous demands of the job. If you are contemplating caring for your mother or father yourself, you might discuss the case first with a registered nurse at a hospital or a visiting nurse in your community, and find out as much as you can about the necessary routines. When your father needs constant care, that means around the clock, 7 days a week. You will be able to take time off, of course, but only if someone else steps in during your absence, and back-up home health services should be considered. Efforts should be made to encourage your father to take care of himself whenever he can: grooming, shaving, feeding, and toileting. But sometimes this is not possible. Beds must be made several times a day, baths and sponge baths given, and medications administered. Special care must be taken of the skin to avoid bedsores—any minor skin condition can be aggravated by incontinence. You may have extra laundry duties and kitchen duties. Nutritious meals, sometimes involving special diets, must be served three times a day, as well as periodic snacks. Orders from the doctor must be followed and reports on the patient's progress turned in to the doctor.

You must also be prepared to offer emotional support to your father. His morale as well as yours must be considered. The life of a shut-in or a bedridden invalid can be endlessly dreary and lonely. Some kind of recreation, such as handicrafts, books, or music, should be provided, and visitors should be encouraged to stop by. Patients can be difficult, discouraged, irritable, demanding, suspicious, or resentful, but caregivers are still expected to treat them with cheerfulness, compassion, and understanding. This is why respite time away from these duties is crucially important.

Helping Those with Dementia

When caring for an older person with some degree of mental impairment, it is essential to have some ongoing psychiatric and medical supervision. Medications prescribed for some agitated elderly patients that could have adverse effects need careful monitoring.

Since too much stimulation and excitement can be overwhelming and confusing, a calm, structured atmosphere with a regular routine is usually the most effective. Body language—of the patient and the caregiver—can often transmit clearer messages than spoken language. A confused older man may not be able to verbalize his fears, but his contorted face and thrashing arms may be caused by some real or imagined terror. An intuitive caregiver will pick up this clue. Spoken words of reassurance may do little to calm your agitated mother, but she may quiet down when the caregiver strokes her forehead and gently squeezes her hand, thereby sending an unspoken message of caring and protection.

If intensive care of a physically disabled parent is a rigorous job, the care of a mentally impaired one is equally taxing, even if it is not performed around the clock. You may find it particularly draining because of your close emotional involvement. Dealing with your mother's confusion, disorientation, loss of memory, or delusions day after day can be nerve-racking, and even though you understand perfectly well that she cannot help the way she behaves, you may still feel hurt when she does not even recognize you.

> *Dealing with your mother's confusion, disorientation, loss of memory, or delusions day after day can be nerve-racking, and even though you understand perfectly well that she cannot help the way she behaves, you may still feel hurt when she does not even recognize you.*

The best approach, which involves an almost superhuman effort for many children, is to remove yourself as much as you can from your personal feelings and try to help her hold on to some threads of reality. Although you find the endless repetition agonizing and frustrating day after day, she may be less confused if you quietly repeat simple, factual statements: "Yes, you've had your lunch," or "No, it's not morning, it's bedtime," or "Today is Thursday. Tomorrow is Friday," or "This is Jane, your sister." Big calendars, large clocks, even photographs of relatives can be ever-present silent reminders of everyday realities. Other compensations for memory loss and confusion are lists of daily activities in clear view, color-coded drawers and cupboards, and labeling of frequently used utensils. Older people with only partial mental impairment frequently suffer brief periods of disorientation, slipping into confusion and then out again. The more concrete clues they have available, the less likely they will be to completely lose their grasp of reality.

The same detached calmness is helpful for older adults with mental impairment who distort reality. Arguing about what is real or imagined will not help, but rather will make these patients more anxious and compound their confusions or delusions. There is no advantage to be gained by a pitched battle with your mother when she anxiously insists, "The mailman has a gun!" or "The delivery boy is a thief!" or "The homemaker is poisoning me!" It's best if you can sidestep what she says and pick up the feelings accompanying her words. When your first impulse is to snap back impatiently, "Nonsense! How can you say that?" try taking a deep breath and saying instead, "You're frightened, aren't you, Mom?" If your father keeps angrily insisting that your husband has a girlfriend and everyone is talking about your own immoral behavior, he'll never believe your denials. But he might respond if you ask him, "You're angry at us, aren't you, Pop?"

Helping Yourself

Despite the demands and frustrations, the care of the very sick can be quite rewarding if it is provided with devotion and competence. But regardless of the success you have with your parent, it is absolutely essential that you arrange for regular periods of relief. Friends and relatives may be willing to take over for you at regular intervals. Public health and visiting nurses and health aides may also be called upon, and can be invaluable in showing you more effective nursing techniques. The importance of respite and support services for family caregivers is finally receiving recognition, resulting in more programs, from day care for older persons to support groups, to ease the relentless burden of long-term care. Fortunately, an abundance of helpful resources is now available for family members caring for older adults with dementia. These are listed in the next section on community services and in Appendix A.

Involving the Family

Even if you are confident that you can manage a caregiving job, with all its physical and emotional demands, one final question must be answered before you take it on: how does everyone else in the family feel about it? Is it possible that, even if you won't resent your demanding job, others will? Their lives will be affected; their freedom will probably be curtailed in some way, too. If you end up devoting all your energies to one member of the family while neglecting everyone else, think of the

additional burden you may then have to carry—your guilt at neglecting them and your resentment that they make you feel guilty!
Moreover, if you don't involve them early on, and simply make a
unilateral decision, they may not pitch in later. When the situation
has been discussed freely in advance and all individuals have been
allowed to say how much responsibility they are willing to accept,
family disruption can be avoided, and the resulting family unity can
work wonders (see Chapter 11).

In their book *Gramp*, photographers Dan and Mark Jury put together a pictorial record of the last years in their grandfather's life—
years during which the old man's health seriously deteriorated and
he became incontinent. Nevertheless, he remained in his home, cared
for by his loving and devoted family. The Jurys admit that they were
able to keep Gramp with them until he died, partly because of the
genuine feelings they all had for him and partly because there were
enough of these loving people in the family, especially young, strong
grandsons, to take turns providing ongoing care. No one person was
victimized or martyred. Great satisfaction can be gained by caring for
a deteriorating, but well-loved relative at home, and that is often
compensation enough for the heavy investment of time and energy
required from everyone. The Jury family and others like them stand
as modern examples of the Iroquois precept: "It is the will of the
Great Spirit that you reverence the aged even though they be
helpless as infants."

What Does the Community Have to Offer?

Fortunately, community services for older people who cannot manage on their own are now available in most parts of the country. This
growth has been stimulated by a number of federally funded programs, supplemented in many states by general revenue funds. Each
state has an state Office of the Aging, usually located in the capital, as
well as local Area Agency on Aging offices established and funded by
the Older Americans Act and augmented with state and local funds.
Title III of the Older Americans Act funds social services, nutrition
programs, case management, and in-home services. In some states,
Medicaid is another source of funds for services to eligible older
adults, based on financial need. Social service block grants, awarded to

states to provide community social services for people of all ages, may also fund some programs for older adults.

This section describes the variety of services for older adults living in the community who cannot manage on their own. They may live in their own homes or family homes—some with support from family and friends. These services are vital to older adults who have no close family and can supplement the care when it is provided by family members—offering respite to burdened family caregivers. (Chapter 10 addresses the circumstances of families who are unable to provide any care for an older relative and must rely on others to provide, manage, and coordinate this care.)

For contact information on the community services described in the following pages see "The Quick Reference Directory to Services in the Community" on page 245 or in Appendix A. As noted earlier, social workers or care managers in the agencies providing these services can often help in making an assessment of your parents' needs and arranging for delivery and coordination of services. It is important to remember, however, that whatever ongoing help has been arranged for your parent, your monitoring of these services is critical to the quality of care they receive. Chapter 10 addresses the monitoring role of the private geriatric care manager when you cannot manage this role.

Information and Referral Services

Some communities have special information and referral services (publicly or privately funded) to guide residents of all ages to appropriate local services. You can find out what services there are and which ones your mother or father is eligible to use. When there is no independent information and referral office, similar information can be found at local sectarian or nonsectarian family service agencies, the area Office on Aging, or local senior centers, whose staffs are usually well briefed on community resources and can point you in the right direction.

An important resource for eligible older veterans is the Veterans Administration, which provides a wide variety of medical and social services. Veterans and their families should contact their local Veterans Administration office for more information on services and eligibility requirements.

Quick Reference Directory to Services in the Community

Geriatric Assessment and Care Managers
American Medical Association
www.amaass.org/go/ doctorfinder
National Association of Professional Geriatric Care Managers
www.caremanager.org

Information and Referral Services
The Elder Care Locator (U.S. Department of Health and Human Services)
Provides local information, referral sources, and contact information for local and state agencies.
www.eldercare.gov
800-677-1116

Mental Health
American Association for Geriatric Psychiatry
www.aagponline.org
301-654-7850
Geriatric Mental Health Foundation
www.gmhfonline.org
301-654-7850

Home Health and Hospice Care
The National Association for Home Care and Hospice

www.nahc.org
202-547-7424

Homemaker, Personal Care, Chore, Home-Delivered Meal, Escort, and Transportation Services
Local or State Office on Aging
www.eldercare.gov ("aging network")

Telephone Reassurance and Friendly Visiting
Friendly Visiting Worldwide (DOROT)
www.friendlyvisiting.org

Adult Day Care
National Adult Day Services
www.nadsa.org
800-558-5301

Support for the Caregiver
Children of Aging Parents
www.caps4caregivers.org
800-227-7294
Alzheimer's Association
www.alz.org
800-272-3900

Elder Law Attorneys
National Association of Elder Law Attorneys
www.naela.com
520-881-4005

Appendix A provides additional listings.

Home Health Care and Hospice

Most communities have visiting nurse services or other home health care agencies that offer skilled nursing, rehabilitation, and home health aide services. These agencies can be a link to other community services and may provide nonmedically related personal care services as well.

SKILLED NURSING CARE

Skilled nursing care in the home—following a hospitalization or when the needs of a homebound older adult are brief and intermittent—is covered by Medicare and Medicaid, and by some long-term care insurance policies. This medically related care can also include physical therapy, speech-language therapy, occupational therapy, and the services of a home health aide, homemaker, or social worker. A physician must certify the need for these services.

HOME HEALTH AIDE SERVICES

Whether covered by Medicare, Medicaid, long-term care insurance, or private funds, home health aide services are critically important to ill and disabled older adults living at home. Trained primarily for patient care, these aides may offer some personal care, such as assistance with bathing, dressing, toileting, feeding, and walking. They may also assume some household responsibilities, such as doing the patient's laundry or cleaning the bathroom. Families must keep in mind that health aides are not professional nurses; neither are they maids or servants.

Hospice care for terminally ill patients, described in Chapter 6, is also provided by home health care agencies. These comprehensive services are usually covered by Medicare and other types of insurance.

Medicare coverage for home health care (other than hospice care) is provided only for a limited period (usually not to exceed 100 days). *Medicaid*, which is state-administered, provides a broader array of home health services to eligible low-income older adults, but they vary from state to state. Personal care services may be covered for extended periods, in addition to skilled nursing care and rehabilitation.

Some *long-term care insurance policies* provide coverage for home health aide services. Other than insurance or Medicaid coverage, the costs of extended supportive care in the home must be borne by the older person and the family. Chapter 8 discusses the financial aspects of home health care in more detail.

Be wary of enlisting the services of a home health aide on your own or through an agency that is not state licensed or Medicare certified and that does not provide professional supervision. While there is no guarantee that an aide will be competent, kind, and dependable, the chances that your parent will receive adequate care are far greater if the home health aide is enlisted through a reputable certified home health agency.

Accreditation by the Joint Commission is a plus for a home care agency and can also offer you reassurance about the quality of its services. The Joint Commission's Home Care Accreditation program accredits more than 3,400 organizations that provide services in the home. Visit http:www.jointcommission.org/AccreditationPrograms/HomeCare. Whatever the qualifications of an agency, it is important for family members to remain involved.

HOMEMAKER, PERSONAL CARE, AND CHORE SERVICES

Even when an older adult does not need nursing oversight, he or she may still need help with household chores or personal care. Homemakers are responsible for shopping, doing laundry, and light cooking. Personal care workers assist a convalescent or a chronically ill individual in bathing, dressing, eating, and walking. Some older people are able to take care of themselves alone, but lack the strength, and sometimes the funds, to maintain their home. They can no longer deal with storm windows, clogged gutters, or lawn mowing. Funds are available in some communities for chore services at reduced cost. In a number of communities, vigorous and capable older men and women volunteer to perform repairs and chores for their neighbors who are incapacitated.

These nonmedical-related services are provided by volunteer agencies on a sliding scale fee structure, by the local Office of the Aging, or under private auspices. Families and older adults are cautioned to be selective in their choice of any agency. Standards for hiring, training, and supervision of homemakers, personal care workers, and even chore workers should be in place to prevent abusive situations.

HOME-DELIVERED MEALS

Malnutrition, which aggravates physical and mental problems, is the fate of too many homebound older adults. Inadequate income is one cause, but another is the inability of frail older people to prepare nutritional meals for themselves, especially if they live alone. Late-life changes in the ability to taste and smell, as well as ill health and certain medications, also tend to depress appetite. One way to address this problem is through home-delivered meals, a long-standing service funded by the Older Americans Act and administered through local Offices on Aging and volunteer agencies. Older adults of all financial means are eligible for what is more popularly known as "Meals on Wheels," in which one hot meal a day is delivered, usually 5 days a week and sometimes on weekends. Home-delivered meals provide not only nutritional benefits for older adults but also a side benefit. The volunteer (or paid worker) who delivers the meal may be the only contact a homebound elder has with the outside world and can serve as a social support. This person can also be a vital link, reporting back to the sponsoring agency on the elder's condition if problems arise.

CONGREGATE MEALS

Low-cost or free, these meals provided in senior centers, community centers, and some churches and synagogues encourage older people to get out of the house, eat well, and enjoy some company. Food stamps are another resource for lower-income older adults whose nutrition is at risk. In some communities, emergency food services and shopping assistance are also available.

Looking in on Your Parent

Who can check on your homebound father if you're at work, out of town, or living far away? Who can provide him with companionship?

EMERGENCY RESPONSE SYSTEMS

Technological innovations are offering new security to the families of older relatives living alone in their own homes. Emergencies, such as a fall or an acute illness, are a constant source of concern, since the older person often cannot reach the phone to call for help. Electronic devices located in the home or worn at all times can be activated to call for help if an older person is in distress. The signal is answered immediately by a trained professional, who speaks with the older person over a speaker system installed with the device. The professional assesses the situation and dispatches help if needed. If there is no response, emergency help is sent immediately. These devices are sometimes referred to as personal emergency response systems, but are also sold under different names. Your local Office of the Aging should have a list of reliable companies in your parent's community.

Other home surveillance systems can actually track an older person's movements within the home, or less invasively, pose daily questions about medication compliance or physical complaints and send help when needed. Some try to prevent emergencies, for example, keeping track of blood pressure or other health indictors. It's important to ask if response systems are monitored 24 hours a day by trained people, with what responders they are linked, if they will be serviced if necessary, and whether others have found them reliable. Consoling as electronic monitors may be for families, however, they can never replace human observation and contact

TELEPHONE REASSURANCE PROGRAMS

The telephone is a lifeline for the elderly person living alone—not only for safety purposes but also for companionship. A daily phone call by a regular caller at a prearranged time can serve as the best reassurance that all is well, for another day, at least. Children often set up their own systems, calling every day at the same time to say, "Hello, Mother, how are you?" and older adults themselves sometimes set up "buddy" systems in which two or more friends will call each other. As a back-up, a volunteer or commercial telephone checking service charging moderate fees can be used instead. Here again, the older person receives an added bonus—the chance to hear the sound of a human voice every day: "Hello, Mrs. Gavin. How are you feeling today?" If Mrs. Gavin does not answer her phone, help will immediately be sent to her home; if she does not answer her door, a neighbor, a friend, or a nearby police or fire station is asked to check in person and see if anything has happened. Lives have often been saved that way. Agencies across the country offer telephone reassurance services.

FRIENDLY VISITING

When friends are few and family is at a distance, older adults must fight boredom and loneliness. And friendly visiting, often described as "organized neighborliness," can be a great comfort to them. Friendly visitors may be university students or older adults, volunteering their services under the auspices of volunteer agencies. These visitors stop in to visit the homebound on a regular schedule, one or more times a week, and do whatever any other concerned guest might do: play chess or cards, write letters, run local errands, make telephone calls, sit and chat, and perhaps most important of all, listen. Family members who cannot visit often may find the friendly visiting service a welcome option. Friendly Visiting Worldwide, founded by DOROT, helps older adults and volunteers around the world find local Friendly Visitor programs.

Getting Out and About

ESCORT AND TRANSPORTATION SERVICES

Because they are often afraid to go out of the house alone—afraid of getting hurt, mugged, or lost—even semi-independent older people may retreat, too soon, to being shut-ins. The recent case of a 101-year-old woman in Queens who was mugged and robbed in the lobby of her apartment house only reinforces their fears. With driving behind them and fear before them, what else can they do? But thanks in part to the advocacy of younger disabled adults, much progress has been made in making public transportation accessible to older adults as well. City buses with steps that lower or with wheelchair lifts are more common, and some areas have responsive route systems that pick up or deliver qualified elders at or near their homes.

Providing safety for vulnerable older people in their own homes has yet to be realized. But escort services help to address this situation when relatives and friends are not available to accompany an older person to the store, the doctor, or an overnight visit with the grandchildren. Escort services for those unable or unwilling to travel alone are available in some communities. Volunteer groups under a variety of different names, such as Dial-a-Bus or Dial-a-Car, and often sponsored by religious and social clubs, make convenient transportation available in private cars or buses. Occasionally, these groups provide vans equipped with ramps for wheelchairs and walkers. Other communities may have special vans that periodically take older people and those with disabilities to shopping centers. Volunteers will drive older patients to medical appointments. When your mother leaves her home with an escort, both you and she will have some sense of security that she is likely to arrive safely at her destination. Your local Office of the Aging will have information about escort services available in your community.

COMMUNITY PROGRAMS

It is one thing to be able to get out of the house; it's another to have somewhere to go. Some communities have a lot to offer older adults in the way of recreational, educational, and social programs. These are most often hosted by senior centers, churches and synagogues, and some schools.

Senior centers, established decades ago under the Older Americans Act to provide social activities and a hot meal, now offer a much broader range of activities and services—some designed to help their members cope with the many challenges of later life. Some offer information and referral services, health prevention programs such as flu shots and blood pressure readings, and care management. Members have a chance to enjoy the companionship of their peers as well as that of younger volunteers and professional staff members. A number of senior centers offer intergenerational programs for young and old together.

ADULT DAY CARE

When a frail or impaired person needs help, but not around the clock, yet is too compromised to manage alone all day, an adult day care center may be the answer. It may also be an answer for older adults receiving around-the-clock care from family members—offering much-needed respite to a spouse, son, or daughter.

The programs vary, but usually provide some or most of the following services: assessment; counseling; nutrition, including a midday meal and snacks; special diets; personal care; health services, including blood pressure monitoring; height and weight checks; medication dispensing; health education; and arrangements for physical, dental, foot, eye, and ear examinations. Many adult day care centers also provide transportation to and from the center, on special outings, and to and from doctors' appointments. These centers, like the at-home services described earlier, make it possible for frail older men and women to continue to live in their own homes or with their families. Day care may be located in their own apartment buildings or in senior centers, churches, synagogues, hospitals, nursing homes, and sometimes mental health centers.

Inoperable cataracts had left 86-year-old Fritz Hoffman with little sight. Nevertheless, he was still alert, well oriented, and able to enjoy his record player, radio, talking books, and friends. Unable to shop, prepare meals, clean his house, or go out alone, he was dependent on others for protection and supportive care. Since he loved getting out of the house, his daughter, who lived an hour away, arranged for him to go to a day care program—funded by Medicaid, for which her father was eligible—at a local nursing home. Every day, a bus picked him up early in the morning and delivered him home in the late afternoon. A homemaker and home health aide came in twice a week to help him with household chores and shopping. His evening and weekend meals were delivered by a Meals-on-Wheels program from a nearby church.

At the day care center, Mr. Hoffman was given rehabilitation services and medical and nursing care when he needed it, as well as the opportunity to have a social life that he enjoyed. All of this could have been provided for him 24 hours a day at the nursing home next door, but it was important for him to preserve some portion of his independence and remain for some part of his life in his own home.

Support for the Caregiver

RESPITE SERVICES

Special attention is being given these days to the importance of relieving the burden on family members responsible for ongoing care of an elderly parent. It is essential that these caregivers have regular time-off periods. Beyond the alternative of day care, some nursing homes and hospitals set aside beds for nonresident elderly men and women who may stay for a short time, making it possible for their families to have time off or even to take a vacation. If no organized respite services exist in a given area, a companion or a homemaker may be found who can take over for the caregiver once or twice a week and provide the much-needed respite. If you are seeking this type of respite, contact your local agency on aging.

CAREGIVER SUPPORT GROUPS

Sometimes elderly people feel alone, but so do those caring for them. Caregiver support groups offer a place to air problems and feelings with others who are similarly burdened. Many are informal gatherings started by caregivers themselves with little or no professional backup. Others, usually guided by a social worker, are established by health and social service agencies, or civic and religious organizations. Whatever their aegis, these groups provide a therapeutic forum where caregivers can vent their fears, frustrations, resentments, guilt feelings—and solutions—with a sympathetic, understanding audience made up of people who are eager to air their own. One woman, the caregiver for her domineering father, gained enough strength from her support group to stand up to him for the first time in her life. She was 75 years old, and her father was 98! Some support groups are specifically targeted—for example, for family caregivers of persons with Alzheimer's disease and other similar conditions. These groups are sponsored throughout the country by the Alzheimer's Association and other organizations, and can be found in most communities. See the "Quick Reference Directory to Services in the Community" on page 245 or Appendix A.

What if They Won't be Helped—by You or Anyone Else?

Finding suitable support for both you and your parents may be just the first challenge you face. One of the greatest barriers to helping your parents can be your parents themselves. Firmly believing that they can take care of themselves, they may shun your advice and reject all help—despite being told that their home is unsafe, or that a physical condition will probably get worse and that you would like to bring someone in to help. Perhaps they just need time to digest this distressing news and to

> Finding suitable support for both you and your parents may be just the first challenge you face. One of the greatest barriers to helping your parents can be your parents themselves.

think through the alternatives. Being pushed or even nagged may only cause further distress. They may even dig in their heels.

"I'm perfectly fine. Stop worrying about me!" an 80-year-old severely arthritic mother may shout at her son for the 50th time. "I can still manage my own affairs," a father ill with emphysema may insist. But he's not fine, and she can't manage. Though some older people ask for too much help and others for too little, some won't accept any. They may refuse to accept the limitations imposed by their age, their physical deterioration, and their financial plight. They may not want "strangers" in their home and refuse to sacrifice any degree of their privacy and control. They will not listen to logic and reason, nor will they be coaxed, bribed, or cajoled into changing their life-styles. Sometimes both of your parents may refuse all offers of help, reject any alternative living situations, and insist on staying right where they are, taking care of each other as they always have done—even though their house is an unsanitary shambles and full of hazards.

If you take matters into your own hands and make arrangements for them, they are legally within their rights to fire summarily any outside help you bring in, and this often happens. Maybe they will let someone they already know help out, but if not, there isn't much you can do except wait for the day an accident or illness incapacitates one or both of them. And then you can step in. Surreptitiously making nursing home or home care arrangements behind their backs or taking bold steps when they are in the hospital may make it easier for you, but may only upset the delicate emotional balance they have been trying to sustain in their lives. Occasionally, if they will not listen to you or anyone else in the family, they may listen to someone they trust who is not a relative: a minister, a rabbi, a priest, a social worker, a doctor, or even a close friend.

It is enormously difficult to tell your father that he is not managing well or can no longer drive his own car safely. But let him know clearly that the status quo is not an option you can accept. Let him also know that you will still be there for him, but will not support his current lifestyle. Let him calmly know how much stress he is burdening you with. (After all, he is your parent and presumably still cares for you and is concerned for your welfare.) It is likely that maintaining a loving relationship with you carries more weight in most parents' lives than their independence. After communicating as clearly as possible with your parents, it is important to give them time to think matters over. You may need to repeat your message several times.

Patience, firmness, and clear communication are in order. Keep in mind that the loss of autonomy is a terrifying prospect to some older people. Try and take steps with them that help them feel that they are in charge as they make necessary changes in their lives. Offering them options—even if limited—provides them with some sense of control.

> Bea and Frank Visconti were not managing. Their daughter knew it and their friends knew it, but they would not admit it. Money was not a serious problem, but no outside help was allowed to remain for long. They were both undernourished, their clothes and bodies uncared for, and their apartment littered. Their daughter went back and forth between her town and theirs, trying to bring order to the chaos and hoping each time to persuade them to accept some compromise. Their son-in-law finally stepped in to settle the situation. He did not give orders, and he was not dictatorial; he allowed Bea and Frank to be involved in their future plans. He gave them three choices and time to decide. All they had to do was select one. "All right, which will it be? Come live with us. Go to a nursing home. Or, stop firing the home health aide."

Most important of all, you want to avoid a power struggle with your parents. Avoid nagging them about minor issues, such as exercising more, not eating certain foods, or letting you clean up the clutter in their home. Save your serious discussions for the big issues: their health and safety. Step back if conversations become heated, and wait to talk again when tempers have cooled.

Although children are urged to give quiet support to their parents' lifestyles, no child should support a pattern that threatens life and health. *And this includes driving an automobile.* Chances are that your communications with them are not clear, and perhaps you haven't really listened to their reasons for their "stubbornness." Understanding their reasons may give you clues about proceeding. "If I don't drive, I'll be stuck in the house all the time." "If a stranger comes into the house to clean, she will boss me around." Reassurance that you will help to offset these fears may be all that is needed.

When Incompetence is the Issue

However, the day may come when your father's mental condition deteriorates to such a point that he is no longer capable of deciding about his future and managing his affairs. He may be too disabled to enter into any contract of the sort described in the previous chapter, such as a power-of-attorney agreement, and the only way open to your family may be to have him declared incompetent by the courts. Incompetency proceedings, like many other legal proceedings, vary from state to state, but they usually involve certification by physicians or psychiatrists of the older person involved, and appointment of a guardian to manage his affairs and provide for his needs and well-being.

Many families find the mere idea of incompetency proceedings too painful to consider. There is still much shame and stigma attached to any kind of mental illness in our society. Some states have enacted conservatorship laws designed to avoid the emotional burden normally associated with incompetency proceedings. These laws provide for the appointment of a conservator to take over the financial affairs of anyone who becomes too impaired because of advanced age, illness, infirmity, or mental deterioration to manage alone. It is also important that the older person's long-term interests are respected. Consultation with an elder law attorney is a first step. For contact

When Parents Refuse Help

- Listen to their reasons.
- Communicate clearly your concerns.
- Share with them the impact on your life.
- Provide them with as many options as possible.
- Avoid unnecessary confrontations—stick with the big issue of care and safety.
- Be patient, but firm.

information, see the "Quick Reference Directory to Services in the Community" on page 245 or Appendix A.

"Managing Well"

An indisputable fact is that families provide the great bulk of care to their older relatives, and many are managing this care successfully, often with support from others. Family care can range from providing around-the-clock help, to providing now-and-then assistance, to providing emotional support and being available at times of crisis. In all cases, however, it is not just the older adult's needs and limitations, but those of the family—especially the primary caregiver—that bear considering. Families are coming to realize that turning to others or to community resources is not a negative reflection on them, but an important means to the goal of "managing well" for everyone concerned.

However, there are circumstances when sons and daughters simply cannot manage this care. Perhaps they live too far away, suffer from poor health themselves, or travel constantly. Or a parent they've been caring for suffers some further debilitation with which they can no longer cope. In that case, much of the "managing" must be turned over to others, and support must be sought in the community or a nursing home—situations discussed in the next chapter. Yet even in these circumstances, family members remain indispensable, for no one else on earth can provide what you and your relatives can—shared memories, the intimate knowledge of who an aging parent really was and is, and the comforts of your love and company.

Bob Morris on "Making Sure That We All Had a Good Time"

I think that my generation is hooked on certain things, and one of them is exercise. And so what do we do? We know that it makes *us* feel better—endorphins, yoga, and meditation—and so we are desperate to push this on to our parents, who don't have the same mental, physical, or emotional makeup. You know, it was all about trying to make my mother's life better when it was going downhill. And it was all about the guilt I felt, and the sadness I felt, that there wasn't anything I could do.

It was a mixed bag. I mean, I think about the walking—going for walks, and always trying to get her walking—I didn't know that it was too hard for her—it had to be done with a sense of humor. But I can still remember being out at that house on Long Island, and being shocked at how weak and listless she had become. And I kept hoping to make her understand that moving around is good for you.

I was so upset that I couldn't help her feel better. Well, guess what I found out after she passed away? That she had had lung problems—it wasn't just a blood condition—and it was just really painful to exert herself at all. Had I known that, would I have insisted on the exercise? Maybe not.

Here's a selfish thing. I don't care for the house I grew up in—never have. So when I could avoid visiting my parents there, I would. I'd say, "It's easier for me to take the train to Cold Spring Harbor—or some pretty area of the North Shore of Long island—let's meet there.

So there were many, many, many Sunday afternoons when that was my way of making sure that we all had a good time. I was setting up something that I would also enjoy, so that it didn't become only service-oriented. And I would leave them feeling good that I'd done something nice. It was always something I could enjoy, too. That way, I wouldn't just be forcing a smile, but I'd actually be happy. I was, again, single. I didn't have a country house to go to that was pulling me anywhere else. So it was spring, and I wanted to get out of the city. I think that the good part was that they knew that this was something *I* wanted to do—my suggestion. It intersected well with what they could do and what I wanted.

So in those years, when I wanted to see them and cheer them up, and not make myself unhappy, I would say, "Meet me," and we'd go driving around all these areas on Long Island that they hadn't seen. That worked for my father, and it worked for my mom. And as importantly, it worked for me.

We could enjoy things together.

10

Stepping Back—When They Cannot Manage and Neither Can You

Myra Fields and her older brother, Ben, knew for many years that if and when their parents needed ongoing care, others would have to provide it. Myra lived a continent away, and Ben did not get along with either his mother or his father. Their parents' decision to enter a life care retirement community was a great relief to Myra and Ben. And the "little" Myra could do through e-mail, phone calls, and a yearly visit meant a great deal to her parents.

WHEN OFF-AND-ON CARE OR AROUND-THE-CLOCK care is necessary for one (or both) of your parents, someone must be available to provide it, but that someone does not have to be you, your younger sister, or your older brother. In many cases, as described in the last chapter, you and other family members will manage on your own or with the help of some community resources. In other cases, a self-reliant but disabled older adult will organize his or her own care. But not infrequently, neither the older adult nor the family can manage; therefore, it is necessary to rely heavily on outside resources.

There are times and circumstances in which you simply cannot provide the care your parents need. Perhaps their health and functioning have significantly deteriorated. Perhaps your own health is compromised, or you're faced with the health problems of a spouse or a child; perhaps you live too far away from your parent; perhaps your job is too demanding; and perhaps the relationship with your parent is not a close one. Given those realities, as in the case of Myra, the most you may be able to offer (and maybe all your parent wants) is an arm's-length supportive relationship. This does not translate into your not being a responsible son or daughter, but it does mean that you have limits to your own capabilities. Accepting this knowledge about yourself may cause pangs of guilt, but it is a reality.

Stepping back and allowing or finding someone else to share the burden is not buck-passing or shirking, no matter how other family members or friends choose to label it. The neighbors may tut-tut when they see a stranger coming in every day to take care of Mrs. Grenville, or an outsider taking Mr. Packer to have a medical test. They may enjoy gossiping about Mrs. Grenville's "unfeeling" daughter or Mr. Packer's "no-good" son. Meanwhile, Mrs. Grenville could be quite content that she has someone to take good care of her, and Mr. Packer may be relieved that his brace can be adjusted regularly without the need to bother his busy son.

It's even possible that someone else might do a better job than you in caring for your parents. In fact, skilled workers who are less emotionally involved may provide much better care. Constant attention to your parent's meals, baths, and medications can be a crushing burden even to well-intentioned families, and the quality of that care may ultimately suffer.

It's even possible that someone else might do a better job than you in caring for your parents.

There are significant roles other than caregiver that family members can fill, which in the long run can be just as beneficial to a parent. They can be supervisor or coordinator of services, financial manager, companion, or simply a loving daughter, son, or grandchild who visits. The type of role your and your family assume is determined by your capabilities, availability, health, and obligations to others. Most important of all, *it will also be determined by what the older person wants.*

Modern sons and daughters, tugged guiltily between careers and children, tend to carry an extra layer of guilt about their aging parents. "I was supposed to drop in on Dad tonight, but after I got out of work late, I had to pick up some supper and then Nick had problems with his math homework, and it was just too late," a daughter might berate herself. As it happened, Dad was fine, engrossed in a rerun of *It Happened One Night*. Children sometimes overestimate their own roles in their parents' lives. Studies suggest that many older people, even those with close ties to their offspring, sometimes prefer a measure of separation. Why else do so many choose, as one report shows, houses or apartments in retirement villages with no extra bedrooms? They may say that the choice was based on cost or convenience, but admit to their peers that it was also to prevent lengthy visits from children and grandchildren. "I'm through hosting Thanksgiving for them all," said one 74-year-old, as she moved into an assisted living apartment. "I've passed the turkey platter to my daughter-in-law."

The Home Care Alternative When You Cannot Manage

When the time comes that your father simply cannot manage on his own and the family cannot handle his care, even with the support of some community services, you and your family need to decide whether to bring outside help into the home on a daily or around-the-clock basis or to seek nursing home care. Keep in mind that the "home" of your parent may be special housing for the elderly or an assisted living facility (described in Chapter 7). These housing arrangements (unless they have special units for older adults needing around-the-clock care) do not include in their services the care that would be provided by a skilled nursing facility. You will have to arrange and pay for additional care.

When the time comes that your father simply cannot manage on his own and the family cannot handle his care, even with the support of some community services, you and your family need to decide whether to bring outside help into the home on a daily or around-the-clock basis or to seek nursing home care.

Care in the older person's home or assisted living facility goes beyond hiring a home care worker who provides crucial assistance. Depending on a parent's condition and needs (which must be assessed), there's the additional need for supervision of the home care worker and someone to coordinate a variety of health-related and other services. Families sometimes take on that job, but for those who can't, the services of a geriatric care manager should be considered.

The Geriatric Care Manager

Vivian Worth—a 50-year-old divorcee—always stopped in after work to help her 81-year-old mother, who had diabetes. Vivian fixed her a light supper, ensured that she took her medications, and assisted her in bathing. When Vivian was offered a promotion to senior buyer in her company, she was elated, but then realized that the new job would involve extensive and frequent travel. How could she accept it when her mother needed her on a daily basis?

Even though Vivian lived near her mother and wanted to help, she could not continue the daily support without making drastic sacrifices in her own life. Her community may have been rich in supportive services for older adults, but she had no idea which would be the right ones for her mother or how she would be able to coordinate and supervise them once she had found them.

The use of geriatric care managers or case managers has become common in publicly funded state and local community-based programs. Care managers are professionals skilled at providing client assessment and case planning as well as finding, coordinating, and monitoring other necessary services. The staffs of some volunteer social agencies include care managers. Care management fees in these agencies are on a sliding scale: services are provided at low or no cost for those who cannot pay and at higher cost for those who can. Schedules are usually crowded; there may be a waiting list, or there may be no care managers at all on the staff of certain social service agencies.

Given the growing need, there has been a rapid increase recently in private geriatric care managers and care management agencies. To date, their fees are not covered by Medicare or other insurance. Vivian Worth did not have enough time to devote to her mother's care, but she did have enough money. Through the local hospital social service department, she located a private geriatric care manager and paid privately for the services provided. If you feel that such an arrangement would be helpful to you and your parents, be sure to check the credentials of the care manager you hire. Anyone who assumes this role should have a professional degree and be state certified or licensed in social work, psychology, counseling, or nursing.

Thanks to geriatric care managers, sons and daughters living far away from their parents can find some peace of mind. Nothing is more alarming for children than getting word that a parent who is far away is in trouble. Whether the trouble is a minor crisis or a major one, it can produce frantic anxiety and family turmoil—should they cancel meetings or take a midnight plane? If you live on the East Coast and your parents are on the West Coast, it's one thing to fly out on occasion to help them. But if their difficulties are ongoing, how can you spend your life in the air shuttling between the coasts? An agency, social service or private, in your own community may be able to put you in touch with a similar agency in your parents' community to find and monitor the necessary help. Although now there are more such agencies nationwide, there is no guarantee that one can be found in every area. When one

Thanks to geriatric care managers, sons and daughters living far away from their parents can find some peace of mind.

Finding a Geriatric Care Manager

- For public or private agencies, call Eldercare Locator at 1-800-677-1116 or go to www.eldercare.gov.
- For private geriatric care managers, check www.caremanager.org.
- Contact the discharge planner at your local hospital.

is available, however, it can help to bridge the painful distance separating concerned children and their parents.

It is especially comforting for older people—and their families—to know that they can turn to the same person when troubles arise. Your mother may speak warmly of "that nice Mrs. Walker down at the agency," the person she calls when she needs help. Professionals are becoming increasingly aware of the need to provide this continuity of connection. They realize that the confusing array of different services and suppliers, and the time it takes to sort them all out, often makes it impossible for families to locate the help they need. A care management agency can cut through the confusion by assigning one worker to an elderly person and whatever family is involved, as well as conduct an assessment, calling on medical and nursing help, social workers, and other consultants as needed. This same worker will pull together the necessary services and provide supervision to make sure they are working out. As the older person's condition changes, the cluster of services being received can be increased or decreased.

Enlisting the services of a geriatric care manager is an ideal way to guarantee consistency and continuity of care in lieu of available family members. Unfortunately, care management and similar agencies are not to be found everywhere, so many families must manage by themselves, making do with whatever scattered services they can find.

The Nursing Home Alternative

When a parent's condition requires 24-hour, around-the-clock care and the family cannot provide this care, even with the sort of home support services described here and in the previous chapter, nursing home placement may be the only option. It may be preferable for other reasons as well. Good nursing homes provide opportunities for socialization that are too often missing in the lives of the homebound.

If your parent is already a resident in a continuing care retirement community that provides multiple levels of care, the transfer to a nursing home can be seamless. However, if you wait until serious trouble strikes to seek an alternative, such as a retirement community or an assisted living facility, you will find your options limited. These residential facilities prefer newcomers to be relatively healthy and independent, and of course, wealthy enough to pay their way. Without recourse to such specialized housing, you will probably have to struggle on with a disabled parent, in his or her home, or yours, or seek nursing home placement, at least initially, on your own.

> The second stroke did not kill 80-year-old Peter Vorman, but it severely paralyzed him. He lived—but he needed care 24 hours a day. Someone had to be there all the time to feed him, bathe him, dress him, take him to the bathroom, and medicate him. Neither his wife, a semi-invalid herself, nor his children, who were married with families of their own, could give him the care he needed. There were only limited community services in the small town where they lived. The family made a careful study of available nursing homes and settled on the one they felt would suit Mr. Vorman best. Once he had moved in and was comfortably settled, his family left, feeling relieved. But Mrs. Vorman could not forgive herself for "abandoning" her husband, and the children never lost the feeling that they had failed their father, "locked him up," "put him away."

The Vorman family is not alone. The very term "nursing home" conjures up a series of unhappy, even terrifying images in the minds of old and young alike. The words suggest coldness, impersonality, and regimentation, and at worst, neglect, mistreatment, cruelty, and loneliness. Alas, these negative images legitimately describe some institutions. But they cannot be applied to all. There are too few excellent nursing homes and too many disgraceful ones, but the majority lie somewhere between these two opposites.

No nursing home can work miracles. No nursing home can make the old and feeble young and vigorous again. No nursing home menu will ever please all elderly palates—sensitivities vary, and taste buds are often duller. No nursing home will solve all the various roommate problems or prevent friction between residents: communal living has its built-in stresses. Dissatisfaction is predictable in some areas of nursing home life.

When nursing home placement is necessary for an elderly parent, realistic sons and daughters must face an imperfect situation and two painful realities: the sorrowful deterioration of a person they love,

When nursing home placement is necessary for an elderly parent, realistic sons and daughters must face an imperfect situation and two painful realities: the sorrowful deterioration of a person they love, and their own inability to care for that person.

and their own inability to care for that person. Placement in a nursing home, although often a sad step, is not tantamount to dying. There still may be some gratifying living ahead. Nor does "institutionalization" necessarily imply family rejection. But those are widely held suppositions often reinforced by the elderly themselves. "No matter what happens," a mother may say to her children, "promise me you'll never put me in one of those places."

It is important to note that placement in a nursing home need not necessarily be permanent After being discharged from a hospital, a number of older adults enter a nursing home for rehabilitation or recuperation. Such short-term stays, which are frequent, are often covered by Medicare, and older adults are able to return to their home in the community. It also happens that some elderly residents change their minds after entering a nursing home and—with help—return to their former homes.

Frank Harmon's stressed wife, Ann, knew that she could no longer manage when her husband, who had a failing heart and had been further weakened by a recent bout of the flu, slipped in the bathtub, and she didn't have the strength to lift him out. Her children agreed: for Mom's sake, Dad should now be looked after in the local nursing home, where she could visit him every day. There Frank recovered some strength—enough, in fact, to allow him to phone his friends constantly and beg them to take him home. Desperately homesick, he even called his lawyer, claiming, "The house is mine. I want a divorce!" He wanted a divorce so that he could get home to his beloved wife of 48 years! Without telling her children, Ann finally agreed to take him home. She arranged for around-the-clock home aides and a visiting nurse, and brought him home, putting up with extra equipment and a shifting population of helpers in their small house. And there, contentedly propped by his own fireside, he spent his final 6 months.

Frank was not only stubborn, but also fortunate. Without sufficient resources for help, his move back home might have been impossible. The family—in this case, his wife—can make the crucial difference.

Statistics about nursing home residency are misleading. While it is true that at any one time only 5% of the members of the over-65 population are living in such institutions, 52% of all women and 33% of all men who are now 65 will spend their last years in a nursing home. It may surprise those who share the prevailing negative assumptions to learn that it's not always the children who "put their parents in nursing homes." A number of older people enter voluntarily; they are not pushed in, cast aside by rejecting relatives, or locked up against their will.

> All four of Maria Vincente's children were horrified when their mother, who was becoming severely disabled by arthritis, announced her intention to enter a nursing home. Why did she need this? Didn't she believe they all loved her and wanted to take care of her? And the grandchildren, too? Why should strangers take care of her when she had family? But Maria, a feisty, determined 80-year-old, could not be dissuaded. As a matter of fact, she had already made all the arrangements.
>
> On the day she was to take up residence, her neighbors dropped by her apartment to say goodbye. To each one, she whispered, with a resigned sigh, "My children are putting me in a nursing home."
>
> Her daughter, overhearing, burst out, "Mama! How can you say that? You know it's not true!"
>
> "I know and you know," Maria replied calmly, "but I have to tell them something they'll understand."

Maria Vincente did not share the popular belief that entering a skilled nursing facility inevitably signifies the end of it all. There are some, but not many, Marias around. In truth, most families have two obstacles to overcome before accepting a nursing home solution: their own aversion and the opposition of the ailing parent.

It is hard to pinpoint the exact moment when institutionalization becomes a necessary move—what provides the tipping point that forces the decision. In cases of severe or sudden incapacity, the need for such a decision is more obvious. But the tipping point may also come from a combination of factors: partial incapacity, combined with inadequate help in the home, exacerbated by increasing personality conflicts. The research shows that the tipping point arrives most often when the family, often burdened with their own problems, is no longer able to provide the needed support. But for most families, whenever the tipping point comes, whether early or late, it is painful to accept. For them, it may represent failure, and for their parents, a tolling bell of finality.

Selecting a Nursing Home

If there is no immediate crisis demanding a solution, there can be time for a thorough review of all possibilities, taking into consideration the preferences and attitudes of the older person involved. Nursing home placements made on the basis of impulsive, frantic decisions usually produce disaster all around. The mother or father in question may feel bewildered, coerced, infantilized, and rejected. In addition, rushed placements allow no time to investigate the quality of an institution or to find the one offering the best rehabilitative, restorative, and supportive services. "Who's got room for Mom right away?" is the only question there is time to ask, rather than, "Which is the best place for Mom? Where will she be happiest?" An essential ingredient in all of this planning is to make sure that Mom is involved at each step. Assuming she is still mentally capable, she has the ultimate right to make the final choice.

Deliberate and careful planning has the advantage of giving both the family and the elderly parent sufficient time to prepare emotionally. The feelings stirred up by placement can be so intense that counseling may be invaluable to everyone during this time. Your mother may need someone to whom she can express her anxiety over the separation that placement will bring and perhaps her feelings of being unwanted. Since placement is usually a less socially acceptable solution than remaining in one's own home, it can create feelings of anger, sadness, and guilt, all of which need to be aired if the transition is to be smooth for all concerned.

Here again, the services of a geriatric care manager can be helpful, not only in providing counseling but also in locating an appropriate nursing home. Counseling can also be provided by other professionals. The following discussion summarizes important steps to follow in selecting a nursing home. It will offer guidelines for the actual admission and provide a brief review of institutional life itself as it affects those inside as well as the relatives who remain in the outside world.

Not knowing where to start is the quandary shared by many families when they first approach the unexplored territory of nursing homes. "How do we go about the whole thing?" they ask helplessly. There are thousands of nursing homes in the country, varying in capacity from 25 to more than 1000 beds. In some areas, the choice is limited; in others, there are dozens to choose from. Keep in mind that there are also three different types of sponsorship:

1. Nonprofit, sectarian or nonsectarian, usually governed by a lay board
2. For-profit
3. Public (very few)

In the wake of past nursing home scandals, public and private agencies in some locations drew up lists of acceptable nursing homes in their particular areas. Local information and referral services, social service agencies, ministers, doctors, and nurses may know if such a list has been compiled for your parents' community. Even if no such list exists, the same sources can usually tell you something about the local nursing homes. Knowing what's available is only the beginning. A series of logical steps must be taken to find the answer to the crucial question: Which is the best home for Mother?

Step 1: Deciding on Location

Proximity is an important issue in the selection of a nursing home. The value of visits by family members and old friends cannot be underestimated. That emotional and social support is important not only for them but also for you, since in many ways the family continues to play a significant role in the life of a nursing home resident. The quality of your parent's care also requires monitoring. If placement far from the family is the only alternative, the services of a geriatric care manager or a loyal friend or companion in overseeing nursing home care may be desirable.

Finding a Good Nursing Home

First decide: should it be near your parent's home neighborhood or elsewhere, perhaps nearer your home? The following resources can provide you with information that can help you decide on this and other questions concerning nursing home care.

Contact your local Area Agency on Aging office. Call 800-677-1116 to find your local Agency on Aging.

Or contact any one of the following:

- A discharge social worker at the area's leading hospital
- A local social service agency, such as the Visiting Nurse Association
- A geriatric care manager or physician
- Your parent's own physician or minister
- Other families with experience with a certain home

The following web sites also provide useful information:

- www.AAHSA.org
- This site for the American Association of Homes and Services for the Aging lists nonprofit nursing homes by region, as well as assisted living, senior housing, and community services.
- www.medicare.gov/NHCompare. This site is a free state and county locator of nursing homes qualified for Medicare and Medicaid. It shows statistics for each on patient care and staff-patient time ratios, compared with state and national averages. Phone numbers for regional ombudsman and state agencies are also listed on the site.
- www.healthgrades.com
- This site rates nursing homes of various types by states, based on state inspections and complaints, showing the history over several years. The cost is $19.95 to compare up to 10 facilities, and $3.95 for an additional 10.

Step 2: Understanding How Money Determines Your Options

Unfortunately, as in every other aspect of the lives of older adults, dollars and cents must be considered in choosing a nursing home. The financial picture today is not as bleak as it was before the establishment of Medicare and Medicaid, but it is essential to determine before choosing a nursing home whether it is approved for Medicare and Medicaid, assuming your parents are eligible for either. *Medicare coverage is limited*, only covering care in an approved skilled nursing facility for up to 100 days post-hospitalization and for specified conditions. Medicaid can cover the cost of care for financially eligible persons in approved skilled nursing facilities for as long as their condition merits it.

unfortunately, as in every other aspect of the lives of older adults, dollars and cents must be considered in choosing a nursing home.

If your parents have no money or assets, several agencies can guide them through the steps that must be taken to apply for Medicaid coverage of nursing home placement (as described in Chapter 8). Nursing homes themselves can be helpful. If there is one particular nursing home your parents prefer, the admissions department can help with the necessary applications.

Families also need to be aware of the regulations governing the time limit in which an older adult can transfer his or her assets to others to be eligible for Medicaid coverage. If assets were transferred to adult children less than 5 years prior to admission (it used to be 3), these assets or an equivalent amount from another resource will have to be tapped to pay for the cost of nursing home care before your parent is eligible for Medicaid coverage of nursing home expenses. The rules governing the transfer of assets are complicated, however, and the counsel of an elder law attorney or local Medicaid office is recommended. See Appendix A for information on these resources.

However, many homes do not accept residents who cannot pay for at least some initial period and therefore will not accept anyone who must be admitted on Medicaid funds from the beginning. When your parents have no money at all or no long-term care insurance, their options are limited in every area of their lives, including nursing home selection. However, a house still in a parent's ownership can be, and often is, sold to support initial nursing home care.

Step 3: Evaluating Quality

In finding the answer to the crucial question, "Which home will be best for Mother?" the most important step is a rigorous review of both the dollars and cents of nursing home costs and the levels of care offered. This involves making a list of possibilities in the desired geographic area, checking the opinions and judgments of knowledgeable people, and then inspecting each one during a personal visit. Even better would be to make several visits, at different hours of the day. If they are able, your parents should be encouraged to share all the steps, including the inspection tours and the final decision.

YOU CAN LEARN A LOT FROM YOUR RECEPTION

While it is true that first impressions are sometimes incorrect and need revising, it is usually possible to sense immediately the attitude of a nursing home's staff toward your visit.

While it is true that first impressions are sometimes incorrect and need revising, it is usually possible to sense immediately the attitude of a nursing home's staff toward your visit. Is there a friendly welcome? Are you encouraged to tour freely, ask questions, and talk to residents and staff? If the staff members seem defensive or reluctant to let you tour, or insist on showing you only what *they* want you to see, you would probably be right in supposing that there is something they want to hide. Openness is usually a clue to quality, and all parts of an institution should be open to you. Potential residents and their relatives are consumers shopping for a way of life. They have a right to know, down to the last detail, exactly what kind of life they are buying.

Since the privacy of residents should always be respected, certain areas of any nursing home may be in use and closed to you when you visit. If you are particularly interested in seeing those areas, you might have to return at another time. Return visits can be time-consuming, but they can pay off in terms of information. If you come at lunchtime, for example, how many residents needing help with feeding are getting that help? Are many residents still in bed? If in the afternoon, are there any activities or amusements available?

WHAT DO OTHER PEOPLE HAVE TO SAY?

Other people's opinions can be extremely helpful. Some families prefer to gather as much information as possible about a specific home prior to a first visit, while others decide to visit cold and check out their impressions with informed people afterward. The families of residents already living in a home can tell you about their experiences, and nursing home staff members are usually willing to suggest names of people for you to contact. Community agencies, physicians, and members of the clergy are all good sources of information and may even be willing to tell you why they prefer one home over another. Another source can be the state agency that licenses the homes you are visiting.

It's best to draw on more than one source of information. When talking to families of residents, always keep in mind that emotions run high when a relative is institutionalized. Sons and daughters may be ruled by strong personal feelings and prejudices not universally shared; so weigh all violent opinions carefully. If a friend says of an institution you are considering, "That snake pit! They killed my father there!" she may possibly be justified, but you would be wise to check further. Similarly, don't accept blindly a daughter's glowing report on Apple Tree Manor. Her views may be colored by her relief that someone else is finally taking care of her difficult, demanding mother. No one person or agency is acquainted with, or even interested in, every aspect of good nursing care. A nursing home shopper has to act a bit like a computer, allowing all relevant information to be fed in, hoping that eventually a definitive answer to the all-important question—"What's the right nursing home for Mother?"—will somehow appear on the printout.

WHAT TO LOOK FOR WHEN YOU VISIT

Prospective applicants and their families often find a checklist helpful during nursing home visits. Because the tours have such emotional undertones, visitors often forget many questions they planned to ask and essential things they wanted to see. A checklist is provided in Appendix D, but you may want to draw up your own list of questions to cover your specific requirements. Some queries on the list can be quickly settled by simple observation, and others can be answered by talking to residents and members of the staff.

You probably will have checked out the home's overall licensing status prior to your visit, but if not, now is the time to review it and to find out whether specific staff members are licensed also. Licensing is crucially important, and if a home is unlicensed, try to avoid it, because you can be sure there is something seriously wrong with it. Some states also require that the administrators be licensed. Always check this qualification, too, because the administrator is the key figure, the one who sets the tone of the entire place. Other personnel on staff—physicians, registered nurses, occupational and physical therapists, dietitians, and social workers—should be licensed or certified as well. It is a plus if the home has been accredited under the Joint Commission's Long Term Care Accreditation Program (www .jointcommission.org/AccreditationProgram/LongTermCare/).

Once the routine items are taken care of, a visitor needs to be alert to three broad areas in each institution: the quality of the medical, nursing, and therapeutic services; the quality of housekeeping and meal services; and finally, the "climate" of the home—its social life and emotional atmosphere.

Medical, Nursing, and Therapeutic Services

- *Medical Service.* Every home should have a physician available in case of emergency, on staff or on call. Some good homes allow residents to be treated by their own private physicians as often as necessary. Other patients must depend on the home's physicians, and it is important to find out how often they visit. (In some states, it is mandatory that all nursing home residents be visited by a physician once a month.) If a resident does not have a private physician and there is none on staff, be sure to find out how the home guarantees regular medical attention.
- *Other specialized medical consultants* should be available—either on staff or within easy call—for psychiatric, dental, eye, and foot care. Those specialties are far from minor or incidental ones, and in fact become more essential with age. Even the best nursing home cannot be expected to serve as a fully equipped hospital, but every institution should have an ongoing arrangement with a nearby hospital for acute illnesses. If there is no hospital nearby, it is important to find out how the home deals with emergency situations.

- *Nursing and Therapeutic Services.* The competence and humanity of the nursing staff probably affect the morale of the place more than any other quality. Nurses and aides have more continuing contact with residents than anyone else on staff, and their attitudes and behavior have great impact. To hear them converse cheerfully, even with withdrawn residents, calling them by name, can be heartening. "Look out the window, Mr. Ames, we got 3 inches of snow!" "Who gave you that pretty new bathrobe, Mrs. Thompson? Was it your daughter?" Yet the opposite atmosphere, where staff members are overstressed, officious, and remote, can be chilling.
- *One or more registered nurses* should be on duty at all times to provide appropriate coverage in a skilled nursing facility (depending on the size of the home). Nurses give medication and directly supervise the care of residents. Licensed practical nurses with at least 1 year of specialized geriatric training should be on duty around the clock on all shifts.
- *Other Services.* Highly competent medical and nursing staffs are essential, but they cannot be responsible for all aspects of an elderly person's care. Other services, some of which may be required by state health codes, are also essential if an elderly resident's ability to function is to be restored or even maintained: occupational and physical therapists, dietitians, and social workers with clinical training.
- *What about the resident with mental impairment?* The care of older adults with advanced chronic brain disorders is a fledgling art. Nevertheless, you have a right to expect that any good nursing home will have a positive approach to those with Alzheimer's disease or other types of dementia or mental conditions. Staff members that show patience, understanding, and warmth toward these residents, formerly written off as hopeless or impossible to reach, are much to be prized. Some therapeutic tools have been developed to deal successfully with the behavioral problems associated with Alzheimer's disease, and ideally, the staff of nursing homes should be trained accordingly. For example, through reminiscence therapy, some residents are helped to recapture some of their memories, and functions lost as the result of a stroke may respond to rehabilitation.

- *Medication.* It is not uncommon for nursing homes to treat the behavioral problems associated with mental impairment with psychotropic medications. If they are not administered properly, your parent may be overmedicated, and family members need to be alert to this possibility. If your father is suffering any serious mental condition, it is particularly important to make sure that the home he enters is equipped to deal with his particular situation. Psychiatrists and specially trained staff members should be available. These situations, and others, such as the use of restraints, have caused great concern among watchdog groups, such as the National Citizen's Coalition for Nursing Home Reform (www.nccrhr.org).

  > If your father is suffering any serious mental condition, it is particularly important to make sure that the home he enters is equipped to deal with his particular situation.

- *Is it all shadow or substance?* Many nursing homes boast a wide variety of special services. Their brochures show an impressive staff of professionals and an array of services to prospective applicants and their families. But visitors are advised to judge for themselves whether the boasted services are actually making an impact and whether the touted professionals are in evidence. Are the residents clean and properly dressed during the day? By what time? Are physical and occupational therapy rooms in use—or empty, showing little sign of ongoing programs? Are residents involved in activities, or are they lined up in rows against the wall, staring into space? Are they responsive to each other and to what is happening around them? Do you feel as if you've walked into Sleeping Beauty's palace and found a perfectly set scene with all the actors fast asleep? Poor nursing homes rely on sleep as a great problem solver, and as noted, often medicate residents heavily to avoid trouble. Even when there are high standards of professional staffing, efficiency, and cleanliness, steer clear of homes where residents spend much of their time in bed and asleep.

Housekeeping and Meal Services

- *How good is the housekeeping?* Every institution must provide room and board for its residents, but they should be provided in an attractive physical setting. Preferably, this includes comfortable rooms; a safe, clean environment; and furnishings appropriate and comfortable for residents with disabilities. An older person can adjust much more quickly to attractive surroundings than to a hospital atmosphere suggesting coldness, efficiency, and sterility. A homelike effect is enhanced when residents are allowed to furnish their own rooms with personal items. There should also be comfortable public rooms and dining halls, recreation rooms, special purpose rooms where residents can have some privacy, and ideally, some opportunity for fresh air and sunshine outdoors. Even urban institutions can provide terraces and roof gardens.

- *How good are the meals?* Although their taste sensitivity and appetite may have diminished with age, nutritious and tasty meals are important to frail older adults. For some, mealtimes take on even great significance since their lives have become more constricted. Whether served in a dining room or by the bedside, tasty and nutritious meals are essential and ideally planned by a trained dietician. Family members should inquire if attention is paid to the needs, restrictions, and preferences of the individual resident. Is thoughtful planning given to the enjoyment of food and the socialization associated with meal time? Some nursing homes have dining rooms where residents and visitors can dine together.

- Some elderly residents have difficulty eating and drinking due to diminished vision and difficulty handling utensils or opening cartons because of hand tremors or paralysis. They require assistance, and here a family member or friend can be particularly helpful by visiting at mealtimes.

Climate

- *Homelike or sterile and repressive atmosphere?* Judging the climate and making an accurate prediction of the prevailing "weather patterns" can be one of the most challenging parts of any nursing home visit. This may be the major factor determining whether your parent will make a reasonably good adjustment to nursing home life or will slip further into emotional or physical decline. Accurate weather prediction is notoriously difficult. Professional facilities and services in one home may meet your highest hopes, but the fine quality may be neutralized by an atmosphere of coldness and repression. That alone might not prevent you from selecting the facility, but should warn you that there could be trouble in the future.

- An ideal atmosphere—one that is warm, respects individuality, and confers dignity—is not easy to achieve. Even though this type of atmosphere may appear spontaneous and undirected to you, it usually is just the opposite, the result of explicit expectations percolating down from the top: from the board of directors and administration through the supervisors and professionals.

PERSONAL PREFERENCES MAY DICTATE CHOICES

In addition to high performance in all of these areas, the best nursing home for your parents may have to meet some particular needs. If your mother is an orthodox Jew, for example, it may be crucial to her to be in a place where the dietary laws are strictly observed and the holidays honored. If she is foreign-born and has difficulty with English, she may need someone available who understands her language. Homes can be found that satisfy quite a range of such individualized demands. Whether or not it matters to you, the particular cultural, religious, or ethnic inclination of a nursing home may matter a great deal to your parent. Equally crucial can be the location and setting of the home—whether in the country, the suburbs, or the city.

> The Farmer family was delighted to find a top-flight home conveniently located in their own suburban town. There were beautiful grounds and a view of rolling hills from every window, and the family fully expected Mrs. Farmer to make a good adjustment there. She had certainly seemed favorably impressed when she visited before her placement. To her children's great disappointment, however, she remained withdrawn and apathetic, while the nurses reported that she slept badly and ate little. Eventually, it was discovered that she hated the country and pined for city sights and sounds. Born in the shadow of the Third Avenue El in New York City, she had lived all her life on a busy main thoroughfare. Fire engines, ambulances, and noisy traffic never disturbed her sleep, but crickets,

bullfrogs, early-rising birds, and the wind rustling in the trees outside her window terrified her and kept her awake. Neither she nor her children had considered that possibility when they selected the home.

When everything else is equal, proximity can be the deciding factor in the selection of one home over another. You may know already that your mother thrives on close contact with you or another one of her children

> When everything else is equal, proximity can be the deciding factor in the selection of one home over another.

Frequent visits will be crucial to her well-being. If so, it may be better for everyone if she selects a home, even if it is imperfect, where you can visit easily without disrupting your life completely. Another place may offer a wider range of services, but those assets may not balance the benefit of family visits. You know your own mother best!

WHEN THERE IS NO CHOICE

It is tragic that, for people in many areas of this country, there is no choice, or only a limited choice. When your mother begins to deteriorate, you may look into all the nursing homes within a wide radius of your community or hers, yet find nothing that meets your standards. If, after following all the steps listed earlier in the search for a nursing home, you are forced to settle for one that does not meet your expectations, it may be cold comfort to know that you are not to blame. You can rightfully blame society at large when you see at close range the narrow, limited, and often inadequate provisions made for the nation's older citizens.

MAKING THE FINAL DECISION

Once all the relevant data have been collected, several nursing homes will emerge as worth considering, each of which probably will have some pros and cons. Even with several possibilities to choose from, most families find the period leading up to a final decision to be a time of anxiety, insecurity, and guilt. Regardless of the degree of planning and the excellence of the institution selected, nursing home placement often symbolizes irrevocable changes in familiar and valued relationships.

This is the moment when families must accept the fact that someone else will be taking care of an ailing parent from now on. For many, it represents the end of a long struggle to maintain their parent in the community. They will have to deal with the guilt they feel by admitting that they are unwilling or unable to continue handling the burden themselves. At this time, when family unity is most desirable, family tensions often run high. Tension may occur between husbands and wives—"If you weren't so selfish, you'd let my mother live with us"—or between brothers and sisters—"We'd love to take Father, but how can we, when we travel so much? Why don't you take him?"

Difficult as this period prior to nursing home placement can be for the relatives, it can be even more painful and more terrifying for the older person involved. After a long series of losses he has already suffered, your father's nursing home placement can represent the ultimate loss—of his household and his role as a householder. All the roles that, in combination, made up his status in society are now gone. At an advanced age, he faces an identity crisis: "Who am I?" and "What am I doing here?" He must now adapt to someone else's routines and regulations because, no matter how caring, intimate, or family-like the nursing home, certain basic routines must be carried out. Even the best home requires the surrender of some independence, and that is a cruel loss for men and women who have formerly prided themselves on their self-reliance and self-sufficiency.

Becoming a Nursing Home Resident

When Moving Day Comes—Admission and Early Adjustment

The transition to nursing home life can be an orderly, carefully maneuvered undertaking, unless the move is made directly from a hospital to the home and a speedy transfer is necessary. But whether the transition is hectic or leisurely, the admission itself is a traumatic process for prospective residents and their relatives as well. There must be room for a variety of feelings at that time: irritation, anger, recrimination, depression, and disappointment. Intermingled with all these painful feelings can be a sense of relief for everyone—both the new resident and the family—that "the worst is over."

To a certain extent, a sense of relief is warranted, because the long, and often wearying, period of uncertainty and indecision is past. But it is certainly too soon to sit back complacently, because a sometimes equally wearying period of adjustment lies ahead. Now, as the nursing home staff enters the picture, a relationship that was formerly two-sided, involving children and an elderly parent, becomes three-sided. A delicate balance must be found between a hands-off, no-interference approach and an overly involved one. The best way to achieve this balance is to aim for it from the beginning.

In Charge of Their Choices

Whenever possible, the older person should be in charge of his or her own move, taking the major responsibility, even if it slows things up and inconveniences everyone a little. Your father should discuss the date of his admission and make the arrangements for the closing of his own home, the handling

Whenever possible, the older person should be in charge of his or her own move, taking the major responsibility, even if it slows things up and inconveniences everyone a little.

of his finances, and the choice of clothing and furniture he will take with him. Most homes today allow residents to bring personal objects with them: a special pillow and blanket, their own clothes, family photos, and sometimes pieces of furniture. All of these provide some continuity for the older adult during a time of often wrenching disruption in their lives.

If your father cannot manage those procedures physically, he should at least direct them and be consulted all along the way. He may even have planned already which grandson would get his walnut desk or which daughter would most appreciate the framed portrait of her grandmother. Deciding about every big and little thing is a process far more time-consuming and less efficient than calling an auctioneer or the Salvation Army, who can remove everything in a matter of hours. To think of his treasured possessions remaining with friends and family rather than going to strangers can be deeply reassuring, offering a kind of immortality. Even if he's indecisive, try not to make decisions for him, but help him make a choice for himself. "Your blue coat is pretty shabby—do you want to take that, or your new brown one?" is a better ploy than "I'm packing your new brown coat; that old blue one's not worth taking." Don't be surprised, either, at the unlikely array of items he decides to bring. "Surely, you're not taking that lumpy old pillow. It's falling apart!" But that lumpy old pillow may hold a lifetime of memories. It may be too precious to leave behind and just the thing that will add a familiar touch to a strange room in a stranger place.

The more involved your father is, the less he will feel as if he has been coerced and treated like a child, and the deeper will be his commitment to his new home. He will be better able, if permitted to disburse and choose his possessions, to cross the shaky bridge linking his former life with his new one. This approach, however, does not always guarantee the desired results, especially with someone who is consistently negative.

> The Gordon family was keenly aware of the need to allow Mrs. Gordon to do things her way. While she was in traction in the hospital, they discussed nursing home placement with her, visited various homes themselves, reported about each one in detail, and let her decide on the one she preferred. Instead of moving her directly to the home from the hospital, they made complicated arrangements to allow her to return to her own house for a week and direct the disposal of her possessions as well as her own packing. The family congratulated themselves because they never told her what to do during the whole difficult period. It came as quite a shock to them, therefore, to hear her frequently refer to that period as "the time you made me give up my house and sent me to this place."

Once They Are in Residence

Each home has its own approach to welcoming a new resident, and it is now that the new three-sided staff-family-resident relationship begins. Some homes treat the admission process with the greatest consideration, assigning trained staff members to help the newcomer, remaining close by his or her side, and helping to orient him or her to the new surroundings. This consideration is especially helpful for the mildly confused or blind person.

Other homes, which are excellent in different ways, are perfunctory about the admission process and do little to acquaint the new resident with the environment. If your mother senses a laissez-faire attitude when she comes in, she may want you to be there with her as much as possible in the early days. Frequently, the home itself will ask relatives to spend considerable time with a new resident, even when staff members are available and ready to help. Other homes prefer relatives to stay in the background in the early days, until the newcomer has settled in.

Your mother may face some dramatic adaptations during her early days in a nursing home. Already exhausted physically from the strains of moving, and exhausted emotionally by the storm of feelings aroused by the move, your mother must now become familiar with new patterns of living: new daily routines, new rules, and new roommates, unless she can afford a private room. As one feisty 90-year-old widow, who could afford a single room, pronounced: "I do not share bedrooms with people I'm not married to." But since single rooms are far and few between, a newcomer may wake up in the night and ask in bewilderment, "What's that strange person doing in my bedroom?" In the midst of all these adjustments, older adults must continue to adapt to the physical disabilities that made nursing home placement necessary in the first place. It's not surprising that it is often a very rocky time.

Your mother may face some dramatic adaptations during her early days in a nursing home.

There May Be Reversals

Many new residents suffer physical and mental reversals during this adjustment period. Although occasionally severe, these may only be temporary setbacks that improve significantly with time. Residents with Alzheimer's disease and other dementias can actually show some improvement in a secure environment. Speedy changes for the better are often seen in the malnourished elderly adult, whose overall condition improves remarkably with a balanced diet. Sociable people, who felt cruelly isolated in their own homes or apartments prior to placement, often flourish when they find companionship again, and those who have made the move independently, without pressure or persuasion from relatives, make the transition more easily.

Marie Cohen had spent 4 years living in her son's extra bed-room. Although she was visited daily by a home health aide while her son and daughter-in-law went to work, it had been a lonely time. When her condition worsened and she became fearful after two nighttime falls, she agreed with her son and daughter-in-law that the best thing to do was to enter a nursing home. Thanks to a sensitive admissions person, Marie was able to share her room with Naomi, a resident who was 4 years older, but equally alert. Naomi filled her in on the place—the "nice" nurses, the favorite mac-and-cheese lunch, the annoy-ing woman at their dining table. They watched *Jeopardy* to-gether and, within weeks, had become good friends. Though Marie sorely missed the big, comfortable room she'd occupied at her son's house, she made a good adjustment, thanks to Naomi.

Everyone Makes Mistakes

In their eagerness to speed up the adjustment or because of a con-tinuing unresolved sense of guilt, families often make mistakes. It is impossible to catalogue the endless variety of human errors made by relatives whose intentions are good and whose judgment is poor, but two common ones should be avoided.

1. Beware of Early Visits Home. Instead of making the adjust-ment process less painful for new residents, weekends away, overnight visits, or even dinner invitations usually do the opposite. Adapting to the strange atmosphere involves a slow, steady progression from one stage to the next. Each day that passes helps to erase the sense of strangeness. Shuttling back and forth between an old life and a new one is confusing, and the physical travel adds stress at an already difficult time. It will be hard to refuse if your mother begs to visit or pines to have Sunday dinner with the family, but one Sunday dinner might set back her adjustment by several weeks. Residents themselves often sense the potentially harmful effects of visits outside and refuse all invitations.

"Not yet, thank you," said one particularly sprightly old lady, repeatedly refusing her relatives' invitations to dinner. "Not while I'm in training."

"Training for what?" they asked.

"I'm training myself to stand the terrible cooking in this place," was the answer, and she waited 4 months before accepting an invitation.

2. Beware of Panic. Nursing home professionals report that it can take as much as 6 months for an older person to make a reasonable adjustment to institutional life. The ups and downs of the period are hard to take, and too often families and staff members are quick to panic—to regret the admission or feel that the resident has been placed in an inappropriate part of the home. This may turn out to be true eventually, but it is not wise to jump to conclusions too early. Patience and helpful support can go a long way toward helping your father return to his former self. Jumping the gun, taking drastic measures, insisting that another home would be better, and moving him will only put him under further stress and compound his problems.

What If They Don't Adjust?

Some residents adapt to nursing home life with a kind of passive acceptance, neither happy nor unhappy, abiding by the daily routines and participating in activities with little enthusiasm. Others are active participants, obviously flourishing, deeply involved, ready to take responsibility, and full of ideas for changes. But then, sadly, there will always be some who never adjust at all, remaining bitterly unhappy and finding no compensations to engage them. They may withdraw or sink irreversibly into mental or physical decline.

Families always hope for a positive adjustment, but it is hard to predict at the outset whether this will happen. Nursing home professionals who have seen hundreds of elderly people and screened dozens of applicants are unable to say who will do well in institutional life and who will not. Even if the outcome could be reliably predicted—if, say, someone devised a test to prove that Mr. Jenkins will never adjust to nursing home living— there still might be no other workable

The families of residents who never adjust have a particularly difficult burden to bear: they must watch their parents' unhappiness and pain, at the same time suffering feelings of guilt and shame for their involvement in the placement.

alternative for Mr. Jenkins, and placement would have to be made anyhow.

The families of residents who never adjust have a particularly difficult burden to bear: they must watch their parents' unhappiness and pain, at the same time suffering feelings of guilt and shame for their involvement in the placement. But blaming themselves will not help, nor will it help to blame the staff or the institution. The difficulties facing older adults often go far beyond their children's help and the help of any institution.

In the ideal situation, the staff, the family, and the resident will emerge after the adjustment period with a smoothly working relationship, a three-sided partnership in which each side assumes different responsibilities. The resident does something that no one else can do for him or her: adapts to a new way of living. The staff offers something that the family cannot: 24-hour-a-day skilled protective care. And the family offers something that the staff cannot: intimate affection, links with the past, and contact with the community outside. While the ideal situation is hard to achieve and all three sides are often in conflict, some kind of workable relationship can usually be developed.

The Ongoing Roles of the Family

Even though they are not involved in much of the daily care of their parents, family members play several important ongoing roles: those of providing oversight, maintaining bonds of affection, and providing a link with the community outside.

Even though they are not involved in much of the daily care of their parents, family members play several important ongoing roles: those of providing oversight, maintaining bonds of affection, and providing a link with the community outside. The oversight role is critical particularly on behalf of residents who, because of physical or mental impairments, cannot speak up for themselves. Even in the best institutions the regular presence of family members signals to staff their ongoing concern for the resident. If family members live at a distance, it is important that someone close by—friend, care manager, or lawyer—fill this role.

Regular visits are very important to most older people, but close relationships can also be maintained in other ways. Cards, letters, phone calls, photographs, and newspaper clippings can reassure elderly men and women that their close ties are still strong and that those they love are concerned about their welfare.

When it comes to the small comforts a parent cherishes, no one understands them better than the family. Only a loving daughter will know what kind of underwear her mother finds most comfortable, what kind of powder she likes after a bath, or which flower is her favorite. A son may be aware of his father's need for a night light and his intense aversion to the only newspaper circulated in the home. Families also are aware of the particular talents of their relatives. Trying not to "stick out" in his new residence, Mr. Fisher may never reveal that he's a talented pianist unless a family member encourages him to play again—giving delight to himself and all around him. These individual needs may seem inconsequential, but when added up, they can make the difference between happiness and unhappiness in the home.

Yet while residents often thrive on family contact, many can also manage to get along without it. Close friends can act as substitutes; other residents and sometimes even staff members step in to fill the gaps left by absent or uninterested relatives. Occasionally, residents previously torn by long-standing destructive relationships use their nursing home placement as a way to withdraw from family battles, turning to new relationships within the home. The extent of your own involvement with your parent will depend on your old relationship and your parent's needs and receptivity. In some cases, old seesaws come into a new balance: domineering parents mellow, and children long fearful of criticism feel freer to be loving in response to a parent's gratitude for their attentions.

Keeping Residents in Touch with Their World

Although some nursing home residents become recluses, most are eager to be kept in the loop by their families—told about the niece who had a baby, the minister's retirement party, and the new supermarket in their former neighborhood. Since older people usually want to be informed truthfully, bad news as well as good should be shared. Understandably, however, many families try to hide bad news from a fragile parent and are particularly reluctant to reveal the death of a close relative, a friend, or even a pet. "Don't let Mother know!" is often the first thought in everyone's mind when tragedy

strikes. But Mother, even though she seems confused and disoriented, is usually quick to sense when something is wrong, which
only adds to her confusion.

It is unrealistic to try to hide the death of a close friend or family
member, and the attempt usually leads
to more trouble. If Uncle Joe used to
visit her regularly, how will she be able
to understand why he doesn't come
anymore? It may be less painful for her
to accept his death than to sit, day after
day, thinking he has forgotten her.
Older adults can often accept tragedy much better than you think
they can—possibly even better than you do. People living into their
70s, 80s, or 90s have had plenty of time and opportunity to experience tragedy. If you deny them the right to hear painful news, then
you also deny them an equally important right: to share in the pain
of the people they love, even to be of help. No wonder that kind of
treatment leaves them feeling excluded. Although no one should live
on a constant diet of bad news, the chance to share in family problems
may be the one thing that penetrates the self-involvement shown by
so many nursing home residents—and older people in general.

> It is unrealistic to try to hide
> the death of a close friend
> or family member, and the
> attempt usually leads to
> more trouble.

People used to turn to Doris Price when they were in trouble.
She was valued as a concerned mother and grandmother and
a helpful friend, until she became ill and entered a nursing
home. There she seemed to withdraw into herself and showed
little interest in anyone else. Visitors were shocked at the
change in her and tried to rouse her with reports of family and
community activities, but only the pleasant ones. She showed
little interest in those and quickly changed the subject back to
her favorite one: herself. One day, her son, overburdened by
his own problems, let slip news of her grandson's arrest on
drug charges. Instead of having the adverse effects everyone
might have feared, that was the news that finally roused her,
and she responded to it with all her former concern and understanding. Afterward, her family members were able to resume their old relationship with her, turning to her with their
troubles and thereby reassuring her that she was still part of
their lives.

When There Is Trouble

Troubles can erupt in a nursing home: some due to the demanding behavior of a resident or family member and some to problems in the care being provided.

The Demanding Resident

Some elderly residents make endless demands on their families: telephoning constantly, insisting on more visits than anyone could reasonably manage, complaining loudly about poor care, and accusing every relative of selfishness and lack of concern. That kind of demanding behavior is sometimes seen right after admission, and if it is out of character and is dealt with calmly by the family, it may subside after the difficult period is over. It may also occur because nursing home residents, forced to give up control in so many areas of daily life, may need to assert themselves in whatever ways they can.

But if people have been demanding, selfish, and resentful prior to admission, they are likely to continue this behavior, and their families will have to learn how to deal with them. Easier said than done, such families will say. If they haven't learned to say no to a domineering mother in 50 years, it's hard to begin. But it is possible for her family, even at that late date, to tell her firmly, without becoming rejecting, just how much they can be expected to do for her. They may even learn to say no at last.

Demanding behavior, whatever its causes, can be used by older residents as a way to trap their relatives. If you spend inordinate amounts of time with your father just because he insists, you are trapped. If you feel guilty when your father complains about the "miserable conditions" in the home, you are trapped. Complaints should be considered and checked for validity, of course, but the worst trap of all is allowing yourself to become involved in a power struggle with the staff over your father's care. He'll never give up behavior that produces just the results he thinks he wants until you set limits on your time and energy. When he realizes that further demands are fruitless, he may gradually begin to focus less on you and more on his involvement with other residents.

> *Demanding behavior, whatever its causes, can be used by older residents as a way to trap their relatives.*

The Demanding Family

Families also resort to demanding behavior. They may disguise their demands by being overly solicitous, by incessant visiting, or by constant complaints and interference with the staff, all of which may put undue emotional strain on their own relatives. There are always reasons for such behavior. A son may be trying to curry his mother's favor, to stay in her good graces. A daughter may be continuing a lifetime of sibling rivalry, still competing with her sisters and trying to prove that she's the best one. Children may be overly attentive to quiet their guilt or to protect their share of an expected inheritance. Excessive behavior from families is as destructive as excessive behavior by residents and becomes even more so if the staff gets drawn in.

> Frances Wilson, a rather simple person herself, had raised three children who grew up to be successful professionals. All of them were very dependent on her and very competitive with each other. When she was 79, she became seriously disoriented, and her children arranged for nursing home placement. They did not really accept her mental decline, which they aggravated by their demands. She deteriorated further after placement, partly in retribution for their action and partly to withdraw from further conflict.
>
> Her oldest daughter took the lead among her siblings, as she always had, and constantly found fault with the staff. She blamed them for not rehabilitating her mother, but at the same time, interfered with their efforts to help. She directed most of her hostility at nonprofessional personnel, the aides and orderlies, whom she snubbed. They reacted with understandable resentment, some of which affected Mrs. Wilson. As the three-way battle continued, her condition regressed to the point where she became incontinent and uncomprehending, and she deteriorated beyond help.

Help for the Troubled Family and Resident

Some nursing homes have social service staffs capable of helping with troubled family relationships. Psychiatric consultation may also be available. The trouble may be recognized first by a staff member who, hearing that a family's behavior is too demanding on a resident or overly critical of personnel, suggests a consultation. Similarly, families who are being drained by a relative's demands, or are in serious conflict with the nurses, may ask for help themselves. When no services are available or additional ones are needed, help can be found outside the institution from social workers, social service agencies, or private psychotherapists. Self-help groups, organized and run by families themselves, are appearing in many nursing homes. The members have much to offer each other—support, information, and above all, the reassurance that they are not alone in facing these problems. (See Appendix A.)

When Things Go Wrong

Things can go seriously wrong with nursing home care, even in the best-run institutions. If you have selected your mother's home with great care, you may find it hard to believe that any criticism you feel (or any complaint she makes) could be valid, and you may wonder at first if the trouble lies in your own unreasonable expectations or in your mother's unreasonable demands. But when you are convinced that a complaint is justified, you have a duty to speak up about it, or even to take drastic action.

A move to another institution, disruptive though it may be, may be the only humane way to escape mistreatment. If you find that your mother's basic needs are constantly neglected—if she suffers from bedsores (decubiti) and seems frightened and withdrawn, and if the staff is callous and neglectful or disregards your concerns—you may be forced to move her. But you have a further responsibility beyond her personal welfare: a responsibility to other residents and an obligation to file a detailed complaint with the proper authorities.

In general, however, the situation is neither drastic nor clear-cut. When things are going reasonably well, you may be tempted to adopt a "don't make waves" or "don't rock the boat" philosophy. But a series of minor incidents, added up over time, can produce major setbacks. Poorly prepared meals, rudeness or callousness from a staff member, missing clothing, beds still unmade or residents still in night clothes at noon: all should be reported. In nursing homes, as in every institution, there is a chain of command, and if you do not find satisfaction at the first level, take your concerns to a higher level, from floor nurse to the nursing supervisor or administrator. Concerns may be aired through resident councils by residents themselves or through relatives' auxiliaries by the families. These groups can exert pressure on the administration to improve general welfare and therefore general morale, but they are not found in every institution; often they exist in name only.

When no such machinery exists, the proper authority can be alerted in a businesslike way by letter or telephone. You can call your local department of health if you have a justifiable complaint that is being ignored. The Older Americans Act made funds available for ombudsmen at the state level to "receive, investigate, and act on" complaints made by elderly residents of long-term care facilities. The Area Agency on Aging will know if your state has such ombudsmen, and if so, how to contact them. The National Citizen's Coalition for Nursing Home Reform (www.nccrhr.org) may be able to refer you to a local helpful resource.

You have a right to expect an answer to a complaint. If no answer is received and the problem continues, repeat the process until you see action. If you run into a stone wall but are reluctant to transfer your parent, there are higher authorities outside the institution that can address complaints. All nursing homes are accountable to a state department of health that licenses them, and there are channels through which families can take legal action. Such drastic steps should not be necessary in homes, where responsible administrators welcome consumer feedback, aware that a constant dialogue, involving staff, residents, and families, produces the most constructive results.

Don't Be Afraid—But Don't Point a Finger

"If I cause a ruckus by going over the staff's heads with my complaints, won't they just take it out on Mom?" a concerned child may worry. In well-run homes, at least, experience shows that a resident who speaks up for his rights or has a vocal and alert family to speak up for him or her usually receives better care. Keeping quiet out of fear only allows a bad situation to get worse. Rather than retaliation, responsible consumer feedback usually leads to improved services. Pity the timid residents who are afraid to complain and have no families to back them up—they are the more likely victims. Growing public pressure to protect the rights of helpless residents resulted in the mandated Resident's Bill of Rights, which every nursing home receiving government assistance must abide by.

It is wise, however, to balance your persistence with tact. Rather than blaming the staff or the home, take responsibility.

When she finally was able to make an appointment with the director of her mother's nursing home, Jean Reynolds was overwrought and angry because her mother had lost a third pair of eyeglasses and her dentures. On the advice of a friend, however, she calmed down, and in her meeting with the administrator, she asked for help in understanding her mother's situation. She also asked what she could do as a family member to be helpful. Relieved that he was not under attack, the administrator agreed to try to resolve the problem.

Other Transitions Can Be Rocky, Too

Keep in mind that moving from one's home to a nursing home is only one of the stressful changes older adults must endure. Consider the following other types of transitions:

- From home to a retirement community or other type of special housing, such as an assisted living facility
- From one level of care in a retirement community to another
- From one room to another in a nursing home
- To and from the hospital for acute care

The physical risks implicit in transitions are of great concern, but so are the mental and emotional risks. For those who are mentally sound—for any of us, in fact—admission to a hospital is particularly upsetting. For those with dementia who cannot process the changes taking place, confusion can be greatly exacerbated. Sometimes, even moving from one hall to an unfamiliar one can cause a setback in physical health and functioning.

The physical risks implicit in transitions are of great concern, but so are the mental and emotional risks.

Sons, daughters, and other family members can do a great deal to ease the stress of transitions for an aging parent. Inform the staff that you want to be alerted to pending moves so that you can, if possible, be present to prepare your mother or father and help them settle in their new surroundings (even if it is the room next door). Giving priority to visiting at such times can be very important including meeting with staff if your parent has been moved to another floor or facility and sharing a little of their background. It will help humanize your parent who is more than the patient in room 12D. It can be comforting to your parent to carry along a familiar object such as a family photograph, a favorite shawl, or music.

> Bob McMurray rushed to the hospital when he was notified by the assisted living facility where his father lived that his father had suffered a mild stroke and was hospitalized. Beyond learning as much as possible about his father's medical condition, Bob did everything he could to make him comfortable, including providing him with some of his favorite music. Bob also engaged the staff by sharing the fact that his father, a former lawyer, loved jazz and at one time played the guitar quite well. The staff members were pleased to have something to talk to his father about.

Hospitalization, as in this case, is often necessary. But is it always? Any move for a frail, very old adult is perilous, and the medical

---

Steps in Easing Any Transitions

- Involve the older person to the greatest extent possible.
- In a hospital or nursing home, ask the staff to notify you (or your surrogate) if any move is being planned, so that you can help prepare your parent and make sure that his or her necessary belongings are packed—especially eyeglasses and dentures.
- Bring along a beloved object or two to provide a modicum of continuity and to comfort your parent during the move—a family photograph, jewelry, or a favorite book.
- Be there (or have someone present) to help your parent settle in to the new environment.
- Introduce your parent to the floor staff and share with them a little of his or her background.

community is now putting a spotlight on multiple and unnecessary moves of patients to and from nursing homes and acute care hospitals. As noted by Dr. Matthew Maurer, a geriatric specialist at Columbia University, "repeated transfers are common and have been described as a 'Ping Pong' pattern." He calls for strengthening the collaboration between hospital and nursing home staffs. Though long overdue, "transitional care"—the special attention older patients require at times of transfer between health care settings—is emerging as an important area of geriatric care.

Striving for a Reasonable Goal

This chapter has discussed those situations in which you cannot manage your parents' care, either in their own home or in a residence, such as an assisted living facility, and those in which the nursing home option may be preferable. The basic steps in nursing home selection have been described, as have procedures likely to make the transition to institutional life less painful for both you and your aging parent; suggested behavior most likely to lead to a satisfying adjustment after placement has also been considered. But steps and procedures, which are easy enough to describe on paper, are not so easily accomplished in real life. On this journey, imperfection and distress invariably crop up at some stage.

Human behavior has its own built-in imperfections, too. When facing nursing home placement with their elderly parents, some children handle the process with total success, while others falter or fail. But in general, well-intentioned children will ride a seesaw between success and failure. You may find it difficult to behave according to the recommendations described in this book. Some recommendations will even run counter to your personality. Patience, understanding, and empathy cannot be produced just because an emergency calls for those qualities, nor can humans maintain them consistently. Your compassion and attention are likely to fluctuate according to other pressures in your life. Given that knowledge, your most realistic goal may be to help your mother or father in the direction of a *reasonably* satisfying adjustment, and in the process, to achieve a *reasonably* peaceful state of mind for yourself. And that's a lot.

Bob Morris on Not Managing, But Trying

My dad was miserable. And into his life walked an aide, provided by a local agency at great expense. I was fascinated by the dynamics he had with her. She seemed like a nice person and was a gentle, quiet soul. My father had a small, two-bedroom apartment in Great Neck, at another assisted living place. And one of my main images of this aide was of a woman in her 50s, quietly sitting in his extra guest room, listening to her iPod and doing crossword puzzles. That's my predominant image of her presence in his life. Now, maybe that was her way of staying out of his way. But once my father was paying for help, he wanted help. And he didn't like the fact that she would go to sleep at 9 o'clock. He was a night owl. He might go to sleep at midnight, and he had nobody to get him in and out of bed at that hour, or he felt bad about having to wake her. But he didn't want to let her go either. He had empathy for her and her situation—in that this was all she could do with her professional life. And she seemed like a kind person, but she was lazy.

And so, suddenly, my brother and I were getting calls from my father, sounding as if he were trapped in a bad relationship, "I don't know how to motivate her. I have to talk to you really quietly, because she's here. I don't know what to do. She won't go get my dry cleaning. She won't deposit my checks." I got the feeling that he had this slow moving person on his hands. But he was becoming increasingly dependent. He ended up in a wheelchair, because he was sitting around all day. She wasn't encouraging him to walk or to rehabilitate at all. And so he ended up getting edema in his legs, and sores, and that just got to be a nightmare because it kept him from getting any exercise at all.

And suddenly, now I'm dealing with a new member of the family—this aide. How do I feel good about being there, on my weekly visits to Great Neck, under the presence of this seemingly quietly judgmental staff person? There were a couple of times when she would say to me—pushing all the wrong buttons: "Your father misses you so much. He wishes you would come out and see him more." Or "Why can't you get here earlier?" I didn't know then that she just wanted to go to bed.

But suddenly, this was all part of the formula of my father and his new incapacitated life—this quiet, but big, presence in the middle of his little apartment. So, I would often come out to visit and say, "I'm taking my dad for a ride," just so that he could vent about her. Can you imagine paying $150 a day for somebody who becomes an emotional source of conflict and turmoil? And so, of course, my brother and I said: "Get rid of her—get somebody else." Not so simple, you know. She did care about him. And she was docile in a way that kept him calm. But she had no energy for catering to all his constant little needs. It was like a brief, bad marriage.

11

Keeping in Step—The Family Task Force

Greg and Sandy Pratt prided themselves on their ability to plan ahead. They had never been caught unprepared. "We're a great team," Greg used to say proudly, explaining that whenever they were faced with a decision they'd always done their homework first and were prepared with all necessary information. Buying a home, finding a summer camp, changing jobs—their decisions were never impulsive or off the cuff. When it came to guardianships for their children, they went all out. They talked over various possibilities with their brothers and sisters, in-laws, lawyers, accountants, and even the minister at their church. They not only worked out careful plans but also created back-up plans. "Sandy even insisted on back-ups for the back-ups," Greg teased.

But when Greg's mother had a stroke, he and Sandy were caught unprepared for the first time. They didn't have the slightest idea what to do next, where to turn for advice, or what help she might need in the future. The whole family was hovering around anxiously, but Greg didn't know which of his relatives could be counted on to help. He wasn't even sure how much responsibility he and Sandy would be willing to shoulder. "She's 82 years old, for God's sake!" Greg burst out desperately to Sandy one day. "We've had years to prepare for this, and we didn't do a thing!"

Americans as individuals tend to think ahead. Just like Sandy and Greg, we spend time and energy planning for future events: vacations, new cars, our children's education, life insurance, long-term career goals. Some of us give more than a passing thought to our own old age. But, like Sandy and Greg, too many of us are caught unprepared when elderly parents begin to fail.

"Taking Steps"—Part 2 of this book—has reviewed the wide range of help available to older people who cannot manage alone. It has also stressed the importance of the family in locating and making use of this help. The underlying theme of the entire book has been that the family is the major support system for its elderly members, but the family turns to the community when more help is needed than it can provide alone. We've come a long way from the days when the family was accused of neglecting or abandoning its aging relatives, and attention has now turned to programs designed to tap the strengths of the family.

We've come a long way from the days when the family was accused of neglecting or abandoning its aging relatives, and attention has now turned to programs designed to tap the strengths of the family.

Many families, however, do not know how to tap these strengths or how to be effective. Even though they are willing, they may be unable to deal with the number of unfamiliar challenges associated with old age. This chapter, therefore, is not concerned with specific problems, but offers families a systematic approach to these problems in general. Many issues raised now have been touched on in earlier sections of the book—they may seem repetitive. But here for the first time they are discussed as essential elements in an overall strategy designed to produce effective—and collective—family action. The strategy to be reviewed may not be of interest to all families. It may not be needed by those who have worked out their own special ways of taking care of their own special problems. Nor does the material that follows have to be taken as an all-or-nothing proposition. Parts of the strategy may seem appropriate to your own family situation, and you may want to incorporate them into your own plan of action; other parts may seem inappropriate, and you may decide to ignore them.

There are families who work together on shared problems—particularly when these involve the older generation. Over time, they develop cooperative patterns that work for them. When Mother begins to fail or Father has a crisis, an army of concerned relatives may rally around. Good, solid solutions may be found. But if all the efforts do not bring reasonable results, it may be because this "army" does not know how to function as a cohesive unit; it may not understand the strategy of collective action.

The mere idea of collective action may seem truly foreign to other families, those who are fragmented by conflicts and whirling forever on a merry-go-round. The members may never have even tried to take collective action about anything in the past. How can they start now, just because Mother is sick? Unable to work together on her behalf, they may find it easier to ignore her problems or to argue about them. Is she or isn't she getting worse? Whose suggestions are acceptable, and whose are worthless? While the arguments continue, Mother's condition is likely to deteriorate further and the family conflicts intensify. If constructive action is ever going to be taken, the merry-go-round must stop its aimless circling.

Getting Off the Merry-Go-Round

It probably will not be easy to stop. The crisis in an aging parent's life is likely to accelerate the speed of the merry-go-round and fragment the family still further. The crisis may even precipitate dissension where there never was any—at least on the surface. Families whose relationships have been reasonably smooth over the years may find themselves in serious conflict for the first time. At the very point when it is essential that close relatives work with each other, they may start to work against each other.

Families who recognize the value of working together are often able to shelve their conflicts at difficult times—at least for a while—and organize their fragmented members into a new unit, a kind of a task force for action.

Families who recognize the value of working together are often able to shelve their conflicts at difficult times—at least for a while—and organize their fragmented members into a new unit, a kind of a task force for action. Instead of circling around problems, they can attack them directly. Forming this task force sometimes requires new behavior patterns. Many people will be surprised to hear that these patterns can be learned, even late in life, when long-standing relationships seem to have solidified forever. Even the old power structure in the family can be modified. In most families, the lines of power were drawn up long ago. Certain members have been recognized by all as the most powerful, and others are seen as submissive. The power may be held by one person or by several wielding their power as a team. The most dominant member may be the oldest child or the youngest, the richest, the favorite, or the one with the closest pipeline to the parents. The power may also be held by the aging father himself—or even by the frail mother.

The less powerful, even though initially willing to try to work collectively, may give up almost before they start, assuming that their opinions will—as usual—count for nothing. "Sam always has to have his own way." "Father won't ever listen to us." "No one can say anything to Mother." But it is a mistake to assume that the power elite will continue to operate forever and that collective action "is not possible in our family." Just because the dominant forces will, naturally, try to exert the most power when collective action is needed, the followers should not assume they have zero power. Actually, the weakest in the group may have the most powerful weapon of all: withdrawal. Once the dominant members realize they are likely to have no followers and may end up carrying all the problems themselves, they may be willing to cede some of their power.

Just as new behavior patterns within the family power structure can be learned, so can other new patterns leading to collective action. The learning process can be seen as a series of steps. If the steps are taken successfully, the result can be a family task force prepared to take action. The steps, to be sure, may not progress in a smooth, straight line. Several may be taken forward, but then one may have to be taken backward—or sideways. There are traps lying in wait along the way that may threaten the success of the entire process. But if families are aware in advance of the possibly rocky road ahead, they will be better prepared to take all steps—forward, backward, and sideways—in their stride.

Step 1: Planning a Family Conference

When the family is in an uproar about the situation of an elderly parent, one member may be tempted to take matters into his or her own hands, bring order out of chaos, and settle everything with a dictatorial announcement: "It's all arranged. Mother's going to move into Fairmont Manor a week from Friday. *I've* made all the arrangements." At the moment, this type of action may seem like a shortcut to sanity, but dictatorial edicts often produce mutinies among the lower ranks. Furthermore, the elderly parent, feeling railroaded into a new situation, may make a poor adjustment.

A family conference is the alternative to dictatorial rule. When successful, it provides the forum for open communication among all members—including, of course, the aging parent. The conference does not have to be a formal affair or even a face-to-face meeting. It can be an informal meeting, with everyone getting together at sister Betty's house on a Sunday morning. Some of those invited may refuse to come—that's to be expected—but the conference can proceed without them. However, a number of family members should attend, or the meeting at Betty's house will end up as a waste of a good Sunday morning. While it is ideal for all involved to meet in person, it is important for family members living far away to be included. Conference phone calls can be arranged whereby relatives, separated by thousands of miles, can talk directly to each other. Once it has been decided to hold a family conference, the next question to be considered is which family members should participate—whom to include, whom to exclude. One person, however, can never be left out of the family conference, and that is the person most closely involved: Mother herself or Father himself.

What Does Mother Have to Say?

This probably seems like an unnecessary question. How could Mother be forgotten? Easily! Many problems must be dealt with when crises arise in the lives of the elderly. Sons and daughters frantically search for solutions while still trying to keep their own lives, their business affairs, and their children functioning smoothly. Although all the confusion may be caused by Mother's crisis, and the purpose of the family conference is specifically to figure out "what's best for Mother," Mother herself may be the forgotten woman. No one may remember to tell her what's going on or to ask her what *she* thinks would be best for her. If Father is alive, even though frail, he also must be consulted. Excluding one or both of the elderly parents, while understandable, may be the very thing that causes carefully made plans to boomerang. Here again, as in most dealings between the generations, shared decisions are likely to produce the best results. Some semblance of a partnership can continue to operate between the generations, even when the older adult may plead, "Tell me what to do." Unless totally incapacitated, elderly family members have a legal and moral right to share in decisions that affect their own lives. If they are unable to attend the family conference in person, they should be kept informed of the proceedings.

Deciding Who Else Is Involved

All sons and daughters—some with greater concern, others with less—are naturally connected to their parents' problems. Nobody can assume automatically that a sister can be left out because she "never visits Mother" or that a brother doesn't need to be consulted because he "never lifts a finger for Mom and Dad." Even though your younger brother may have lived far away for years, the rest of the family living nearby should think twice before plunging ahead with their own decisions just because he's called long-distance to say, "Go ahead. Do what you think best." Even if he shows little interest in the plans as they are being made, he may appear months later and tell your mother, "If I'd been around, I'd never have let them do this to you," thereby torpedoing any adjustment she may have begun to make to her new situation.

In this electronic age, long-distance relationships are easily maintained by telephone and e-mail, and with the availability of telephone conferencing, all adult children can be involved. A sister who has offered financial support should be brought in, even if she lives far away and cannot oversee in person how her money is spent. Her opinion should be considered, or she may feel unappreciated later on and may even withdraw her support. Sons and daughters who live far away are still your parents' children and may even be the very ones to whom your parents always turn for advice. This is a somewhat bitter pill to swallow for the family members on the spot who take everyday responsibility.

Other family members, such as sons- and daughters-in-law, may be concerned and involved. Your parents may still be very close to their own brothers and sisters, or to nieces, nephews, grandchildren, cousins, and all the variety of step-relatives brought into the family by divorce and remarriage. Four criteria can be used to decide who should sit in on the family conference and become members of the family task force once it develops: Who is most concerned? Who is most affected? Who has a relationship with the older relative? Who has resources to offer?

The family conference may break down at its first session if the wrong people are included and the right ones left out. Just because your brother Jim is difficult and argumentative, he should not be excluded. He may be particularly influential with your mother. Furthermore, once he's blown off steam, he may be willing to play an important role in the task force. Even if it is assumed in advance that your sister Lily will be Mother's caregiver, Lily should be given a chance to discuss the job and how it would affect her life. The title should not be conferred on her in absentia. Cousin Millie, on the other hand, whose main function is giving advice and criticism, should be excluded. She contributes nothing in terms of time and energy. Meaningless plans may result if unconcerned relatives share in decisions that will in no way affect their lives.

Giving the Floor to All

It is essential that all those attending have a chance to speak their minds, lay their cards on the table, and explain their own personal situations, capabilities, intentions, and preferences. Suggestions and options from each one should be considered. If the floor is monopolized by the loudest members, the most articulate, or the most powerful, then valuable contributions from the meeker participants may never be heard. Care must be taken to ensure that family members who are on the phone are given the floor and that others identify themselves when speaking to the person on the phone.

While the task force is only in its infancy at this stage and is far from arriving at solutions to the problem at hand, this first go-around lays the groundwork for full family participation. Trial balloons will be floated, and a grab bag of ideas shared. Many of these may be discarded later, but some may eventually become part of a workable plan.

At this point, a new leadership may begin to emerge. The former family dictator is not likely to remain as leader—brother Sam, for instance, who has held the power for years, or sister Flo, who has controlled the purse strings. Rather, the power may shift to brother Jo or sister Peggy, who are trusted and respected by everyone or who have specific skills and understanding. Sam, though unseated, need not feel excluded. He may still give the soundest legal advice or have the best understanding of money. Flo's role cannot be discounted either—her resources are important. The new leadership does not necessarily become another dictatorship; it may be shared, with different leaders taking over different tasks or at different stages.

The early sessions of the family conference—even with well-chosen membership—may be stormy. This may be the first time these concerned relatives have been forced to communicate with each other in a group rather than on a one-to-one basis. Sparks may fly and old conflicts be rekindled. But a word of warning must be given here: a family conference of this type is not going to resolve these old conflicts surfacing from the past. Nor should it be used for this purpose. It cannot be allowed to develop into a shouting match or a free-for-all that would prevent everyone from tackling the problem at hand. What happened years ago in the nursery is not relevant here. What *is* relevant is Mother's welfare or Father's disability. Anyone who goes off topic should be brought back by one of the new leaders or by anyone with a steadying hand—or with the least involvement in the confrontation.

But even if everyone stays on target, the participants may discover things about each other—and about themselves—that they never knew before. You may come to see that your friction with your husband over your parents' care was not caused, as you kept insisting, by *his* unreasonable jealousy or *his* hostility or selfishness, but by *your* disregard of his feelings and *your* neglect of the children. If you are the caregiver for your mother, you should be given an opportunity to list your complaints about the burdens you carry alone. The others should listen. But if you are willing to listen to them in return, you may learn that your behavior has seemed autocratic and that you have rejected their offers to help. It may begin to dawn on you that they have not been doing their share because you have not allowed them to. The stormy sessions may be painful, but they can clear the air by helping to clarify the strengths and weaknesses of each member.

Step 2: Identifying the Problem

Before the problem can be identified, there is work to be done. More information may need to be gathered about the elderly parent's condition and situation. Professionals—doctors, nurses, psychiatrists, or geriatric specialists—may need to be consulted to make a full assessment of your parent's condition and situation. Helpful information may be found in books: a review of the earlier chapters of this book might prove useful. Information gathering is a necessary process because the problems of older people often present a confusing picture.

When a problem arises for a family in its earlier stages—mother, father, and growing children—it is easier to define not only *who* is involved but also *what*, precisely, the problem is: Carol is doing badly in school. Johnny has nightmares. Father is drinking too much. Mother is depressed. Each one of these problems, naturally, has deeper ramifications, but each one offers a starting point. With the elderly, the picture can be much less clear. There may be general agreement that Mother is not doing well, although there may be some in the family who continue to deny that anything is wrong. Mother herself may be the loudest in her denials. But even when everyone agrees that Mother needs help, there may be complete ignorance about what, specifically, her problem is and what, specifically, can be done about it.

Eighty-one-year-old Charles Denver was obviously slipping, and his family was concerned. His hearing and eyesight were failing. He was withdrawn, apathetic, forgetful, and weak. He was losing weight and had fallen on several occasions. His daughter wanted him to see an eye doctor. His son thought he needed psychiatric help. Luckily, Charles's sister suggested a general checkup with her own internist, who discovered that Charles was severely malnourished and anemic. Although he was not blind, his deteriorating sight made it increasingly difficult for him to cook for himself, as he had done since he was widowed a few years before. He cooked less, bought less food, ate less, and therefore grew weaker. He became depressed, and his appetite diminished further. Once the basic problems had been identified, Charles's family was able to start working on concrete, specific solutions. Instead of agonizing—"We must do something about Father"—they could move ahead, knowing that they "must do something about Father's diet and failing hearing and eyesight."

Families tend to panic and stand still when problems seem overwhelming. Once specific trouble spots are identified, they know better where to direct their energies to find specific solutions. Charles Denver's family was able to pinpoint his main problem with comparative ease, but the process is not always this straightforward. Sometimes the basic problem is buried too deeply. Obvious surface difficulties may become red herrings, leading families in the wrong directions. More time and effort and further information may be needed before the true root of the trouble is isolated. This may be the point where outside professionals have to be brought in or consulted—doctors, nurses, and social workers.

Once identified, the problem may not be as easy to cope with as Charles Denver's malnutrition. It may have many levels and require more complicated solutions. In such cases, it may help to break down the problem into manageable components, taking care of the most urgent first.

Amanda Heller was 82, widowed, and living alone in a small, but comfortable apartment. Her income, though modest, was adequate to cover some household help, but she refused to have any. This worried her two sons, but they admitted that she seemed to manage well enough until she had a severe bout of the flu. During her illness, she allowed her sons to bring in a practical nurse, but as soon as she felt a little better, she fired the woman.

After her recovery, the family was alarmed by what seemed to be serious changes in her personality and living habits. Formerly methodical and meticulous about her home and her appearance, she gradually lost interest in both. She had once prided herself on her cooking, even when alone, but in a short time, she stopped cooking completely and lived on tea and crackers. She became increasingly suspicious of everyone—even her sons and their wives. Despite her frail condition and formerly frugal spending habits, she started going on buying sprees, piling up large bills for clothing she never wore, but left lying around in boxes. Neighbors reported on several occasions that they'd seen her giving money to people she hardly knew. Whenever relatives visited, they found personal papers, checkbooks, and bankbooks strewn carelessly around. One day, her older son retrieved some uncashed dividend checks from the trash can.

She ignored her sons' concern and refused to allow her daughters-in-law to help her in the apartment. The family felt helpless, overwhelmed by Amanda's steadily deteriorating condition. They seemed incapable of doing anything until a friend, who had been through a similar situation himself, advised against searching for an overall solution. He suggested approaching things one by one, attacking the most pressing problem first.

It was obvious that there was an urgent need to conserve Amanda's dwindling finances, so her sons' first move was to consult a lawyer to learn what legal steps could be taken. While a conservatorship was being arranged, they prevailed on their mother to see a geriatric specialist, who began an overall assessment of her physical and mental condition. Then, the family turned to the living situation and hired a homemaker to maintain the apartment and help Amanda with her daily routines—meals, dressing, and personal hygiene.

The process was time-consuming, but breaking the situation into manageable segments enabled the family, no longer overwhelmed, to take effective action.

Step 3: Making Commitments

Encouraging progress will seem to have been made when a specific problem or set of problems is identified. The situation will begin to develop greater clarity. The family now knows what's wrong, and may even have some idea of the necessary solutions. It is probably less clear how these solutions will be put into operation, and by whom. How much responsibility will each family member be willing to take?

This is a kind of zero hour for everyone. All involved are now forced to face squarely how much of an investment they are honestly willing to make as individuals in providing the solutions for a parent's problem. It can be a painful experience and usually involves admitting personal shortcomings and inadequacies. Charles Denver's daughter, who had always devotedly claimed, "I'd do anything in the world for Father," may now have to ask herself whether she is willing to cook her father's dinner every night to be sure he has a balanced meal. Her claim of devotion may seem less impressive when she is forced to admit to herself, and everyone else, "I'd do anything in the world for Father, *except* cook dinner for him every night." Self-confrontation may take place now or later on, as the situation continues or deteriorates, but whenever it takes place, it can be a disillusioning experience, and as a result, one or more of the members may drop out of the task force temporarily, or even permanently.

Roadblocks to helping will differ. A son obviously cannot take on any daily responsibility in his mother's life if his job requires him to travel constantly during the week. He may, instead, commit himself to taking his mother for physiotherapy every Saturday morning. A daughter who works full time cannot take care of her disabled father's housekeeping as well as her own, but she and her aunt may alternate weekend housekeeping while others share responsibility for

> *All involved are now forced to face squarely how much of an investment they are honestly willing to make as individuals in providing the solutions for a parent's problem.*

the weekday chores. A certain amount of trial and error may be necessary before a plan begins to mesh well and move along smoothly. Even when things seem to be running perfectly, family members must be open to change and revision of the plan according to new developments.

Setting Your Priorities

At this point, it is necessary for everyone to step away from the extended family and the collective process. All individuals and couples need to move back into their own family units and examine the other commitments in their lives. Helping your father or mother is not likely to be the only commitment you have. There are undoubtedly plenty of others already, and these must be considered. If you take on a new one, how will this affect other people, other activities, and even other pleasures that may be important to you? How much are you prepared to give up? It's a difficult choice to make, and it's a rare person who can choose easily without guilt, conflict, or regret. The new commitment may be easier to accept—or to refuse— if you see it in relation to others you have made already. It might help to ask, "If I take on some major responsibility for my mother's care, how will this affect my children? My grandchildren? My husband? My wife? How will it affect my community activities, my work, and my health? How will it affect the time I need for myself or to spend with my friends?"

The priority you give to helping your mother may be determined not by other commitments but by the relationship you have had with her through the years. Your feelings—discussed in Chapter 2—may decide the priority. It will not help to watch with awe and envy as your neighbor, who has as many commitments as you do, still manages to devote part of her life to her mother. Their relationship with each other is probably quite different from yours with your mother. Despite the similarity in your lives, when it comes to mothers, there's no similarity at all. You may feel cold-blooded and heartless—"a thankless child"—if it turns out that you cannot give your mother's needs the highest priority in your life. But better to admit this now—out loud—than to make a commitment you cannot sustain. Better to announce in advance the limits of the help you can be counted on to give. At least you can be counted on for something.

Others in the task force may refuse to be counted on at all and vanish completely.

Step 4: Agreeing on a Plan

If the task force has been able to take the first three steps with a certain amount of success and has not lost too many members along the way, it should be ready for the fourth and last step: to make an agreement. Discussion has been essential through the earlier steps and is equally essential at the fourth, but at some point, talk must stop. Decisions must be made, and an agreement must be reached. Only when the agreement is accepted will the task force be able to take action. The agreement may not be completely satisfactory to everyone. It may require compromise and sacrifice from many members. But once accepted, it will represent a group commitment binding on all individuals.

The final agreement reached at step 4 may surprise everyone and be totally different from anything ever dreamed of at step 1, when the family conference was being planned.

> Even though she had two brothers and several aunts, Sonia Kepple had always taken care of everything for her disabled father. She was in daily touch with him, and despite having a part-time job, she visited him several times a week and supervised the homemaker who took care of him in his apartment. Every weekend, when the homemaker was off, she brought the elderly man to her home in the suburbs.
>
> She and her husband never had time alone with each other or their children and felt worn out by their endless routine. Finally, in desperation, she called her brothers and her aunts to her house and accused them all of shirking responsibility and leaving everything to her. She was amazed to learn after her outburst that she wasn't the only one who felt ill-used. She found that everyone assumed that she enjoyed taking charge of everything and that the others resented her for not allowing anyone else to be close to her father. It dawned on her for the first time that the others had not been doing their share because she had not permitted them to.

When the air cleared, everyone offered to help. Sonia's aunts committed themselves to supervising the weekday home-maker, and her brothers agreed to rotate weekends with her. But on the first weekend with his younger son, the 86-year-old man, waking up in a strange place, became confused, turned on all the lights, woke the children, and tried to get out of the house in his pajamas. On the second weekend, the older son went out to pick up his father, but on the way, skidded on wet leaves and drove his car into a ditch.

The new weekend plan seemed doomed to failure. Sonia's brothers were unable to follow along in the pattern that Sonia had established. But the family refused to admit defeat. They were stumped for a time. So they stepped back and began to retrace their steps. They reassessed the problem and realized that their elderly father was more confused than they had realized. Too much moving around only increased his confusion. They then revised their original commitments and came up with a different agreement. Rather than moving their father every weekend, the brothers decided that they would share the cost of a weekend homemaker and would take turns super-vising things at their father's apartment on Saturdays and Sundays. Sonia would still continue to take her father to her home when it was her turn because her place was familiar to him.

By not insisting that things had to be done her way, and allowing her brothers to try something different, Sonia was able to spend two out of three weekends alone with her family.

Beware of Traps Along the Way

Progress is rarely smooth from step 1 through step 4. Few families can take all four steps in stride and arrive at the finish line without stumbling along the way. Unpredictable, unavoidable roadblocks may appear at any time and must be dealt with. Other traps are more predictable, and if the task force is aware of these in advance, it may be able to avoid them completely. The four that follow are the most common.

Keeping Secrets

Honesty is an essential ingredient if the family task force is to function efficiently. Members of the

Honesty is an essential in-gredient if the family task force is to function efficiently.

task force may be tempted to keep secrets—from each other and from their parents. Some secrets may have been kept for years out of guilt, shame, or pride. A sister, for instance, may not want to admit to the rest of her family that her marriage is in trouble and that one of the causes of conflict with her husband has been her close relationship with her mother through the years. Instead of admitting why she cannot be counted on to take her place in the task force, she may keep her secret and agree to participate. When her husband walks out on her several months later and she has to take a full-time job, the task force can no longer function according to its original agreement. It must regroup and form a new plan.

Families often keep secrets for more altruistic reasons and because facing the truth can be painful.

Margaret Frank's children never came out and told her why it would be impossible for her to remain alone much longer in the big house where they'd all grown up. They knew how much she loved it, so they circled around the truth, singing the praises of a small apartment in a retirement complex nearby. They tried to convince her that she'd be happier there, less lonely, and that she'd have more activities to fill her time. But Margaret refused to be budged.

What her family did not tell her, because they did not want to worry her, was that her older son Bill had developed a back problem and could no longer take care of his mother's house and garden repairs. Her son-in-law was in line for a promotion that would require relocation, so her daughter, Jess, would not be able to help her mother with the domestic chores as she had in the past. Most important of all, Margaret's doctor had told the family that she should no longer be climbing stairs because of a deteriorating heart condition. The family stalemate occurred because one side kept secrets and the other side, therefore, saw no reason to make any changes in her life.

Hiding Feelings

This is closely related to keeping secrets and is often intertwined with it. As discussed in Chapter 2, negative feelings about close relatives—particularly parents—are often uncomfortable, and many people prefer to keep them hidden. Their behavior is predicated on what they think they *ought* to feel rather than on what they *do* feel.

> Polly Taylor had always enjoyed her role as "good girl" in the family. Everyone with a problem turned to Polly and knew that she could be counted on for help. When Polly's father became blind, the rest of the family automatically assumed that she would act as caregiver. Polly herself dreaded the thought. She'd always been ready to pitch in to help others through a crisis, but the idea of taking ongoing, permanent responsibility terrified her. Furthermore, she secretly felt that she had never been fully appreciated by her father, and resented him for this. But Polly could not admit her feelings, and with apparent willingness, agreed to be her father's caregiver. If she had refused, she would have had to give up her role of "good girl." As a result, she took on the responsibilities, performed them badly, and eventually had to give up both roles—caregiver and good girl.

Polly was aware of her true feelings and knew she was hiding them from the others, but some people manage to hide their feelings from themselves. These feelings may have been buried for so long that they no longer seem to exist. They may only surface again and disrupt carefully laid plans when there must be renewed involvement and close contact with an aging father or mother, or with the family as a whole. When these feelings do surface, plans may have to be completely revised.

Promises, Promises

One of the most dangerous traps of all is the hastily given promise. While unrealistic promises may be made on the basis of the two previous traps—secrets and hidden feelings—they also may be made out of honest

One of the most dangerous traps of all is the hastily given promise.

intention, prompted by the emotions of the moment. People who make these promises may genuinely believe *at the time* that they expect to keep them. Deathbed promises to a dying parent, such as the one mentioned in Chapter 7—"Of course, I'll bring Dad to live with us"—can produce the greatest problems. Having to back out of such a promise is truly traumatic. It's guilt-producing enough to break a promise to the living; how much more guilt is involved when the broken promise has been made to the dead.

But promises are not always made at the deathbed. The task force can find itself boxed in by a promise made too hastily to a living parent.

"You won't ever go to a nursing home. We promise."

"You'll never have to give up the house. We promise."

"We promise we'll visit you every day."

"If you don't like living at Greenfield Manor, you can leave. We promise."

The words "but we promised Mother" can paralyze the entire task force and prevent it from taking further action. Words like *every, never, ever,* and *always* are equally dangerous. A revised version of the promises discussed earlier would keep the future looser and the plans more open to revision:

"We know how you feel about nursing homes, Mom, and we feel the same way. Let's see how you get along when you come home from the hospital. We promise to help you as much as we can."

"You and Dad can't go on paying those terrible heating bills. We know how much you want to stay in the house, so we've all decided to chip in to help. But with the way oil prices are skyrocketing, we can't promise to do it forever."

"Don't worry—we won't let you be lonely. We'll all visit you as often as possible. We promise."

"It's going to be hard getting used to being at Greenfield Manor, but we promise we'll all be around a lot at the beginning, until you feel more at home."

Jumping the Gun

Although the best plans are usually made through slow, thoughtful analysis, the task force often must take speedy action because of a crisis: "Mother's going to be discharged from the hospital in a few days. Who's going to take care of her? Where's she going to go?" Often there is no time to deliberate because there's a deadline to meet. Some arrangements will obviously have to be made for a week from Tuesday. But here again, families tend to overestimate their immediate problem, thinking that the arrangements made for that Tuesday must last a lifetime. That would be an overwhelming challenge. A delaying action that allows for further investigation is likely to produce better results. Instead of trying to deal with the *long-term* future—especially at a time of crisis, when no one can think clearly—it's usually possible to make arrangements for the *immediate* future: "Mother's going to a convalescent home for a few months when she leaves the hospital. We'll see how she does there." The task force that takes this route will now have the next months free of pressure. During this time, it can watch how things go, consider possible solutions for the future, review them with Mother, and as the months pass, develop a clearer idea of which options are realistic.

Speedy action, however, is often demanded by an impatient task force—or an impatient member. Each member has an individual life to lead, a family to care for, problems to cope with, work to do. It's understandable why many may be eager to arrive at an agreement that permits them to return to their own affairs. There's a real danger that the impatient ones may try to hurry up deliberations to reach some agreement—any agreement. The elderly parents themselves may be the most impatient, rushing impulsively into arrangements that are unrealistic for the future and likely to lead to further problems. If your parents are intent on giving up their apartment and moving to Florida, you and the rest of the family might admire their independence and quickly support their idea, especially if they had been increasingly demanding of everyone's time and attention recently. You may all breathe a sigh of relief and wish them well. However, it would be wise if one of you were to point out the potential hazards of their move, reminding your father that your mother's arthritis has been getting progressively more severe, and that while she could manage now in Florida, she might not be able to remain there if she became incapacitated a year from now. Then, where would they go? The quick agreement made by an impatient task force, or railroaded through by an impatient member, is likely to cause further time-consuming problems for everyone in the future.

When There's an Impasse

The task force is likely to come to a dead stop—not once, but possibly several times—as it tries to move ahead to an agreement. An impasse is to be expected. It may come about for any one of a number of reasons. The task force may exhaust all its resources without reaching a workable agreement that is reasonably satisfactory to all. A power struggle may develop in which the question to be answered is not " 'What's best for Mother?" but "Who's head of the family?" Less outspoken relatives, after trying and failing to have any real say in the deliberations, may throw up their hands in despair and vanish from the task force—at least temporarily.

But an impasse does not mean failure. The whole process of getting together and trying to form a task force is likely to be a novel experience in many families. Learning how to talk to each other honestly, without hiding behind old masks and postures, can be an uncomfortable experience—as bewildering as learning a new language. When the impasse is reached, things may stall for a while, but can get moving again if the task force realizes that all is not lost—that it can step back briefly, take a breather, regroup, and then start again. Landing on the dreaded box "back to home plate" in the old board game Parcheesi does not mean that the game is over, unless some poor sport slams away in a huff. It just means starting over.

The second attempt may be quite different from the first. The lines of power may have started to shift. Mother may be getting feebler, less able to assert her authority over herself and everyone else. A powerful brother may be eager to return to his own affairs and may be more receptive to collective, rather than unilateral, action. The breather may have given everyone a chance to regroup, gather more information, consult more experts, and gain fresh insights. It may also give some members an opportunity to exert informal pressure on particularly rigid members. The original impasse may have occurred because a younger brother took a strong stand and refused to be budged. He may fear he'll lose face if he gives in to an older brother, his lifetime rival. Continued confrontation by the task force en masse is likely to harden his position still further, thereby creating the impasse. In such a situation, it may turn out that he is more reasonable in private than in public if he is approached informally and diplomatically by someone in the family whom he respects. This chapter has stressed a process made famous by President Woodrow Wilson when drafting the peace treaty of World War I— "open covenants, openly arrived at." But this openness does not preclude some diplomatic behind-the-scenes persuasion. It may be just what's needed to break the impasse and start the process moving again.

A family who finds it difficult to gather momentum after the planning process has stalled may get the push it needs from an outsider—someone whose ideas are more objective and less emotionally charged. This outsider can be a respected friend; a more distant, uninvolved relative; or a professional trained in family counseling. The effect of this outside intervention may be to cut through tangled feelings and clear the way for further action. Family counseling, originally considered effective mainly for the family in its early years, is now proving successful in dealing with troubled families at any age. Instead of working only with the nuclear family—parents and their growing children—counselors now look to the more extended family and bring in any members who are closely involved with the problem or likely to contribute to the solution. It is particularly important, however, that the family counselor or therapist consulted has experience in working with older adults and their families. (See Appendix A for suggested resources.)

Looking to the Future

Even when all steps have been taken, all traps avoided, all impasses broken, and all agreements accepted, the family task force cannot assume that it will move along smoothly forever. Nor do the members need to fear that they have locked themselves into situations from which there is no escape. Life will go on, and as it does, the problems of the elderly parents are not likely to remain constant. Things may deteriorate—or improve. The task force must be ready to adapt its original agreement accordingly. The composition of the task force membership may change because of death, illness, relocation, divorce, or abdication. Replacements will be needed and responsibilities reallocated.

But if the family task force has been able to function smoothly for a time, it will not be destroyed by setbacks. The family will have discovered that working together produces the most effective action. It will then be willing to regroup, revise, readjust, and move on. As noted in Chapter 7, deathbed decisions sometimes fall on the shoulders of family members, particularly when the dying parent has not left a directive regarding the prolongation of life. Effective family collaboration in these difficult situations can help to assuage the pain associated with difficult decisions.

There is much to be gained—for you and your aging parent—from doing the best you can, in collaboration with other family members. A secondary gain, particularly for family members who have drifted apart over the years, can be a renewed and strengthened relationship with siblings and other family members as a result of working together on behalf of an aging parent and sharing mutual concerns and worries.

Bob Morris on His Brother "The Decider"

My brother was the decider.

It's good when somebody takes a stand—someone who happens to be able to put his money where his mouth is, literally. In all scenarios, in all situations, in all cases, in watching my parents get old and die—I had it easy . . . very easy. There was nothing that disrupted my life and tore me apart. And so I'm sure I sound very privileged and spoiled in talking about this, but my brother could make the decisions that required money that my parents might not want to cough up. And he just did it—because he knew it would be best for them and best for us. So I trusted all of his decisions and knew that no matter what the expense, he always had their best interests at heart.

That said, there was a general difference between us. As a man of affairs, and a successful businessman, my brother did believe that he could monitor, oversee, and control doctors. And I wasn't sure that some of the tension that that engendered—a child questioning doctors—would, overall, be healthy for my mother, who was already being treated by a top specialist in New York. My brother spent a lot of time researching, and questioning, and going with my mother to the doctor—and making decisions about the kinds of treatments that would be helpful. Ultimately, he couldn't do much about her medical treatment or her condition, but he tried and I deferred.

I knew that I needed to appreciate the fact that somebody was putting more effort in. And so, you know, as egomaniacal as I am, I was not foolish enough to let my ego get invested and give him a hard time about anything—even if I disagreed.

Basically, when there's love between two siblings—as there is between us—there's still a tremendous amount of fun to be had in working together, even in the worst scenario. If you share a sense of humor, as we did—and a tremendous, relentless cynicism — about the foibles of your parents, whom you love but find so aggravating, then even in the worst scenarios, as for us, there is something that you can laugh about together.

But I firmly believe that if one sibling is doing more, then the other one needs to respect that. When it came to the major decision about ending my mother's life—when she was really in terrible shape and seemed unfixable—I broached the topic, but we made that decision together ultimately.

I took the lead, and I took a lot of guff for it. My brother was very aggressive in saying that it was a decision that I was making for my own convenience. But I knew it was time for my mother to die. She wasn't going to get any better, and there was no point in fighting. Years later, my brother was at peace with that.

Part III
Extra Steps

WRITTEN IN COLLABORATION
WITH KIM WALLER

12

Taking Heed—An Rx Alert

When 81-year-old Tony failed to answer his daughter's daily phone call, she rushed to his apartment and found him semiconscious. Had he had a stroke? Fortunately, she scooped all his pill bottles into a plastic bag as they left for the hospital. From the bottle labels, she and the staff were able to determine the medications and doses prescribed for her father. No, Tony had not had a stroke: it was a problem with his drugs that had caused his collapse. After several days in the hospital, his condition was stabilized under a revised medication routine, and his strength and alertness returned.

TONY'S EMERGENCY IS NOT UNUSUAL. ALTHOUGH HE was still able to live on his own, he had a number of conditions common in the elderly. Over the years, his physician had prescribed medication for an erratic heartbeat, a diuretic for poor circulation in his legs, and an anti-inflammatory for his arthritis. Since the death of his wife, Tony had become depressed and was sleeping poorly, so he was also prescribed an antidepressant and a sedative. Whether the amounts or types of these prescriptions reflected questionable judgment on the part of his doctor, or whether Tony himself was taking too much or too little of some, the net result was the same: extreme weakness and confusion. "You can bet that when I took Dad home from the hospital, both of us had a clear list of the adjusted medications and doses," said his daughter. "His copy is tacked up right by the breakfast table—in large type!"

Without question, all of us benefit enormously from modern medicine. From our childhood on, prescription and over-the-counter drugs have gifted us with better health and an enhanced quality of life. Not surprisingly, those who benefit the most—and take the most—are older adults. People over age 65, who represent only 12% of the population, buy 30% of all prescription drugs and 40% of all over-the-counter drugs. Controlling cardiovascular conditions, such as high blood pressure and high cholesterol, adds years to many lives. Infections and many diseases are cured or managed. Pain is mitigated, allowing more active days. Drugs are a blessing, a boon. Why, then, should one be wary about all those little bedside bottles?

A Silent Epidemic

There is a flip side to the blessing. The more drugs an older person is taking, the greater the chance of undesirable reactions. Every medication, after all, comes with some risk. Some drugs have rare or minor side effects; some have potentially dangerous side effects. And sometimes upsetting interactions occur between one drug, or class of drugs, and others, or between drugs and certain foods or beverages. Sometimes, too, less informed physicians prescribe drugs or dosages that are wrong for older adults. There is also the risk that, for various reasons, people simply won't take their medications or won't take them as prescribed. According to the Sloan Epidemiology Center in Boston, Americans over age 65 take four prescription drugs daily: at age 75, the average is eight prescription drugs daily. And that's not counting various over-the-counter drugs that are usually added to the mix.

As a result, a serious health problem has erupted in this country, called by some "a silent epidemic." How serious is it? As Janice Feinberg, Pharm., J.D., Research Director for the American Society of Consultant Pharmacists Foundation, pointed out in the winter 2000/2001 issue of *Generations*, "Medication-related problems may be the third or fourth leading cause of death in the over-65 age group. And, just as important, medication-related problems can cause unnecessary disability resulting in loss of independence from confusion, depression, gait disturbances and falls." She notes that older adults are twice as likely as younger people to be treated in an emergency room for a drug reaction.

Most at risk are those being treated for several chronic illnesses. Sometimes, too, an unrecognized drug-related symptom is treated with yet another drug. As if these pitfalls weren't scary enough, two recent studies identifying drugs that are not advised for older adults concluded that between 14% and 40% of older patients were receiving just such medications. As in John's case, "any symptom in an elderly patient should be considered a drug side effect until proven otherwise," warns Jerry Avorn, M.D., Professor of Medicine at Harvard Medical School.

Let's face it: we live in an optimistic, pill-pushing culture. We want to believe that most problems, including health problems, can and should be "fixed." After all, so many now are—whether it's simple cold relief from an over-the-counter decongestant or a sophisticated medication that suppresses rejection of an implant or transplant after surgery. We even jokingly apply mechanical metaphors to our bodies, such as "getting a tune-up, "repairing the plumbing," or "going in for an overhaul." And every year, more and more drugs to treat health ailments common to the elderly, among others, are developed and energetically marketed.

Older Bodies Are Different

> Alice Nelson, 75, had been taking the same daily dose of thyroid medicine for years with no apparent problem, even though she had lost about 5 lbs since turning 70. When she suffered dizziness and a racing heartbeat, her current physician realized that the dosage of her thyroid medicine had not been adjusted for a long time. Reducing the dosage gradually brought her system back into balance.

We can all identify the obvious alterations of age in ourselves and our loved ones—in the mirror, in the aches. What is less obvious are the ways in which older bodies become more sensitive to drugs and

We can all identify the obvious alterations of age in ourselves and our loved ones—in the mirror, in the aches. What is less obvious are the ways in which older bodies become more sensitive to drugs and dosages. dosages. Because of changes in water content (less) and the proportion of muscle (less) and fat (usually more), as well as slowed action of the kidneys and liver, many medications linger longer in aging bodies. Dosages that are just fine for a 50-year-old are often too high for an 80-year-old, and can even accumulate in the system to dangerous effect. Unfortunately, the tests on which drug companies base their suggested dosages tend not to include the frail elderly.

Another change to be aware of is the increased effect of almost all drugs on the brain. An antihistamine pill that can make someone feel a bit draggy at age 40 can cause the same person to drive off the road at age 78. This happens because the protective barrier between the bloodstream and the brain becomes less exclusive, less efficient, with age. Notes Mark Beers, M.D., editor-in-chief of the *Merck Manual of Geriatrics*, in *Generations* (2000/2001), "The list of medications that cause confusion or changes to the central nervous system in older people is very long."

Fortunately, as physicians have become more concerned about the ravages of this silent epidemic of many medications, a cautious mantra about prescribing for older adults has evolved: "Start low and go slow."

Psychotropic Drugs: A Special Case

Heaven knows, our aging parents have plenty of real reasons to feel anxious or sad. They suffer grief and loneliness from the loss of friends and spouses, and can also experience a loss of energy, mobility, and independence. They worry—about money, about the future, about small matters that suddenly loom large in their minds. More often than not, they hurt. And we who love them suffer for them.

In decades past, such problems were considered the inevitable companions of age. Increasingly, however, they are being treated with psychotropic drugs. This large class of medications is aimed directly at the central nervous system and includes antidepressants,

Symptoms of a Possible Drug Reaction

- Confusion, depression, delirium
- Weakness, lethargy, falling
- Insomnia, loss of appetite
- Changes in speech
- Changes in mental alertness or memory
- Rash, nausea, or other signs of allergic reaction

Remember:

- "Any new symptom should be considered drug-related until proven otherwise."
- Not all reactions show up immediately; some drugs and drug interactions take a while to build up.

anti-anxiety medications, pain medications, and sedatives for insomnia. Specifically designed to alter brain function, they can result in changes of mood, perception, consciousness, and behavior.

The need—and demand—for psychotropic medications is certainly significant. From sleep disorders to severe agitation, they have become the treatment of choice, sometimes in combination with psychotherapy. Depression, for example, rendering an elderly parent unable to cope with existence or savor its remaining pleasures, is not only heartbreaking but also can be potentially life-threatening. Anyone who has witnessed the gradual lifting of that dark cloud from the life of a loved one and seen them once again take up painting or enjoy companionship and music must certainly feel a deep relief. Yet psychotropic drugs carry special risks, especially for older adults. The more fragile balance they experience between cognitive functioning and emotional states can be upset by the improper choice or dosage of an antidepressant. Changes in the way an aging body absorbs or discharges drugs can lead to such side effects as mental dullness,

Psychotropic drugs carry special risks, especially for older adults. The more fragile balance they experience between cognitive functioning and emotional states can be upset by the improper choice or dosage of an antidepressant.

poor balance resulting in falls and broken hips, or new sleep disturbances—sometimes the very opposite of the desired effects. And some drugs have no effect at all on the problem they were meant to address.

Narcotics prescribed to relieve pain can become addictive and less effective as dependency increases—initiating a vicious cycle. On the other hand, relieving and preventing pain is extremely important. As noted by geriatrician Harrison Bloom, M.D., of the International Longevity Center, "Addiction is less of a concern than appropriately treating pain. In the proper hands, the use of narcotics can be very helpful to patients."

More than any other class of drugs, psychotropic medications loom the largest in surveys of inappropriate drugs prescribed for the elderly. The most fragile members of this age group—often those in nursing homes—are also the most likely to be afflicted by sadness, sleeplessness, and agitation. It is no wonder that they are increasingly treated with psychotropic drugs. Of particular concern are anti-anxiety and antidepressant medications that linger in the body long after they are discontinued. Some are known to be harmful to the elderly or reactive with other medications the older person is taking. How widely is it known that ibuprofen (Advil) and fluoxetine (Prozac) together create a risk of internal bleeding?

For another example, serotonin toxicity, a difficult-to-diagnose syndrome with a wide range of disturbing symptoms, can be caused by the use of multiple drugs that enhance serotonin—from some antidepressants and antipsychotics to certain migraine drugs, anti-parkinsonian drugs, pain relievers, and even weight-loss drugs—and together can have the effect of raising serotonin to toxic levels. In fact, the older the patient and the more additional drugs he or she is taking, the greater the risk from psychotropic drugs. Too often, these drugs are not being prescribed by well-informed psychiatrists or psychopharmacologists but by other physicians trying to be of help. In their effort to keep up with many types of drugs, their information sometimes comes from promotional material.

Even when doctors do "start low and go slow," there is an ongoing need for the effects of any psychotropic drug to be monitored closely—and an equally important need for patients or their caregivers to promptly report any undesirable reactions.

Taking Heed with Over-the-Counter Drugs

Although over-the-counter drugs are accessible to all, they "are real medicines with real risks if misused," said Linda A. Suydam, president of the Consumer Healthcare Products Association *Although over-the-counter drugs are accessible to all, they "are real medicines with real risks if misused."* in a December 12, 2006, interview in the *New York Times*. Although most are intended for only short-term use, overuse and misuse of over-the-counter drugs is an alarming part of the silent epidemic afflicting older adults. Walk the aisles of today's drugstores, and the choice of remedies—for constipation, colds, allergies, aches, or upset stomach—goes confusingly on and on. Only 30 years ago, 700 current over-the-counter products were unavailable with their current ingredients or dosages, except by prescription. We no longer have to visit a doctor to get them; now we can buy them like milk or butter.

But these drugs, as well as the old standbys, such as aspirin, can be potent indeed. For people taking blood thinners or a steroid medication, for example, taking something as seemingly simple as aspirin could result in internal bleeding. Ibuprofen and other nonsteroidal anti-inflammatory drugs can increase the risk of bleeding by themselves. Moreover, the same changes in aging bodies that affect how prescription drugs are absorbed and excreted tend to amplify the side effects of some over-the-counter drugs as well. The idea that "if some is good, more is better," leads to danger. For example, nasal decongestants can be harmful for people with high blood pressure or asthma. Some constipation remedies are too harsh and dehydrating for some older adults. In addition, some over-the-counter products should not be used with certain prescription medicines.

Although the U.S. Food and Drug Administration (FDA) has deemed over-the-counter drugs safe for consumers, they are the cause of thousands of hospitalizations annually. There is particular alarm about common pain-relieving drugs containing acetaminophen, and the nonsteroidal anti-inflammatory agents, such as ibuprofen and naproxen, which have been shown to increase cardiovascular risks. As a result, the American Heart Association is now urging that pain sufferers first try such nonmedical interventions as exercise, diet change, and weight loss. Only then should low doses of low-risk drugs be tried. The FDA recently recommended that labels include much stronger and more complete cautions, a proposal that has been in the works for years and hopefully will result in better label warnings. But will they be more readable? That remains to be seen.

Herbs, Supplements, and Vitamins—Easy Magic?

Also of concern are the vast quantities of herbal remedies and dietary supplements bought by older adults to promote well-being or address a symptom. A *New England Journal of Medicine* study estimated that one in three Americans used some form of alternative medicine in 1990 to relieve chronic health problems—and paid almost $14 billion for them. Despite the fact that herbal medicines have been used for centuries and are promoted as "natural," they should be used with caution, especially by those taking other prescription medications. The FDA categorizes botanical remedies, as well as vitamins, minerals, and supplements such as glucosamine (popular among osteoarthritis sufferers), as "foods," and therefore they do not require FDA approval to be marketed. Nor are their contents or promotional materials regulated for accuracy, though they are prohibited from claiming to be "cures" for specific conditions.

Herbal aids needn't be avoided. Yet, gentle as they tend to be, they behave as drugs. Some can have unsuspected side effects and adverse interactions with other medications. St. John's wort, for example, touted as a relief for minor (but never major) depression, can seriously affect how other drugs act in the body, particularly digoxin, warfarin, and prescription antidepressants. Other herbal extracts, sometimes combined in elixirs, teas, or tablets, can cause allergic or digestive problems. In fact, a significant number of adverse reactions to glucosamine, echinacea, melatonin, and vitamins were reported between 1983 and 2005, according to the American Association of Poison Control Centers, as reported in the *New York Times* on February 6, 2007. And some may just be a waste of money.

"My friend Maggie swears by echinacea, and now I take it whenever I get a cold. The nice clerk at the health store recommends it, too." In the absence of solid studies, these are common reasons why older people turn to alternative remedies. Now, however, the National Institutes of Health is overseeing scientific testing of a number of popular herbal and dietary supplements under its National Center for Complementary and Alternative Medicine. NIH's answer about echinacea? "It *may* help boost the immune system. But it *won't* cure a cold once you've caught it." (Visit www.nccm.nih.gov.)

Americans also swallow commercially produced vitamins in huge quantities. Some consider them a kind of cheap health insurance; others feel that taking a fistful of vitamin pills every morning will somehow make up for a guilty lack of fruits and vegetables in the diet. The truth is, *vitamins are not foods* at all, but catalysts that aid in the metabolism of food. Even *Webster's Dictionary* points out that vitamins "do not provide energy or serve as building units." And taking excessive amounts, especially of fat-soluble vitamins, can be dangerous: vitamin K, for example, which aids in blood clotting, should be avoided by people who are taking blood thinners.

This is not to say that specific vitamin supplements suggested by a physician or trained nutritionist have no value for the elderly. But does that pill actually contain what the bottle label declares? In some cases, no. A recent study of 21 multivitamins by ConsumerLab.com found that only 10 met the claims on their labels or satisfied other quality standards. One guide to buying vitamins is to look for a stamp on the label from USP, NSF (the National Science Foundation), or go to www.ConsumerLab.com to ascertain whether a brand has been submitted to testing. Better yet, most nutrition experts agree that the most reliable source of vitamins is not a pill at all, but a varied diet including plenty of fruits, vegetables, and grains.

In America's vast over-the-counter pharmacopoeia, how does one know what to choose? The first answer is: read all the label warnings—if you can—and use any drug or supplement in moderation. The second answer for making safe choices and avoiding adverse reactions with other drugs is this: inform the doctor of just which over-the-counter medications or supplements your parent takes, and in what quantity and frequency. They belong on your master list of medications.

Inform the doctor of just which over-the-counter medications or supplements your parent takes, and in what quantity and frequency. They belong on your master list of medications.

Keeping the Medications Straight—Who's in Charge Here?

Most of us assume that if an older relative is seeing a physician fairly regularly, his or her medications are being properly managed. That's the doctor's job, right? Unfortunately, a simple "yes" no longer serves. Many entities—from the pharmaceutical companies that produce and promote the medications, to the various types of physicians who may be prescribing for your parent, to the pharmacists who dispense the drugs—have responsibility in today's silent epidemic of muddled medications. And all have an important role in reducing the chances of a medication-related problem. It behooves older adults, as well as family members, to be aware of how these complex roles can work for good or ill.

Physicians Aren't Perfect

The key player in balancing and keeping track of an older person's medications is usually the primary doctor, often an internist or general practitioner. One hopes, of course, that this doctor is up to date enough to avoid inappropriate drugs and turn to better ones. It's also important that he or she not be so overburdened that he or she hasn't time to really listen to your Dad's symptoms, inquire about allergies to foods or medicines, and review his records and all his medications thoughtfully. Yet one recent survey reported in the January 6, 2007, issue of the *New York Times* found that patients over age 65 got an average of 16 minutes of the doctor's attention—enough to discuss one problem, perhaps, but rarely three.

A physician with experience treating many older patients is a real plus. Best of all are geriatricians, medical specialists trained to evaluate and address the individual, and often complex, needs of an older patient.

A physician with experience treating many older patients is a real plus. Best of all are geriatricians, medical specialists trained to evaluate and address the individual, and often complex, needs of an older patient. So far, unfortunately, such specialists are few and far between. In some parts of the country, in fact, other common medical specialties are scarce as well, putting even greater

What to Ask the Doctor When Medication Is Prescribed

Questions to Ask the Prescribing Doctor

- What is the name, type, and purpose of the drug?
- How often is it taken?
- Should it be taken with food or on an empty stomach?
- How should the medication be stored?
- Is it okay to drive or to have an alcoholic drink?
- How soon should its benefit be felt?
- What side effects may occur?
- Which side effects warrant calling the doctor?
- Have you reviewed all other current medications?
- Are all of the other medications still necessary?
- Will this medication interact with any other prescription or over-the-counter medications being taken?

Remember

- Prepare a list of questions in advance.
- Have someone close to you or your parent take notes on what the doctor says, and ask again about anything that is not clear.
- Make sure the doctor's prescription is legible.

At the Pharmacy

- You can ask the pharmacist many of the same questions you might ask the doctor.
- Request a printout on the drug.
- Make sure the pharmacist has an up-to-date list of all the patient's medications.
- Check the label on the bottle—is it the right drug, the right dose?
- Can the label be read?
- Can the patient open the bottle easily?

burden on the shoulders of the general practitioner, who has to be all things to all people.

Of particular concern is the treatment of older patients with emotional problems There is a blurred line today between the practice of internal medicine and psychiatry. Even when psychiatrists are available in the community, medications for depression or anxiety are most often being prescribed by general doctors and internists, whom studies show to rate poorly in choosing appropriate drugs. If possible, such drugs should be prescribed by psychiatrists.

"Psychiatrist? That's for crazy people," says Aunt Ella. "I'm certainly not a loony! I'm just a bit down since my son moved away." After all, she was raised to keep sorrows to herself and to soldier on as best she can, even when impaired. Like Ella, quite a few older people fear the stigma of "mental problems" and will adamantly refuse the suggestion to consult with a psychiatrist. For concerned family members, it can be very hard to overcome such ingrained fears. They can, however, arm themselves with some information and ask their parent's primary care physician about the possible side effects of psychotropic medications. If the answer is an unsatisfactory blank stare or a dismissive "no problem," they should consider taking the next step and seek a psychiatrist for a consultation on the matter. Psychiatrists are specialists trained to identify serious mental difficulties, and if necessary, to treat them with medications and monitor their use. They also, along with other mental health professionals, can provide psychotherapy—"talk therapy"—and indeed may suggest that it is a better option for a depressed or anxious senior than psychotropic medication. Either way, a simple prescription for an antidepressant or another type of psychotropic drug from an internist shouldn't be the first and last word on your elderly mother's mental health.

The Specialist Merry-Go-Round

Say your parent does see some specialists, either recommended by the primary physician or even by a friend who swears by his own cardiologist or urologist. Your parent may very well get an accurate diagnosis and a state-of-the-art treatment plan. So where's the catch?

Andy's primary doctor suggested that he be evaluated by a well-regarded cardiologist for an irregular heart rhythm. The earliest appointment available was in 3 weeks. "We'll send them your records," promised the assistant. But when Andy arrived for his appointment, the cardiologists' office still didn't have his records or a list of his existing prescriptions. And the next available appointment was in 5 weeks. "Oh, just go right in," said the assistant, "I'll have the records faxed over now." Now turned out to be an hour after Andy's consultation was over. Andy was able to tell the cardiologist the names of some of his drugs, "though I forget the dosages," he admitted. Fortunately, that didn't satisfy the cardiologist, who carefully reviewed the faxed records. Noting that Andy periodically took prednisone for asthma, this alert physician called the patient and suggested he also see an ophthalmologist, since prednisone can be a factor in causing glaucoma—something his primary physician had never mentioned. Only then did the cardiologist mail Andy a new heart medication prescription.

Andy, you were lucky. But you or a family member should have called the specialist's office ahead of time to make sure your records had arrived. It never hurts to check and, if necessary nag! If the specialist hadn't consulted a complete list of your medications, any new prescription could have interacted badly with those you were already taking. And by a complete list, remember that you might also see a dentist or podiatrist who may have prescribed medication.

Ideally, before prescribing any new medication, a new physician will be aware of *all* the medications the patient is taking, as well as his or her allergies and general physical condition. Ideally as well, the specialist will inform the primary doctor of the diagnosis and treatment. That way, the patient's records, including reports of electrocardiograms, blood tests, and X-rays or other tests, are complete and up-to-date in both offices. Ideally. This communicate-and-coordinate game becomes particularly critical when an older person who is taking

Ideally, before prescribing any new medication, a new physician will be aware of all the medications the patient is taking, as well as his or her allergies and general physical condition.

multiple medications is seeing multiple doctors, thus exponentially increasing the possibility of unwanted drug interactions. As a safety check, patients or their caregivers should also request that copies of all test reports be sent to them for their personal records.

Death by Handwriting

A few days after Luz Rodriguez' home health aide picked up some newly prescribed pills for her client's high blood pressure, Mrs. Rodriguez suffered violent sieges of vomiting. The aide summoned a visiting nurse, who noticed that the new pills were actually a chemotherapy drug—and Mrs. Rodriguez did not have cancer! An immediate call to both the prescribing physician and the pharmacist revealed that the handwritten prescription the pharmacist had tried to translate had been misread. The quick call did not save Luz Rodriguez several days of misery, but it did save her from being hospitalized.

Physicians who scrawl hasty, illegible prescriptions must assume that all pharmacists can read the Rosetta Stone. Did the doctor mean 1500 mg or 150 mg? Celexa or Celebrex? Is that 3 × or 5 × a day? According to the National Academies of Science, sloppily written prescriptions, resulting in wrong dosages and wrong medications, kill some 7000 people and injure 1.5 million every year. This is a terrifying scandal that doesn't need to happen, especially in the age of computers.

Currently, insurance companies, such as Aetna, and Internet companies, such as Google, are uniting to make confusing handwritten prescriptions a thing of the past. Doctors who have access to the Internet—and that's 90% of them—will be able to select an accurate prescription and dosage from a free online menu, requiring no special software or hardware. They don't actually *write* a thing. The concept, known as the National e-Prescribing Patient Safety Initiative (NEPSI)—or, more simply, eRX—will also provide checks for potentially harmful drug interactions and can be downloaded—lucidly—by the pharmacist.

Just check here. The mouse is stronger than the pen (www.erx network.com/).

Pharmacists Step Up

We all rely on the accuracy of pharmacists to package and label our prescription drugs, as well as on their advice about use. Take with or without food? Avoid alcohol? Oh, a printed information sheet? Fine. Now, however, thanks to their specialized knowledge and the use of computerized records, pharmacists are positioned to become increasingly important partners in preventing prescription mishaps in the years to come.

Already Medicare prescription drug plans are required to provide, for certain eligible patients, a coordinated supervision plan linking pharmacists and health care providers. The goal is to more firmly oversee and control drug safety, appropriate choices, and costs. By catching conflicting prescriptions, improper dosages, or problems with patients who either don't understand or don't take their medications, hospitalizations attributed to these causes can be greatly reduced. So far, these interdisciplinary plans relying on pharmacists, known as medication therapy management services (MTMS), cover only high-risk participants in the Medicare Part D drug plan, especially elderly patients who have multiple chronic conditions and are likely to incur at least $4000 in annual drug costs. But in various forms, the idea is catching on, not only with Medicare and some Medicaid health plans but also with hospitals, clinics, private health plans, nursing homes, and community pharmacists. Hospitals, too, are major culprits, according to the Institute of Medicine of the National Academies of Science. Their drug errors may kill 1.5 million people a year, yet as reported in the *New York Times* on February 25, 2007, only 6% use computer drug systems to ensure that the correct medication is given at the correct doses.

For physicians, giving pharmacists increased responsibility is a win-win situation. In some cases, MTMS programs might use specially trained pharmacists to oversee patients who need frequent monitoring, such as those taking blood thinners or diabetes medicines. Other participating pharmacists will be able to answer questions that might otherwise require a call or visit to the doctor.

Even without participating in an MTMS program, you and your parent can improve drug safety by *using one pharmacy to centrally record all prescriptions from various doctors.* Also, before you leave

Even without participating in an MTMS program, you and your parent can improve drug safety by using one pharmacy to centrally record all prescriptions from various doctors.

the drugstore with a new bottle of pills, examine the label carefully. Check to make sure that it can actually be read by the patient and that it is exactly what the doctor ordered. Can Mom's arthritic hands open that tricky childproof cap? If not, request an easier one. And, if you thought of some questions you or your parent forgot to ask the prescribing doctor, go ahead and ask the pharmacist now: "What side effects might occur? What if Dad misses taking a pill one day? Will his morning grapefruit juice affect how this medication is absorbed?" When it comes to drugs, all information is healthy. (Helpful guides to prescription and nonprescription drugs are listed in Appendix B.)

"I Won't Take That Big Yellow Pill"

Growing old is a process full of sad ironies. One is this: the more frail people become and the more medications they take, the more challenging it becomes to keep them all straight. Forgetfulness intrudes. Poor vision leads to confusion. Directions—"Is it the little red pill or the white one I take after dinner?"—get muddled. After all, *some drug regimens older adults follow would be daunting, even for a 40-year-old.*

Emergency room attendants have far too many scary stories of elderly patients who have somehow messed up their medications. In fact, a sound drug regimen that is not followed can be as much the cause of trouble as an unsound drug regimen.

The reasons for noncompliance can be as simple as a pill that is too big to be easily swallowed. Lois choked once on a large pill and simply stopped taking it. If her physician had known about her swallowing problem, he might very well have been able to prescribe the same medication as a liquid, or in smaller, multiple tablets. But he didn't know.

Another reason why patients fail to comply with a drug regimen is that they simply don't understand it. Perhaps the doctor used big medical words that were unfamiliar to your father, or maybe he didn't "get" the directions or even the purpose of a certain prescription when the doctor described it. Others misread or misinterpret the directions on the label. Researchers call this "poor health literacy," and it's a cause of error for patients of all education levels. An elderly person who visits the doctor alone should not just sit there mumbling "Yes, uh-huh," when unfamiliar words are used, but should take notes on what the doctor says, then repeat back what he or she has been told. Better yet, the older adult should take an alert companion or family member along to take notes and share in all stages of the consultation—not just sit in the waiting room.

More seriously, many older people simply cannot afford to continue to take the medications they need. In 2006, the prices of 200 drugs commonly used by older people rose 6.2%, almost twice the rate of inflation. Perhaps some found enrolling in the Medicare Part D drug option far too complicated, or have used up their cost allowance. Others, whose medications require periodic monitoring and adjustment, tend to shun the inconvenience or cost of appointments or find it physically difficult even to get to a doctor without a helper.

If an older relative is unable to sort and take prescribed medications correctly, others must step in to help. A home health aide, visiting nurse, or reliable neighbor can organize a week's

If an older relative is unable to sort and take prescribed medications correctly, others must step in to help.

medications in a pillbox divided into sections for days of the week and times of day, and then check regularly to see if the correct pills were taken. Even alert, independent people can benefit from memory aids. Some turn the bottle they've just used upside down, in case the phone rings or the teakettle whistles and they forget which of the three morning pills they've already taken. If Dad is supposed to take his second diuretic pill at 6 o'clock but tends to forget because the evening news is on then, a special alarm clock can be set to ring 15 minutes earlier to remind him to take the medication.

And then there are some older persons who medicate themselves—choosing not to follow prescribed doses, but taking medications according to how they feel. Very often they are noncompliant about other medical directives as well. If your parent is cognitively intact, the most you can do is provide as much information as possible about the dangers of misuse of medications and hope for the best. If a medical crisis occurs due to your mother's noncompliance, she may be sufficiently frightened to follow your advice. But, then again—maybe not.

The Advertised Cure

Wherever one turns today—from the Internet to the newspaper to the bus—ads for prescription medications are ubiquitous. We are bombarded with promotions for strong drugs to relieve pain, enhance sexual functioning, and reduce cholesterol, bone loss, blood pressure, and anxiety. Major pharmaceutical companies have discovered the power of marketing directly to consumers (something no other country but New Zealand permits), and they spend close to $4.5 billion a year to capture our attention. That figure doesn't include the undisclosed amounts spent to promote their drugs directly to physicians and other providers. The industry's goal is to maximize profits; and profits, the companies assert, underwrite the development of newer and better drugs.

Aids to Compliance

Remembering when to take what medication can be a challenge. Try these tips.

- Post a highly visible master list of drugs and times of day to take them.
- Coordinate doses with a daily ritual, such as eating breakfast or watching the evening news.
- Group pills in a special pillbox with sections for the day of the week and the time of day. (A helper or family member can fill and check this container weekly.)
- Keep at least one pill in the original labeled bottle, to avoid confusion about which is which.
- Label the top of each bottle with the time or times a pill should be taken.
- Set an alarm clock after each daily dose to signal when it is time for the next dose.
- Subscribe to a telephone reminder service.

Although the main side effects of medications are disclosed in public advertisements, and always include the cautionary reminder to "talk to your doctor," these promotions overtly encourage consumers to pressure their doctors. As such, they are both cause and proof of the greater role that consumers play in the health care scenario. The plus side of these expensive campaigns is that people have more information about available drugs—if they heed them. But the combination of the quality of promotional information, and up to now, the lax oversight of drug ads by the FDA, has raised concerns that have recently been addressed by Congress.

Although the main side effects of medications are disclosed in public advertisements, and always include the cautionary reminder to "talk to your doctor," these promotions overtly encourage consumers to pressure their doctors. As such, they are both cause and proof of the greater role that consumers play in the health care scenario.

Aggressive, competitive advertising is, after all, a hallmark of our society. Yet when it comes to medicines, critics accuse the pharmaceutical industry of using raw political power and distorting information in its advertising—downplaying some serious side effects or attempting to prop up a profitable drug that may have been superseded. In some rare cases, doctors have been led to use a drug for conditions for which it has never been tested or approved—"off-label" prescribing.

A recent cautionary tale concerns Vioxx, a nonsteroidal anti-inflammatory drug used to relieve pain from osteoarthritis and rheumatoid arthritis. When postmarketing trials showed a significant increase in strokes and heart attacks in patients taking it, the producer voluntarily withdrew the product from the market in 2004. The result? Pharmaceutical advertising directly to consumers dipped for a year. Then it surged again.

What consumers don't know is that safety data are often drawn from limited clinical trials in selected groups. Since 1997, drug safety tests have been required by the FDA to include older adults, but that subgroup tends not to include "those who are very old and frail." Other well-known prescription drugs went on the market before testing procedures were tightened. Some known side effects remain unpublicized by the drug companies; others are not known until the drug has been in use for some time.

Millions of people in this country suffer from insomnia. To advertise the three top-selling sleep medications (known as sedative hypnotics), drug companies spent just under $200 million in 2005 and 2006. Yet recent reports indicate that the most popular sleeping pill, Ambien, can have such bizarre side effects as nighttime eating binges or episodes of driving when the patient is asleep. Afterward, patients have no memory whatsoever of their actions. These rare but dangerous reactions usually occurred when the patient had also been drinking alcohol. Though warnings about mixing this drug and other similar insomnia medications with alcohol were shown on the labels, the FDA is sufficiently alarmed to now require much stronger warnings—on labels, in advertising, and on new inserts to come with the medications.

Why only now? Postmarketing trials, which follow up on how actual patients are reacting, have been both rare and costly for the chronically underfunded FDA. Since the Vioxx scandal threw light on these problems, the 2007 Congress has raised urgent calls for greatly increased oversight of drug safety. An outcome of this increased diligence was the levying of hefty fines in May 2007 on the manufacturers of OxyContin for failing to fully report the addictive potential of this drug.

There is no doubt that high-powered advertising campaigns add considerably to the cost of brand-name medications. Along with new consumers won, let us not forget those forced to stop using their drugs because of higher prices—not only to support research and development but also to cover advertising and promotional costs.

The Informed Consumer

This brings us back to the consumers—you and your aging parent. The benefits of modern medicine and the medications that are a critical component of patient care are both life saving and life-extending. Medications are a powerful tool in improving and maintaining health, but the flip side of the coin is that their potency can be dangerous. Consumers must rely on their own vigilance as well as that of their health care providers, and take heed!

Bob Morris on His Father's Noncompliance

My father was such an iconoclast, and such a control freak, that he liked to experiment with his prescriptions. You know, take a little bit of this, a little bit of that: "I'll have half of this, and I'm not feeling right today, so maybe I'll try that." He really had a salad bar approach to his prescriptions. For awhile he was convinced that chocolate was the answer to a cough he had. And guess what? Recent studies are finding it can actually be a cough suppressant! And God forbid you should sneeze in front of him—then he would be pushing his prescriptions on you as well.

My brother and I used to joke about that all the time, and it gave us some laughs. Unfortunately, one day, he ended up in the hospital because he took something that sent his blood pressure spiraling down. So they found him on the floor at his assisted living place. This was before his last year, actually. There are a lot of medications that have to do with blood pressure levels. Children should be aware of what these effects are.

I would go and visit him and be alarmed at his listlessness, thinking, "Oh, well, I need to make you more alert. You have to drink coffee—he hated coffee. Or you're losing your mind, or something." And it wasn't that—it was just low blood pressure because of Lasix, or whatever it is that is so commonly prescribed.

It wouldn't be bad to get a handle on the effects of drugs seniors take. My brother was very good at being on top of all of that, and there were a million pills for both my parents. My prescription was coffee. I know that that's not medicine. But, to me, when I could get a little coffee in him, that would help counteract the meds. It wasn't always easy—but what's the point of being listless and drowsy all day?

No, I think he took what he wanted, and we didn't have much control over it. And, again—*it became the same old argument. Do we sweep in and try to control him?* Or do we let him live the life that he wants to lead? With the pill taking, he didn't do that much damage. And we even began to wonder who knew better than he did what was working—and what was making him feel better?

It was very hard. Because when my mother was just completely incapacitated—even at the assisted living place—there were still pills to be taken at a certain time of day. And there wasn't a full-time nurse there to tell her when to take this and that. So we had to lay them out in those little pillboxes, with the date on them, and make sure that that got done. And we could not rely on my father to do that effectively. So we had to keep emphasizing to him to just make sure that she got her pills. And it was a lot of pills. It was like a still life—those baskets of pills. And when you started to get them out it sounded like maracas. You could shake those bottles, and each one sounded different. Big ones, little ones. You do the hokey pokey and you turn yourself around. That's what it's all about!

13

Taking a Stand

Kitty Braden dropped out of college before her first child was born and went back to finish after her youngest child reached junior high school. In her first semester, her mother died, and Kitty, unable to let her nearly blind father live alone, brought him to live with her. Kitty dropped out of college for the second time.

Vince Phillips, a science teacher with three children—one in college already and the other two in high school—learned last year that his mother, after a long struggle with cancer, had used up all her health insurance benefits and her money and could no longer pay for the medical and nursing care she needed. Vince and his brothers now share those expenses. Vince moonlights on the evening shift at the Lomax plant.

Elaine Murphy, although sad and lonely in the early days after her father's death, was a little ashamed of the thoughts that kept running through her head: "No more Medicare forms to fill out . . . no more frantic scrambling for homemakers and nurses . . . no more emergency calls in the middle of the night . . . no more visits to that terrible old neighborhood . . . no more canceling our plans because Dad has another attack . . . . Thank God, all that's over."

T HESE THREE FAMILIES—AND MANY OTHERS LIKE them—belie the popular belief that "children in modern society neglect their old parents." Such families know they do everything they can for their parents under the circumstances. The only thing they do not do is try to change the circumstances.

If adequately supportive alternative living arrangements had been available for their fathers, Kitty and Elaine would not have had to disrupt their own lives. If adequate insurance coverage for chronic illness had been available for his mother, Jack would not have had to moonlight. None of these children would have loved their parents less, but they would have had to sacrifice less of their personal lives. Even today, when it is a generally accepted fact that most families with elderly relatives are doing their best to help, society is calling on them to do even more, as evidenced by the plethora of advice books for family caregivers with the implicit message, "Are you taking good enough care of your elderly relatives?" Perhaps it is finally time for those generations to call society to task for its shortcomings, with the message, "*You* are not taking good enough care of your elderly citizens."

The Glass: Half-Full and Half-Empty

Society itself has been trying to "care enough" for its elderly. But if a visitor from another planet were to ask how America treats its older citizens, the answer would depend on the respondent's point of view. The optimist, always seeing the glass as half-full, might reply, "Life is much better for older people than it used to be. Look how far we've come in the 72 years since Social Security began, and in the 42 years since the passage of the Older Americans Act. Look at the decline in poverty among the elderly, falling from 35% in 1959 to 10.1% in 2005. Look at Medicare, Medicaid, and SSI! Look at the millions who are being helped to live better." But the pessimist, always seeing the glass as half-empty, might counter with, "Look how much still needs to be done!"

Both these statements are true in part. This book has reviewed many of the federal and other programs throughout the nation that benefit older Americans: income benefits; financing of health care; protection of rights, including laws preventing discrimination against older workers; and a proliferation of research studies on aging; federal supports for state and local organizations providing services for older men and women. Indeed, many older Americans are in fine financial shape, thanks to pensions, private investments, and annuity plans, in addition to Social Security checks. Current economic statistics reveal that the over-50 population is actually better off than those under 50. A new acronym has even been added to the list of demographic epithets, such as WASP and yuppie: the *woofs*— "well-off older folks"!

But the fact that older adults today have more support than their parents and grandparents did does not mean that they have *enough* support. If some, like the woofs, live visibly well, enjoying comfortable surroundings and travel (often to the resentment of younger folks), others live marginally and are invisible. Society still too often fails its elderly who are frail, dependent, and incapacitated, and have limited income.

The fact that older adults today have more support than their parents and grandparents did does not mean that they have enough support.

How long will independence last for an older man who is determined to take care of himself, but who has little income, substandard housing, and minimal health protection? The poverty figures may show a dramatic decline, but too many still live below the poverty line, and many more count as near-poor. This latter group includes some formerly self-supporting people, such as Vince Phillips's mother, who is poor for the first time because her resources were drained away in her old age by long illnesses.

If your community lacks home services, you may, like Kitty Braden, feel obligated to reorganize your life to take your widowed father into your own home. Or, if that is not possible, he may be forced to accept institutional placement. And what if that initial placement provides poor care or has to be closed down? The search begins all over again.

In the current economic pinch of state and federal budgets, there is an ever-present threat of cutbacks in existing benefits and services, including the outright closing down of some hospitals, clinics, senior centers, and meal programs. Whenever there is a need to save money, the most obvious place to look for cuts is frequently funds for the most vulnerable, among them older Americans.

Social Security—Where Is It Headed?

Even more ominous than the shortfall in services to the most vulnerable elderly is the growing threat to those stalwarts of support for the majority of older Americans: Social Security and Medicare. Keep in mind that more than 48 million Americans today (two thirds of them seniors) receive checks from the Social Security system. In 2006, the average monthly payment to these individuals was $955.

Social Security constitutes more than half of the incomes of nearly two thirds of retired Americans, and for one in five, it is their only income. Yet in 2007, the annual raise of 3.3% was greatly offset by a parallel raise in Medicare deductions. In fact, many of those participating in the Medicare Part D benefit for drugs actually saw their Social Security checks *reduced*—for the first time in history.

Even more dramatic changes may be in the air. Shortly after the presidential elections of 2004, aggressive steps were taken to attempt to privatize the then 69-year-old Social Security program. Some warned of the fund's bankruptcy within 50 years as baby boomers, reached their elder years. Under this plan, younger workers could chose to divert their Social Security taxes to private savings and investment accounts, and manage them themselves, just as they would any investments. Yet many distrusted both the prediction and the plan, and believe that adjustments can be made to the present system that would forestall a shortfall in the years to come.

Although the efforts toward privatization proved unpopular, and were stalled, there are still sharply differing opinions about this initiative along the political divide. For example, in "Twelve Reasons Why Privatizing Social Security Is a Bad Idea," Greg Anrig of the Century Foundation maintains that addressing Social Security's potential long-term financing challenges by taking the extreme step of diverting its payroll taxes to private savings accounts will have dire consequences for federal finances and also for present and future retirees and persons who are disabled. He notes that if the plan were to go into effect, it would be extremely costly both to the trust fund itself and certainly to individuals incurring brokerage and management fees. Those favoring private accounts—including such conservative think tanks as the Cato Institute—point to the salutary benefits to individuals in controlling their own investments and believe that the long-term reduction in Social Security payments will maintain the solvency of the trust fund. Whatever your political persuasion, it is incumbent upon you, for the sake of your parents and your own future, to be well informed and proactive. The reform of Social Security remains a live issue—though changing, it is regarded as a "third rail" for politicians. To ensure that changes are for the better, and not for the worse, adults of all ages need to stay informed and let their voices be heard.

The Train Has Already Left the Station

Unlike Social Security, the privatization of Medicare is already under way. Since its inception in 1965, when over 19 million older persons were enrolled in the program, it has grown to over 42 million enrollees in 2005. Whatever its flaws, Medicare has provided universal coverage for older adults, rich and poor, and has contributed significantly to the increasingly healthy lives of older Americans.

Unlike Social Security, the privatization of Medicare is already under way.

It would seem in the best interests of all Americans, young and old, to preserve this system and to be alert to changes that are taking place and being proposed. For philosophical or cost-cutting reasons, privatization efforts go back a number of years. One attempt at private options—known as Medicare+Choice—was introduced in 1997, but after several years, these Medicare-funded private plans began withdrawing as government payments and profit margins diminished. But more recently, enrollment in these plans as a result of extensive marketing has dramatically increased. Subsidized by the federal government, these plans cost the taxpayer more than Medicare, and according to a May, 7, 2007, *New York Times* article, they promise more than they can deliver.

In 2003, a major restructuring of the traditional Medicare program took place with the passage of the Medicare Modernization

Act. It relies exclusively on private plans to deliver the new Part D prescription drug coverage, begun in 2006. Yet it seems that even such positive reforms come with glaring inadequacies.

As underscored in Chapter 8, this coverage has been, to say the least, a challenge to older adults—and even to their helpful families—because of the baffling array of private plans to choose from, each different from the other. To add to the confusion, more plans were being added in 2007. In many cases, initially available drugs have been withdrawn from a plan's formulary, and prices of others have gone up considerably. And speaking of prices, critics denounce the fact that Congress in its initial legislation protected the drug companies from negotiating competitive prices with private Medicare D plans—as the Veterans Administration is permitted to do. This provision is being challenged by Congress. The deficiencies in Medicare coverage—such as no coverage for long-term care, dental care, or hearing aids, and little in the way of vision rehabilitation—have been outlined earlier chapters.

Just as troubling are continuing threats that would undermine the provisions now in place that benefit many millions of older Americans.

Let's Hear It from the Families

Older people are not taking these threats lying down. In fact, the most militant opposition to cutbacks and the greatest pressure for additional help have come, until recently, from older adults themselves. Increasingly vocal, the over-65 population has become adept at organizing and protecting their own well-being. Advocacy from such groups as the Gray Panthers, the American Association of Retired Persons, the National Council on the Aging, and the National Active and Retired Federal employees Association has led to new legislation and appropriations to aid the elderly. Their efforts have now been joined by professionals, young and old, active in the field of aging, and not to be overlooked has been the powerful influence exerted by disability groups, whose advocacy has benefited people of all ages.

But what of that other potentially powerful group—the families of older adults? So far, they have tended to hover on the sidelines, struggling with immediate demands, settling for stopgap measures, complaining among themselves about their problems—but rarely making their collective voices heard.

There are understandable reasons for this. Most of us tend to regard our older relatives as family responsibilities, rather than public ones. "Washing your own laundry" is a proud frontier ideal ingrained in many American families. But seeking positive social change hardly constitutes abandoning our own caring input. Should the day ever come when all elderly men and women are well supported, well fed, well housed, and well nursed, parents with close relationships will still turn to their children for the affection, under-standing, and intimacy no one else can provide. When public support comes in the door, private relationships will *not* fly out the window. Never have. Never will.

When public support comes in the door, private relation-ships will not fly out the window. Never have. Never will.

When it comes to effecting change, a public chorus is far more effective than a solo sung in the shower. For proof, one need only note what has been accomplished by the family caregivers of older adults with Alzheimer's disease. Bearing the burden of 24-hour care and the emotional turmoil caused by this devastating disease, family members organized over 27 years ago to bring public attention to the devastating effects of the disease and the burdens of family care-giving. They founded the Alzheimer's Association, which now has chapters throughout the nation that provide information and support to family caregivers. In addition, they play an important and effective advocacy role and have succeeded in increasing funds for Alzheimer's research.

Whether or not sons and daughters provide direct care, they can behave responsibly to their parents—and themselves—by pressing for social action. The future arrives for everyone. As the baby boom of the 1950s becomes the geriatric boom, the over-65 population is expected to reach 71.5 million by the year 2030. At some point later in this century, a full quarter of Americans may be 65 and over. Society may have been able to consider 13% of its citizens as outside the mainstream, but 25% will not be so easy to ignore.

The children of the elderly, sandwiched between older and younger generations, are forced to give in two directions at the same time. They receive no compensation for that double burden, and they are usually the most heavily taxed. They have a right to stand up and shout, "We need help, too! Pay attention to us!" They also have a right to expect that someone will listen.

Society's Unfinished Business

Attention Legislators, Insurance Underwriters, and Employers!

Despite recent gains, there remains a great deal to be accomplished in caring for our elderly. The inequalities of the Social Security system, particularly as they affect elderly women, need to be evened out, so that becoming a widow does not also usually mean becoming poorer. Although there are no longer restrictions on earned income for those who want to work after the age of 70, age discrimination in the workplace remains a fact of life. Too many older adults are thwarted in their efforts to earn additional income, along with the psychic income that comes from feeling productive. Actually, able older workers should be prized for their experience and maturity! Yet many who prefer and seek part-time work are told, "That arrangement just doesn't fit our corporate structure."

And then there are disabled and frail older adults. Throughout this book, we have described the variety of community-based services needed by older adults if they are to live safely, and to the extent possible, enjoy healthy lives in their own homes. While these services have increased dramatically in number since the first edition of *You and Your Aging Parent* in 1976, much more is required—particularly coverage for long-term care in the community.

And what of the children of older adults who are willing to care for a disabled father or mother, but find themselves, like Vince Phillips, financially crushed by the burden? They have a right to financial assistance, in the form of either tax deductions or some type of government subsidy, to help defray their outlays of time and effort. So far, such assistance reaches only the most overwhelmed families. Unreimbursed medical expenses that exceed 7.5% of an adult child's gross income are tax-deductible. (If siblings are sharing in this cost, the expenses can be aggregated and attributed to one child.) And an aging parent whose income is less than $3200 annually, *and who is living in a child's home,* may be declared a dependent.

Even solutions for those with more financial resources, such as buying private long-term care insurance (preferably well before the need arrives), offer questionable coverage in an age of soaring costs. And too often, those in the middle-income brackets, saddled with mortgages and college tuition, simply can't afford it. When the first edition of this book was published in 1976, it stressed the urgent need for major public and private financing of long-term illness. Now, more than 30 later, the need is *still* urgent and *still* unmet.

Attention Planners, Builders, Architects—and Legislators Again!

GETTING AROUND

> When Amy Freers, 79, whose legs are essentially crippled by peripheral vascular disease, gets into her electric wheelchair for an outing in the city, her miniature poodle Bebee jumps up into her lap. Amanda snaps on the leash, they take the elevator to the lobby of her apartment building, and then off they go together, summer and winter, rolling easily over the low curbs. Perhaps they'll go to the grocery store or the park. Or, taking a public bus with a wheelchair lift, they'll travel to a midtown bookstore for an author's reading. Bebee gets her walk, and Amanda returns to her apartment building with pink cheeks, an autographed novel, and the pleasure of feeling part of the outside world.

The Americans with Disability Act, passed in 1990, is a landmark piece of legislation requiring accessibility for person with disabilities in public accommodations and transportation. Fueled by the political action of younger disabled persons, including veterans, it has greatly benefited older adults as well. Accommodations for wheelchair users, including lowered curbs on city street corners and ramps into public buildings, have made theaters, restaurants, and churches open at

The Americans with Disability Act, passed in 1990, is a landmark piece of legislation requiring accessibility for person with disabilities in public accommodations and transportation.

last to those formerly left at the bottom of the stairs. Technology enabling people with impaired hearing to use telephones and large print signs with good contrast for those who are visually impaired are also cases in point. The impact of this legislation is immeasurable—many disabled persons, old and young, are now far more independent.

Amy is particularly lucky to live in a city where the assists she relies on are at hand. But in countless rural and suburban communities, there is little in the way of public transportation for the frail and disabled. In rapidly gentrifying neighborhoods, even those who used to walk to the cleaners and greengrocer are seeing their familiar shops replaced by big box national chain stores that are less accessible to them.

The law helps many, if not all. But there is no law yet that requires architects or interior designers to incorporate many other environmental changes—some quite simple—that would make life a lot better for older and younger adults with impaired vision. For example, people with failing or partial vision see even less well in glaring lighting. For them, signs, stairs, and doorways without strong color contrast are confusing or perilous. That was the problem when 81-year-old Leslie Arnold, who has macular degeneration, went to meet a friend for lunch. On her way to the restroom after lunch, she was stopped by three descending limestone stairs that blurred together in her sight. "I was forced to ask a stranger's help," she said. "So I told the restaurant owner that his steps were dangerous and unacceptable, and that he had to have black lines painted on the treads. I'm not shy anymore about speaking up!"

And speaking of speaking: when will those electronic wizards, who now have masses of younger people phoning their friends and downloading files by tapping tiny spots on tiny, palm-sized devices, wake up to another growing market? All it takes to get more hip elders on board is a choice of simpler and visually accessible equipment. A case in point is the recent introduction of cell phones designed for older adults. Leslie would go for that.

WHERE CAN WE LIVE?

In Horton Foote's poignant play and movie *The Trip to Bountiful*, elderly Mrs. Watts has no choice but to live with her well-meaning but repressed son, Ludie, and her bossy daughter-in-law, Jessie Mae, in the couple's cramped apartment in Texas. Jessie Mae is constantly irritated by having her mother-in-law on her hands. Feeling always in the way, and homesick for her past life on the prairie, Mrs. Watts stages an escape: she runs away and takes a bus to Bountiful, her rural childhood village. It's all but a ghost town now. Her best friend has died, and the house she grew up in is an abandoned wreck. But Mrs. Watts once more takes the nourishing soil of her roots in her hands. Then she returns with Ludie and Jessie Mae to live out her days in their apartment.

Like Mrs. Watts, there are some older men and women who are trapped in a stressful living situation because they can't afford a separate rent. Others soldier on in sub- standard housing, in decaying neighbor- hoods, with landlords who have no interest in their welfare. There is a crying need for adequate low-cost housing in this country, not only for the old but also for young families who are priced out of the market. Government subsidies, now lagging seriously, are unlikely to meet this need in the near future, so only small numbers will benefit for many years.

> *There is a crying need for adequate low-cost housing in this country, not only for the old but also for young families who are priced out of the market.*

> Why should Ellen Vorst—retired after 30 years of teaching in one small, affluent community—be forced to move to another town when her house becomes too big for her to manage alone? She would like to stay where she is, but zoning in her town forbids apartments, so she has no choice. Why should exile be the reward for years of dedicated community service?

Many older people want to remain right where they are. They see no reason to trade familiar scenes and neighbors for alien territory. But their own communities may not offer appropriate housing—small enough, affordable enough, manageable enough. Those who con- tinue, out of choice or necessity, as tenants in their previous living quarters could be offered rent reductions or subsidies instead, while tax rebates could be available to homeowners. There is a trend in this direction in some communities but so far, no nationwide pattern. In some regions, older homeowners who don't want to budge but are short of funds can tap into the current equity in their homes with a reverse bank mortgage, as discussed in Chapter 8.

Even those willing to "sell up" and move have very different requirements. Some put a warm climate first; some want to be near museums, restaurants, and theaters. Some are happiest in age-segregated communities offering new friendships among their own age group. Others dread such exclusive ghettos and look instead for integrated communities where they can enjoy living near children, teenagers, and young adults as well. Clearly, such different goals need various choices.

Today, retirement communities for the well-heeled, with comfortable housing and meals and nursing and medical care, are springing up in many areas, and some are quite luxurious. But what about those elderly who also require security and support but can't afford the first-class ticket? Legislators, builders, city planners, architects, and church groups must confront this need and find a range of workable solutions. And the sooner, the better.

Attention Educators, Physicians, Nurses, and Social Workers!

Adequate health care, like adequate housing, is predicated on adequate funding. A lack of funds, however, is not the only roadblock to good health care. Given the awesome number of physiological and psychological ills that threaten human life, health care professionals have not been able to give high priority to the special problems of the elderly—among them, chronic conditions that defy healing, so often the fate of the old. Is it possible that these professions are reflecting the same fears and denial about the subject of aging that is so prevalent in our society at large?

The second edition of this book, published in 1982, suggested that the medical professions were in the process of realigning priorities and recognizing the need to better understand the physical and emotional needs of older people. Although health care in general has been one of the fastest growing areas of employment, that optimistic projection of 25 years ago has not yet been realized. Yet the fact is that the elderly segment, though only 13% of the total population, accounts for more than 36% of physician time and more than 40% of acute care hospital admissions. Despite these realities, there are still far too few geriatric specialists coming out of medical schools. The

American Public Health Association reports that only 150 physicians a year complete fellowships in geriatric medicine or geriatric psychiatry, and that 500 physicians in all have completed fellowships in either specialty.

There remains an urgent need in the allied health fields as well—for geriatric nurses, social workers, physical therapists, dietitians, and speech therapists. Public support is necessary if funds are to be found to underwrite continuing development in these fields of health care, all of which are essential to the well-being of older adults. The shortages are serious now, but they may assume crisis proportions unless health care professionals step up to the challenge before the baby boom generation reaches old age.

Public support is necessary if funds are to be found to underwrite continuing development in these fields of health care, all of which are essential to the well-being of older adults.

Join the Action

If adult children want tax relief in return for the support and services they personally offer their elderly parents, they will have to organize to demand it. If they suffer because their community is poor in services for older adults, they are more likely to get those services—and respite from daily caregiving routines—if they work for them together.

There is nothing new about advocacy on the part of families. Families of patients suffering from such devastating diseases as AIDS, cystic fibrosis, muscular dystrophy, and cerebral palsy—as well as such disabling conditions as severe mental illness—have been effective in bringing public attention to these conditions. Parents of children with intellectual disabilities have worked hard to make the goal of their children's full inclusion in the educational system a living, breathing—if not always easy—reality. Young mothers and fathers, unable to find local nursery schools or day care centers, have begun their own, even if they started taking turns in each other's playrooms.

However eager they are to "do something," not all families have experience in community action. They may never have organized anything before and are baffled about how to get started. A good way to begin would be to take a look at what other people have been doing and examine established programs that are working successfully elsewhere. All across the country, in scattered locations, small effective programs can be found that may benefit only a limited number of older people. Those can be used as models and duplicated again and again, thereby helping an increasing number of older people. Caregiver advocacy groups are proliferating, and national organizations have sprung up. One of these is the National Family Caregivers Association (twww.nfcacares.org), which details state-funded programs in every state and offers links for more information.

For example, transportation, companion and escort services, or respite and recreation programs can be started by small groups in communities where there are few formal programs. Preliminary informal meetings can give families a chance to discuss their common problems, raise possible solutions, and begin to discover, perhaps for the first time, that they are not alone with their struggles. It soon becomes apparent that combined voices carry over greater distances than a single voice.

Transportation, companion and escort services, or respite and recreation programs can be started by small groups in communities where there are few formal programs.

The same kind of informal family organization can make a significant difference to the elderly in nursing homes as well as in the outside community. "Watchdog groups," such as the National Citizen's Coalition for Nursing Home Reform (www.nccnhr.org), have been organized to monitor nursing home operations, protect patients' needs and rights, and push for improved services. Similar groups need to be organized in every community across the country. Adult homes, boarding homes, and residences are being exposed every day for providing substandard living conditions. Fires are not uncommon because of inadequate safety systems. Medicare and Medicaid funds have been misused by doctors and health care providers. Similar abuses will creep into any new programs that are established for vulnerable populations, such as the frail elderly. Unless there is careful surveillance by public agencies and alert family consumer groups, home care services will end up participating in a new version of the nursing home scandals.

What Can You Do?

Act Nationally

Lend your support to national organizations that advocate, educate, and lobby for the interests of older people and their families. Appendix A lists some of their web sites. Some prominently effective examples are:

- The Gray Panthers
- The American Association of Retired Persons
- The National Citizen's Coalition for Nursing Home Reform
- The National Council on the Aging
- The National Family Caregiver's Association
- The Association of Retired Federal Employees

Or you can support a professional group, for example, of retired teachers, or an organization devoted to a specific disease.

Also support political candidates who advocate for the elders, and urge your state and national representatives to support legislation significant to older Americans and their families.

Act Locally

Many communities with active and willing retirees as well as younger people have initiated local support groups. State grants may be available for some projects (visit www.caregivers.org to learn what is available in your state). Others agencies are partly or entirely staffed by volunteers. Here are just a few ideas for how you can contribute your efforts to improve the lives of older people:

- Drive homebound elders to doctors' appointments.
- Deliver meals to the homebound.
- Volunteer as a friendly visitor.
- Read to someone with failing eyesight.
- Organize a bus service to make nearby shopping possible.
- Start a senior lunch and social center, or exercise group, at your church or temple.

[contd.,]

(continued)

- Join a chore service, employing screened students and unemployed adults, who can provide help in housekeeping, groundskeeping, repairs, or other tasks that have become too much for elderly homeowners. (In one small town, fundraising, as well as clients who pay full fare, subsidize those who can pay little or nothing for this service.)
- Create a neighborhood list of able-bodied people who are available to check on elderly neighbors when storms, floods, and power outages occur.
- At a local nursing home, help serve meals and aid those who are frail in eating. Or serve as an ombudsman, representing patient needs to the administration. Or join a watchdog group to monitor the facility's standards.
- Does your town need affordable housing? An assisted living facility? Can land or architectural services be donated? Ask around, and talk it up.

New Images for Older Adults

Images resonate. And negative images have a tendency to stick. In our youth- and beauty-worshipping culture, how easily the term "65 and-over" slips mentally into an image of "old, ugly, and sick," stirring up anxieties that come out in jokes! Well, jokes are fun, and probably older folks tell most of them on themselves. But unfortunately, the same negative images also cast a very real gray cloud over the still-glowing capacities of older people. The result is that too many valuable resources are wasted, too many skills are abandoned, too much knowledge is unused, too many talents are buried, and too much initiative is stifled.

Unfortunately, the same negative images also cast a very real gray cloud over the still-glowing capacities of older people.

Today, a lot of older people aren't buying into that. They are proving that contentment, creativity, understanding, and self-reliance can actually be greater in the later decades. They are proud, not ashamed, of their age, and want the world to know it: "What can I do for you today, young lady?" asked the jovial salesman. "First, you can stop calling me 'young lady,' " replied his elderly customer, "because I'm an old woman. Then you can show me a nylon hairbrush." Other, less forthright, people move toward age with dread and denial. Victims of the stereotype, they allow themselves to feel useless, dependent, and finished. Perhaps they haven't heard of the 75-year-old doctor who is still practicing, or the couple who met on a dating web site and married in their 80s. Said the happy groom, with a chuckle, "We're a perfect match—I don't see very well, and she's a bit deaf!" Or perhaps the anxious older adults haven't met the woman in an assisted living facility, who, confined to a wheelchair, used her time to write her family history for the benefit of her children, grandchildren, and great-grandchildren. Perhaps they haven't heard of Lora.

> Once a week, Lora Hays meets with her film editing seminar at New York University. Her professional history goes back to the early days of film documentaries; the numbers of her now-successful former students are legion. Each week, she brings a currently in-demand film editor to address the class. Lora is 96. Early on Sunday mornings, if it's not too rainy or windy, she can be found pedaling along the bike path by the river.

Though Lora may be an exception among nonagenarians, the creative potential of older adults deserves—and is getting—more and more attention. Lora's case gives credence to the potential of expanded creativity in the later years.

Public and private attitudes have definitely been changing, as more people with intact abilities move into their later years. But stereotypes will need to change more dramatically. The up-to-date outlook on aging sensibly emphasizes diversity. It urges public concern for older people who are sick, helpless, and needy. It does not leave out the old who are cantankerous, difficult, rigid, repetitive, resentful, or eccentric. Nor does it omit the old who are useful, optimistic, resourceful, involved—and romantic!

The generation in the middle, today's baby boomers, have redefined middle age as we once knew it. They can and will undoubtedly fight these negative images. Just notice how often these images

One hoped-for result is that society will find less cause to avoid those who have arrived at old age already.

are false! One hoped-for result is that society will find less cause to avoid those who have arrived at old age. Once we all acknowledge the endless possibilities available for those 65 and over, we will have less reason to dread the years ahead ourselves. The new images may not take hold in time to help our parents, but they may take hold in time to help someone else's parents—or perhaps ourselves and our children.

Bob Morris on Muscling Our Way Through

These days the system is so heinous that you're spending $6000 a month for care. I can't even begin to address how hard it must be for people who really have very little means. But, you know, if you don't want to spend all that money to make it easier on yourself—by putting your parents in a nice assisted living place, with a full-time aide—then, I suppose, you're more in the trenches.

But I don't believe that there are a lot of economically strong societies, like ours, in which this situation happens—where care is so privatized. I don't know what's going on in Denmark right now, but I imagine it's not what's going on here—where you have to pay for every single thing to keep parents comfortable. I know the Scandinavian countries have a very advanced way of thinking about their social problems. And, certainly, people don't have to think about the cost of pills. Right? That doesn't exist.

My political ideas about all of this—which I do think are political, to some extent—is that *we don't want to take care of what took care of us*. We want to put all of our lives into aspiration—the aspiration of raising children, or building businesses, or climbing up to achieve professional success.

But, here's what I actually think is going to happen. The baby boomer generation is a force that is equivalent to a tidal wave. And that whatever we do—wherever we are—we will strong-arm the society into doing what we need.

The fact is that, right about now—in the next 5 years, and some of my friends are now close to 65 and retirement—there will be all kinds of new words in the language that have to do with seniors and the elderly.

I wonder if people are going to start to look at *The Golden Girls* on television and say, "You know what? That's a working scenario, and there should be some economic way of making that work better for everybody." We are a generation that likes the idea of communities. Right now, for example, people are building communities for gays— you know, senior gays. And there's a community in Pasadena that is for people who worked in the arts—and they're living together and making movies and shows. And maybe, because our generation is very nature-oriented, they may start buying up tracts of land to create senior utopian communities. Who knows?

We boomers do have buying power—and we have voting power—and we will make the government sorry if it continues to marginalize old people.

I think that we are such a selfish generation, and so used to having things our way, that it's entirely possible that any day now the government is going to stop messing with Medicare benefits. Now, I don't know that Social Security is going to survive—I can't predict that—but there'll be many class-action lawsuits, if they try to mess with people like me 10 years from now. And it won't even be that I'll have to spearhead it. It simply will be the force of numbers. *We'll just muscle our way through it.*

Epilogue
Looking Back

RARELY DO THE MEMORIES OF OUR PARENTS FADE AFTER death. Our recollections are colored by the same range of feelings toward them that we experienced when they were alive: feelings carried over from childhood, new feelings that emerged in our adult years, and the often conflicting feelings that accompany their increased dependence in old age. In looking back, an opportunity is afforded us to explore the totality of our relationship with our parents: fondly recollecting the good times; for some, regretting the bad times; and perhaps appreciating how we grew as persons when our parents increasingly needed our care.

Bob Morris, in looking back, describes the impact of his parents on his life:

> After my mom had died, my brother's son, who was about 8 or 9 at the time, was biking with my brother and me on this beautiful peninsula in Florida, and the sun was setting. My mother was a big fan of sunsets. She loved nature. To her, the greatest deal on earth was that all these beautiful spring flowers, sunsets, and stars were free.
>
> We sat and watched the sunset together. And this little nephew of mine said, "I wonder if you're thinking about Grandma." And my brother and I said, Why do you ask?" And

he said, "Well...I guess you miss her. But, you know, think about how great it'll be when you see her again." And then he said, "Like it'll probably be as great as when you were first born, and you looked at her face and saw her for the very first time." And, after that, we went off to play video games. But I will love him for that for as long as I live.

Plenty of songs remind me of my dad, and I'm glad I have that, too. I also have his terrible habit of mixing all kinds of ridiculous concoctions, just the way he did. It made me laugh. He was the original person to pour orange juice into his hot tea—or to pour raspberry sweetener all over a dessert that my mother had prepared so lovingly. He'd walk around with packages of Sweet'N Low, and salad dressings, and he was always making concoctions and pushing them on people. And I always was so repulsed by it, and I let him know how hideous it was—and now I'm doing the same thing myself. But what is an ice-blended mocha at Starbucks but an invention that my father would have made 10 years ago? He was a futurist in beverages. So it's nice to have these memories and all the memories of tropical vacations and singing together at the end. It's great if people can be aware, when they're having these experiences, that these are things that you can take with you.

I think your parents make you whole. It's very hard when you're in the middle of a crisis. But I would imagine that if a concerned child is having it really, really hard, it would help just to remember you only get one father and one mother in your life. And I think that a lot of people are wrenched, and regretful, and remorseful because they feel that they blew it, and when they're gone and it's too late. Maybe I was close to blowing it a lot, but I always had one foot in there in my parents' last years. This was really a growth-inducing, tremendously humanizing experience for me. I just got to grow as a person. Maybe it's easy to say after it's over, but I think I felt it even then: this is an opportunity.

Appendix A
Helpful Resources

A large and ever-increasing number of resources for older adults and their families on a variety of important topics can be found online, as well as in offline publications, such as those given in Appendix B. The Internet is flooded with web sites and blogs on every imaginable subject, and so listed here by topic are just some of the web sites (as well as phone numbers) that may be especially helpful to you. Note, though, that "here today and gone tomorrow" is the plight of some good web sites or subsections of web sites, and so there is no guarantee that all of the sites given here will still be available to you in the years ahead. Nor is this list in any way intended to be exclusive. Many other legitimate resources will certainly come to your attention as you browse the Web.

Caution: When you surf the Web, searching on your own for helpful information, beware of sites that provide inadequate, misleading, or incorrect information. Powerful and popular search engines such as Google or Yahoo only identify frequently used web sites—not necessarily reliable ones. You may want to check out: www.consumer webwatch.org, sponsored by Consumer Reports. Its mission is to "investigate, inform, and improve the quality of information published on the World Wide Web."

General Information and Referral

Administration on Aging: Elders and Families
www.aoa.gov/eldfam/eldfam.asp
202-619-0724

Administration on Aging: Aging Internet Information Notes
www.aoa.gov/prof/notes/notes.asp
202-619-0724

American Association of Retired Persons (AARP)
www.aarp.org
888-687-2277

American Society on Aging
www.asaging.org
800-537-9728

Eldercare Locator (U.S. Department of Health
and Human Services)
www.eldercare.gov
800-677-1116

National Association of Area Agencies on Aging
www.n4a.org
202-872-0888

National Council on the Aging
www.ncoa.org
202-479-1200

National Institute on Aging
www.nia.nih.gov
800-222-2225

National Institutes of Health Senior Health
www.nihseniorhealth.gov

Senior Net
www.seniornet.org

U.S. Department of Labor
www.dol.gov
866-4-USA-DOL (866-487-2365)

Physical Health

American Cancer Society
www.cancer.org
800-227-2345

American Diabetes Association
www.diabetes.org
800-342-2383

American Geriatrics Society
www.americangeriatrics.org
212-308-1414

American Heart Association
www.americanheart.org
800-242-8721

American Lung Association
www.lungusa.org
800-586-4872

American Parkinson Disease Association
www.apdaparkinson.org
800-223-2732

American Physical Therapy Association
www.apta.org
800-999-2782

American Stroke Association
www.strokeassociation.org
888-478-7653

Arthritis Foundation
www.arthritis.org
800-283-7800

Consumer Reports Guide to Health
   Web sites
www.HealthRatings.org
DisabilityInfo.Gov
www.disabilityinfo.gov

FamilyDoctor.org from the American Academy of Family Physicians
www.familydoctor.org

Mayo Clinic
www.mayoclinic.org
The Merck Manual of Geriatrics, 3rd ed.
www.merck.com/pubs/mmgeriatrics/

National Association on HIV Over 50 (NAHOF)
www.hivoverfifty.org
617-233-7107

National Cancer Institute
www.nci.nih.gov
800-422-6237

National Health Information Center
www.health.gov/nhic
800-336-4797

National Osteoporosis Foundation
www.nof.org
800-223-9994

WebMD
www.webmd.com

Mental Health

Alzheimer's Association
www.alz.org
800-272-3900

Alzheimer's Disease Education and Referral Center
www.alzheimers.org
800-438-4380

Alzheimer's Foundation of America
www.alzfdn.org

Alzheimer's Resource Room
www.aoa.gov/alz

American Association for Geriatric Psychiatry
www.aagponline.org
301-654-7850

Geriatric Mental Health Foundation
www.gmhfonline.org
301-654-7850

National Institute of Mental Health
www.nimh.nih.gov
866-615-6464

National Institute of Neurological Disorders and Stroke
www.ninds.nih.gov
800-352-9424

National Mental Health Association
www.nmha.org
800-969-6642

Sensory Loss

American Academy of Ophthalmology
www.aao.org
415-561-8500

American Foundation for the Blind
www.afb.org
800-232-5463

Better Hearing Institute
www.betterhearing.org
703-684-3391

League for the Hard of Hearing
www.lhh.org
917-305-7700

Lighthouse International
www.lighthouse.org
800-829-0500

Medications

Consumer Lab
www.consumerlab.com

Consumer Reports Best Buy Drugs
www.bestbuydrugs.org

eMedicine World Medical Library
www.emedicine.com

eRX Network
www.eRXnetwork.com

National Center for Complementary and Alternative
  Medicine
www.nccam.nih.gov
888-644-6226

Home Health Care and Hospice

National Association for Home Care and Hospice
www.nahc.org
202-547-7424

National PACE Association (Programs of All-Inclusive Care
  for the Elderly)
www.natlpaceassn.org
703-535-1566

Visiting Nurse Associations of America
www.vnaa.org
800-426-2547

Professional Services

American Association for Marriage and Family
  Therapy (AAMFT)
www.therapistlocator.net
703-838-9808

American Medical Association
www.ama-assn.org/go/doctorfinder
800-621-8335

Employee Assistance Program Directory
www.EAP-SAP.com

National Association of Professional Geriatric Care Managers
www.caremanager.org
520-881-8008

National Association of Social Workers Find a Licensed Social
  Worker
www.socialworkers.org
202-408-8600

Financing Health and Long-Term Care

Centers for Medicare & Medicaid Services
www.cms.hhs.gov
877-267-2323

Department of Veterans Affairs
www.va.gov
800-827-1000

GovBenefits
www.govbenefits.gov
800-333-4636

Medicare
www.medicare.gov
800-633-4227

Medicare Plan options
www.medicare.gov/choices/overview.asp

Retirement and Financial Planning

Employee Retirement Income Security Act (ERISA)
http://www.dol.gov/dol/topic/health-plans/erisa.htm
866-487-2365

Financial Planning Association
www.fpanet.org
800-282-7526

National Active and Retired Federal Employees Association (NARFE)
www.narfe.org
703-838-7760

National Association of Personal Financial Advisors
www.napfa.org
800-366-2732

National Center for home Equity Conversion
www.reverse.org

Pension Rights Center
www.pensionrights.org
202-296-3776

Social Security Administration
www.ssa.gov
800-772-1213

Supplemental Security Income
http://www.ssa.gov/notices/supplemental-security-income/
800-772-1213

Elder Law

Elder Law Answers
www.elderlawanswers.com
866-267-0947

National Academy of Elder Law Attorneys
www.naela.com
520-881-4005

Housing, Assisted Living, and Nursing Homes

American Association of Homes and Services for the Aging
www.aahsa.org
202-783-2242

Assisted Living Federation of America
www.alfa.org
703-691-8100

Continuing Care Accreditation Commission (CCAC)
www.ccaconline.org
866-888-1122

CCAC recently became a part of the Commission on
  Accreditation of Rehabilitation Facilities (CARF).
www.carf.org

Health Grades
www.healthgrades.com

Joint Commission's Long Term Care Accreditation
  Program
www.jointcommission.org/AccreditationPrograms/
  Long TermCare/

Medicare's Nursing Home Compare
www.medicare.gov/NHCompare
800-633-4227

National Long Term Care Ombudsman Resource Center
www.ltcombudsman.org
202-332-2275

Naturally Occurring Retirement Communities
  (NORCS)
www.norcs.com
202-785-5900

Community Services and Programs

Alliance for Children and Families
www.alliance1.org
414-359-1040

DOROT (Friendly Visiting)
www.friendlyvisiting.org
212-769-2850

The Joint Commission's Home Care Accreditation Program
www.jointcommission.org/AccreditationPrograms/HomeCare/

Local or State Office on Aging
www.eldercare.gov (click on "The Aging Network")
800-677-1116

National Adult Day Services Association
www.nadsa.org
800-558-5301

National Meals on Wheels Association of America
www.mowaa.org
703-548-5558

Retired and Senior Volunteer Program
www.cssny.org/rsvp/

Support for Family Caregivers

Alzheimer's Association
www.alz.org
800-272-3900

Alzheimer's Foundation of America
www.alzfdn.org

Children of Aging Parents
www.caps4caregivers.org
800-227-7294

Family Caregiver Alliance
www.caregiver.org
800-445-8106

National Family Caregiver Support Program
www.aoa.gov/prof/aoaprog/caregiver/caregiver.asp
202-619-0724

National Family Caregivers Association (NFCA)
www.nfcacares.org
800-896-3650

Advocacy

Center for Medicare Advocacy
www.medicareadvocacy.org
860-456-7790

Gray Panthers
www.graypanthers.org
800-280-5362

Medicare Rights Center
www.medicarerights.org
212-869-3850

National Citizen's Coalition for Nursing Home Reform
www.nccnhr.org
202-332-2276

Protect Social Security
www.socialsecurity.ourfuture.org

Appendix B
Suggested Readings

Memoirs

Burack-Weiss, Ann. *The Caregiver's Tale: Loss and Renewal in Memoirs of Family Life*. New York: Columbia University Press, 2006.

Cowley, Malcom. *The View from 80*. London: Viking Adult, Penguin, 1980.

De Beauvoir, Simone. *A Very Easy Death*. New York: Pantheon, 1985.

Hyman, Helen Kandel. *More Than Meets the Eye*. Washington, DC: AARP, 2005.

Nuland, Sherwin B. *Lost in America: A Journey with My Father*. New York: Alfred A. Knopf, 2003.

Olsen, Tillie. *Tell Me A Riddle*. Piscataway, NJ: Rutgers University Press, 1995.

Perspectives on Normal Aging

Butler, Robert N., and Myrna I. Lewis, *The New Love and Sex After Sixty*. New York: Ballantine Books, 2002.

Butler, Robert N. *Why Survive? Being Old in America*. Baltimore, MD: The Johns Hopkins University Press, 2002.

Carter, J. *The Virtues of Aging*. New York: Ballantine Books, 1998.

Cohen, Gene D. *The Creative Age: Awakening Human Potential in the Second Half of Life*. New York: HarperCollins Publishers, 2000.

Rowe, J. W., and R. L. Kahn, *Successful Aging*. New York: Pantheon, 1998.

Guides (in addition to the online information in Appendix A)

Avorn, Jerry. *Powerful Medicines: The Benefits, Risks, and Costs of Prescription Drugs.* New York: Knopf Publishing Group, 2005.

Carmen, Richard. *The Consumer Handbook on Hearing Loss and Hearing Aids: A Bridge to Healing.* Sedona, AZ: Auricle Ink Publishers, 2004.

Delehanty, Hugh, and Elinor Ginzler, *Caring for Your Parents: The Complete AARP Guide.* New York: Sterling Publishing Company, Inc., 2006.

Griffith, H. Winter, and Stephen Moore, *Complete Guide to Prescription and Nonprescription Drugs* (2007 Edition). New York: Perigee Trade, 2006.

Hochadel, MaryAnne. *The AARP Guide to Pills: Essential Information on More Than 1,200 Prescription & Nonprescription Medications, Including Generics, Side Effects & Drug Interactions.* New York: Sterling Publishing Company, Inc., 2007.

Mace, Nancy L., and Peter V. Rabins, *The 36-Hour Day: A Family Guide to Caring for People with Alzheimer Disease, Other Dementias, and Memory Loss in Later Life* (4th ed.). Baltimore: The Johns Hopkins University Press, 2006.

Medicare and You. Baltimore: Centers for Medicare and Medicaid Services, 2007. (Available: http://www.medicare.gov/publications/pubs/pdf/10050.pdf or by calling 1–800-MEDICARE).

Merck and Co., Inc. *The Merck Manual of Health and Aging: The Comprehensive Guide to the Changes and Challenges of Aging—For Older Adults and Those Who Care for and About Them.* New York: Ballantine Books, 2005.

Mogk, Lylas G., and Marja Mogk, *Macular Degeneration: The Complete Guide to Saving and Maximizing Your Sight.* New York: Ballantine Books, 2003.

Morris, Virginia. *How to Care for Aging Parents.* New York: Workman Publishing, 2004.

Rosenthal, Bruce P., and Kate Kelly, *Living Well with Macular Degeneration: Practical Tips and Essential Information.* New York: New American Library, 2001.

Appendix C
Penny's Personal Papers Inventory

NAME: _____

DATE OF BIRTH: _____

SOCIAL SECURITY NO.: _____

ADDRESS: _____

_____

TELEPHONE: _____

WILL: YES ☐　NO ☐	Executor of Will:
Location of Will:	Address:
Address:	
	Telephone:
Telephone:	Attorney:
Preparer of Will:	Address:
Address:	
	Telephone:

Telephone:	Financial Planner:
Bank(er)	Address:
Address:	
Telephone:	Telephone:
Power of Attorney:	Guardian:
Address:	Address:
Telephone:	Telephone:

PPI ITEM	2007	2008	2009	2010
Birth Certificate Location:				
Naturalization Papers Location:				
Green Card				
Other INS Documentation				
Foreign Passport/Entry Visa No.: Location:				
Marriage Certificate Location:				
Separation/Divorce Location:				
Adoption Papers Location:				

PPI ITEM	2007	2008	2009	2010
Social Security No.: Card Location:				
Medicare Card No.: Part A Part B				
U.S. Passport No.: Location:				
Military Discharge Papers Location:				

Lease
  Location:
  Name of Landlord:
  Address:
  Telephone:				

Mortgage/Title/Coop/Condo Agreement, Closing Papers, Deed Location:				

Cemetery Plot
  Cemetery Name:
  Plot No.:
  Deed Location:				

Safety Deposit Box
  Box No.:
  Location:
  Location of Key:
  Joint Owner:
    Address:
    Telephone:				

Income Sources Self-Employment Amount: Employment Amount: Consulting:				

PPI ITEM	2007	2008	2009	2010
Name of Firm:				
Telephone:				
Amount:				
Name of Firm:				
Telephone:				
Amount:				
Name of Firm:				
Telephone:				
Amount:				
Social Security				
Amount:				
Pension				
Amount:				
IRA				
Amount:				
IRA				
Amount:				
Annuity				
Amount:				
Annuity				
Amount:				
Other Income Sources				
Amount:				
Financial Accounts				
Savings				
Bank & Branch No.:				
Location:				
Account No. & PIN No.:				
Bank & Branch No.:				
Location:				
Account No. & PIN No.:				
Checking				
Bank & Branch No.:				
Location:				
Account No. & PIN No.:				

PPI ITEM	2007	2008	2009	2010
Bank & Branch No.: Location: Account No. & PIN No.:				
CDs Bank & Branch No.: Location: Account No.: Bank & Branch No.: Location: Account No.: Bank & Branch No.: Location: Account No.:				
Investment Accounts Type: Broker's Name: Telephone: Type: Broker's Name: Telephone: Type: Broker's Name: Telephone:				
Retirement Benefits Type: Company: Location: Telephone:				
Credit Card Accounts Card Holder: Card Name: Card No.: Cust. Serv. Telephone:				

PPI ITEM	2007	2008	2009	2010
Card Holder: Card Name: Card No.: Cust. Serv. Telephone: Card Holder: Card Name: Card No.: Cust. Serv. Telephone: Card Holder: Card Name: Card No.: Cust. Serv. Telephone:				
Lost Credit Card Insurance Co.: Telephone:				
Health Benefits Insurer: Address: Telephone: Identification No.: Group Name: Group No.: Location of Policy: Benefits Office Phone (if through work):				
Long-Term Health Insurance Insurer: Address: Telephone: Identification No.: Group Name: Group No.: Location of Policy:				
Health Care Proxy/Health Care Directives Location of Proxy:				

PPI ITEM	2007	2008	2009	2010
Medic Alert Information Company Name: Company Telephone No.				

Life Insurance
  Insurance Co.:
  Type:
  Amount:
    Face value:
    Cash Value:
  Policy Number:
  Location of Policy:
  Broker's Name:
  Broker's Address:
  Broker's Telephone:				

Homeowner's Insurance
  Company:
  Co. Telephone:
  Broker:
  Broker's Address:
  Broker's Telephone:
  Type:
  Amount:
  Policy No.:
  Location of Policy:				

Mortgage Insurance
  Company:
  Co. Telephone:
  Broker:
  Broker's Address:
  Broker's Telephone:
  Amount:
  Policy No.:
  Location of Policy:				

PPI ITEM	2007	2008	2009	2010

Disability Insurance
    Company:
    Address:
    Co. Telephone:
    Broker:
    Broker's Address:
    Broker's Telephone:
    Amount:
    Policy No:
    Location of Policy:				

Automobile Information
    Title (in name of):
    Location:
    Car Loan: Yes ☐   No ☐
    Name of Bank:
    Address of Bank:
    Telephone:
    Amt. Remaining:
    Insurance Co.:
    Co. Telephone No.:
    Broker:
    Broker's Telephone:
    Policy No.
    Location of Policy:				

Other Outstanding Debts & Loans
    Educational Loans
        Lender:
        Lender's Telephone:
        Amount of Loan:
    Homeowner's Loan
        Lender:
        Lender's Telephone:
        Amount of Loan:
    Other Loans:				

PPI ITEM	2007	2008	2009	2010
Business Agreements Location:				

Special Contacts
  Name:
  Address:
  Telephone:
  Name:
  Address:
  Telephone:
  Name:
  Address:
  Telephone:				

Organ Donation Information
  a. Any needed organ parts: _____
  b. The following organ parts:
    1. _____
    2. _____
    3. _____
    4. _____
  c. Limitations/exceptions:
    1. _____
    2. _____
    3. _____
    4. _____				

PIN Nos.:				
Computer Access Passwords and PINS				
E-Mail/Web Site Information				
Miscellaneous				
Additional Comments & Final Wishes				

Source: Designed by Dr. Penny Schwartz, Mount Sinai Medical Center, New York, NY.

Appendix D
Checklists for Evaluating Services

Checklist for Evaluating Nursing Homes

I. Where to start
  A. Get a list of nursing homes in your area from:
    1. Hospital social service departments
    2. Local departments of health and departments of social services
    3. State department of health and department of social services
    4. County medical society
    5. Social Security district office
    6. State and local Office of the Aging
    7. Physician, clergyman, relatives, and friends
  B. Visit several before making a decision.

II. What to notice about the general atmosphere
  A. Are visitors welcome?
    1. Are you encouraged to tour freely?
    2. Do staff members answer questions willingly?
  B. Is the home clean and odor free?
  C. Is the staff pleasant, friendly, cheerful, and affectionate?
  D. Are lounges available for socializing?

III. Is attention paid to the patients' morale?
    A. Are they called patronizingly by their first names or addressed with dignity as "Mr.," "Mrs.," or "Miss"?
    B. Are they dressed in nightclothes or street clothes?
    C. Do many of them appear oversedated?
    D. Are they allowed to have some of their own possessions?
    E. Are they given sufficient privacy?
        1. Are married couples kept together?
        2. Are "sweethearts" given a place to visit with each other in privacy?
    F. Is good grooming encouraged?
        1. Are the services of a beautician and a barber available?
    G. Is tipping necessary to obtain services?

IV. What licensing to look for:
    A. State nursing home license
    B. Nursing home administrator license
    C. Joint Committee on Accreditation of Hospital Certificate
    D. American Association of Homes for the Aging
    E. American Nursing Home Association

V. Location
    A. Is it convenient for visiting?
    B. Is the neighborhood safe for ambulatory residents?
    C. Is there an outdoor garden with benches?

VI. Safety considerations?
    A. Does the home meet federal and state fire codes?
        1. Ask to see the latest inspection report.
        2. Are regular fire drills scheduled?
    B. Is the home accident-proof?
        1. Is the lighting adequate?
        2. Are handrails and grab bars available in the halls and bathrooms?
        3. Are corridors free of obstructions?
        4. Are rooms free of scatter rugs and easily tipped chairs?
        5. Are stairway doors kept closed?

VII. Living arrangements
    A. Are the bedrooms comfortable and spacious?
    B. Is the furniture appropriate?
        1. Is there enough drawer and closet space?

2. Are doors and drawers easy to open?

3. Can residents furnish their rooms with personal items?

C. Can closets and drawers be locked?

D. Is there enough space between beds, through doorways, and in corridors for wheelchairs?

E. Are there enough elevators for the number of patients?

1. Are elevators large enough for wheelchairs?

VIII. Food services

A. Is there a qualified dietitian in charge?

1. Are special therapeutic diets followed?

2. Are individual food preferences considered?

B. Are you welcome to inspect the kitchen?

C. Are menus posted?

1. Do the menus reflect what is actually served?

D. Are dining rooms cheerful?

1. Are patients encouraged to eat in the dining room rather than at the bedside?

2. Is there room between the tables for the passage of wheelchairs?

E. Are bedridden patients fed when necessary?

1. Is food left uneaten on trays?

F. Are snacks available between meals and at bedtime?

1. Are snacks scheduled too close to meals to accommodate staff shifts?

2. Is there too long a period between supper and breakfast the next morning?

IX. Medical services

A. Is there a medical director qualified in geriatric medicine?

B. Are patients allowed to have private doctors?

C. If there are staff physicians, what are their qualifications?

1. Is a doctor available 24 hours a day?

2. How often is each patient seen by a doctor?

D. Does each patient get a complete physical examination before or upon admission?

E. Does the home have a hospital affiliation or a transfer agreement with a hospital?

F. Does each patient have an individual treatment plan?

G. Is a psychiatrist available?

H. Is provision made for dental, eye, and foot care as well as other specialized services?

I. Are there adequate medical records?

X. Nursing services
 A. Is the nursing director fully qualified?
 B. Is there a registered nurse on duty at all times?
 C. Are licensed practical nurses graduates of approved schools?
 D. Is there adequate nursing staff for the number of patients?
 E. Is there an in-service training program for nurse's aides and orderlies?

XI. Rehabilitation services
 A. Is there a registered physiotherapist on staff?
    1. Is there good equipment?
    2. How often are patients scheduled?
 B. Is there a registered occupational therapist on staff?
    1. Is functional therapy prescribed in addition to diversionary activities?
 C. Is a speech therapist available for poststroke patients?
 D. Is the staff trained in reality orientation, remotivation, and bladder training for the mentally impaired?

XII. Group activities
 A. Is the activities director professionally trained?
 B. Are a variety of programs offered?
    1. Ask to see a calendar of activities.
 C. Are there trips to theaters, concerts, and museums for those who can go out?
 D. Are wheelchair-bound patients transported to group activities?
 E. Is there a library for patients?
 F. Is there an opportunity to take adult education courses or participate in discussion groups?

XIII. Social services
 A. Is a professional social worker involved in admissions procedures?
    1. Are both the applicant and the family interviewed?
    2. Are alternatives to institutionalization explored?

B. Is a professional, trained social worker available to discuss personal problems and help with adjustments of the patient and family?

C. Are social and psychological needs of patients included in treatment plans?

D. Is a professional, trained social worker available to the staff for consultation:

    1. On social and psychological problems of patients?

    2. On roommate choices and tablemates?

XIV. Religious observances

A. Is there a chapel on the grounds?

B. Are religious services held regularly for those who wish to attend?

C. If the home is run under sectarian auspices, are clergy of other faiths permitted to see patients when requested?

XV. Citizen participation

A. Is the Patient Bill of Rights prominently displayed and understood?

B. Is there a resident council?

    1. How often does it meet?

    2. Does it have access to the administrator and department heads?

C. Is there a family organization?

    1. How often does it meet?

    2. Does it have access to the administrator and department heads?

D. Do the patients vote in local, state, and federal elections?

    1. Are they taken to the polls?

    2. Do they apply for absentee ballots?

XVI. Financial questions

A. What are the basic costs?

    1. Are itemized bills available?

    2. Are there any extra charges?

B. Is the home eligible for Medicare and Medicaid reimbursement?

    1. Is a staff member available to assist in making application for these funds?

2. Is assistance available for questions about veterans'
pensions? Union benefits?

ᴄ. What provision is made for the patient's spending money?

Checklist for Evaluating Home Health Care

1. Does the agency from which you are seeking services have
legal authorization to operate? Is it licensed or certified?
2. Is the agency accountable to a regulatory body (government
agency, national council, or board of directors) that monitors
the quality of the services?
3. Does the agency have written personnel policies, job descrip-
tions, and a wage scale established for each job category?
4. Does the agency provide you with the services of a homemaker
or home health aide and a supervisor who makes periodic visits
to check on the care given?
5. Is a professional person (registered nurse or trained social
worker) responsible for a plan of care?
6. Does the agency provide in-service training for the homemaker
or home health aide?
7. Is this training provided by qualified professionals?
8. Is the agency eligible for Medicare and Medicaid reimbursement?
9. Does the agency make regular reports to the community and to
certifying bodies?

*Adapted from the "National Standards for Homemaker-Home Health
Aide Services" established by the National HomeCaring Council, 1981*

Index

abandonment issues, 23, 24, 142, 143, 147
acceptance, by adult children: of acceptable
  parental involvement, 38; of caregiver
  status, 34–35; of guilt feelings, 27; of
  negative feelings towards parents, 20; of
  parent's aging, 30–31; of remarriage by
  parent, 131, 137; of self aging, 31–33
acceptance, by elderly parents: of help/care
  from children, 55; of institutional living,
  94; of money from children, 94; during
  mourning process, 128; of social losses, 88
accidents: from alcohol consumption, 103;
  automobile, 50; fearfulness of, 82; as
  inspiration for self-concern, 229; as
  precipitation of crisis, 224; from
  underestimation of disability, 233
adaptations: adult-to-adult differences in
  capabilities, 86–87; capabilities of older
  adults, 77–78, 80–81; of physical
  environment, 84
Administration on Aging (Dept. of Health
  and Human Services), 7
admissions: by children: of inability to take in
  parent, 183; of mistakes, by adult children,
  37; of not listening to parents, 137; of
  opposition to parent's remarriage, 131; of
  parent's deterioration, 267–68; by parents:
  of keeping children from overnight stays,
  263; of need for help, 115; of sexual
  failures, 136
adolescent rebellion, protracted, 41–42

adult children: acceptance: of caregiver status,
  34–35; of parent's aging, 1, 30–31; of
  self-aging, 31–33; admission of help needed
  for parents, 262; aid/support of mourning
  parent, 127–30; avoidance of parents, 38;
  choice of caregiver, 54–60; dealing with
  own children and parents, 36; denial
  issues, 39–40; drawn into parent's post-
  retirement issues, 114–15; effect of
  parent's death, 126–27; emotional tug-
  of-war of, 44–46; fault-finding by, 38–39;
  fear of abandonment at parent's death,
  143; feelings of, 19–29, 30–31, 35–37;
  forgiveness of self, vs. resentment of
  parents, 37; ignoring of own family for
  parents, 47–48; need for medication
  vigilance, 346; obstacles to caring for
  parents, 18–19; oversolicitousness/
  domination by, 38; possible escape from
  parent care, 4; psychological demands
  placed on, 94–95; saying no to parents,
  171–73; seeing self in parents, 32–33;
  solicitous behavior towards parents, 52–53;
  understanding parental behaviors, 22;
  worries of not doing enough, 17. See also
  caregivers; families; siblings
advance directives, 157–59
advertising, by pharmaceutical companies,
  344–46
agencies: AARP, 205, 207, 211, 218; Area
  Agency on Aging offices, 213, 217, 218,

CHESTNUT HILL